WO18

Applied Basic Science and Clinical Topics

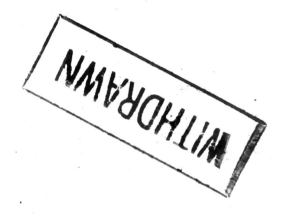

MRCS

Applied Basic Science and Clinical Topics

Stephen Parker BSc DipMedEd MS FRCS (Gen)

Consultant General Surgeon
University Hospitals of Coventry and
Warwickshire NHS Trust
Coventry, UK

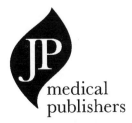

JP
medical
publishers

London • St Louis • Panama City • New Delhi

© 2013 JP Medical Ltd.
Published by JP Medical Ltd
83 Victoria Street, London, SW1H 0HW, UK
Tel: +44 (0)20 3170 8910
Fax: +44 (0)20 3008 6180
Email: info@jpmedpub.com
Web: www.jpmedpub.com

ISBN: 978-1-907816-43-7

British Library Cataloguing in Publication Data
A catalogue record for this book is available from the British Library

Library of Congress Cataloging in Publication Data
A catalog record for this book is available from the Library of Congress

JP Medical Ltd is a subsidiary of Jaypee Brothers Medical Publishers (P) Ltd, New Delhi, India

Publisher:	Richard Furn
Commissioning Editor:	Hannah Applin
Senior Editorial Assistant:	Katrina Rimmer
Design:	Designers Collective Ltd

Typeset, printed and bound in India.

Preface

MRCS Applied Basic Science and Clinical Topics has been written as a resource for candidates who are preparing for postgraduate surgical examinations, in particular Parts A and B of the Intercollegiate MRCS Examination. It has its foundation in my experience as a general surgical consultant with a strong interest in medical education. The content has evolved over time, shaped by feedback from previous candidates who have identified what they would have wanted when preparing for their examinations.

The book aims to fill the gap between large surgical textbooks and smaller revision aids. This has necessitated a selective approach to the topics included and the depth in which they are discussed: the basic science topics have been chosen for their direct bearing on clinical practice and the clinical topics are those commonly encountered both in the wards and in postgraduate surgical examinations.

Each chapter presents the basic science and clinical topics in a consistent format, in accordance with the MRCS syllabus. The clinical chapters aim to cover the whole breadth of surgical special-ties at a level appropriate for the MRCS examination. Variations in surgical practice will inevitably mean that there will be disagreement with some of the views and recommendations that are presented. In potentially contentious areas I have attempted to include opinions that are not too extreme, are supported by current research evidence and will hopefully satisfy most examiners.

Within the space available, the book cannot hope to be exhaustive. Nevertheless, I hope that it will be a useful tool when working in and studying a particular surgical speciality, as well as serving as a revision tool and *aide-mémoire* immediately prior to the examinations.

Stephen Parker BSc MS DipMedEd FRCS(Gen)
October 2012

Contents

The MRCS Examination

The Membership of the Royal College of Surgeons (MRCS) examination is a summative assessment of candidates in the generality of surgery, whether in core surgical training or outside a training programme. Its purpose is to determine that a trainee has acquired the knowledge, skills and attributes required for the completion of core training and for those trainees following the intercollegiate surgical curriculum programme, to determine their ability to progress to higher specialist training. Passing the MRCS is mandatory to progress from ST2/CT2 to ST3/CT3.

Format of Part A

There is one 4-hour examination consisting of two 2-hour multiple choice question (MCQ) papers that are sat consecutively. Paper 1 tests applied basic sciences and has single best answer (SBA) questions. Paper 2 tests principles of surgery-in-general and has extended matching questions (EMQs). Candidates score one mark for each correct answer. To pass Part A the overall pass mark has to be met. The pass mark is set using a modified Angoff method. A score of at least 50% on each paper has to be achieved. Candidates can have an unlimited number of attempts at this part.

Format of Part B

Part B is now in an objective structured clinical examination (OSCE) format. There are 16 stations and four rest stations, each of 9 minutes. Candidates start at different points in the circuit. The stations assess knowledge and skills in five main subject areas:

- Anatomy and surgical pathology
- Surgical skills and patient safety
- Communication skills
- Applied surgical science and critical care
- Clinical skills

Twelve stations test generic knowledge and are compulsory for all candidates. To allow for differences in training, there are four speciality stations. Candidates select their speciality context at the time of application. In each of the five subject areas, six domains are tested:

- Clinical knowledge
- Clinical skill
- Technical skill
- Communication
- Decision making and problem solving
- Organisation and planning

Most of the stations have surgeon examiners and all examiners must have completed a training course. The marking scheme is a matrix in which the stations are marked using several domains. There is a structured mark sheet for each station. The mark sheet includes a holistic judgement of the candidate. Candidates must reach the overall pass mark set for Part B. They must also achieve a minimum score in each of the domains. A variant of the contrasting groups method is used for setting the overall mark.

Glossary

AAA	Abdominal aortic aneurysm	CNS	Central nervous system
ABPI	Ankle brachial pressure index	CO	Cardiac output
ACE	Angiotensin converting enzyme	CPAP	Constant positive airway pressure
ACTH	Adrenocorticotrophic hormone	CPP	Cerebral perfusion pressure
ADH	Antidiuretic hormone	CRF	Chronic renal failure
AF	Atrial fibrillation	CRP	C reactive protein
AIDS	Acquired immunodeficiency syndrome	CSF	Cerebrospinal fluid
		CSOM	Chronic secretary otitis media
ALI	Acute limb ischaemia	CVA	Cerebrovascular accident
ALI	Acute lung injury	CVP	Central venous pressure
ALP	Alkaline phosphatase		
ANDI	Aberrations of normal development and involution	DCIS	Ductal carcinoma in situ
		DIC	Disseminated intravascular coagulation
ANS	Autonomic nervous system		
APACHE	Acute Physiology and Chronic Health Evaluation	DIND	Delayed ischaemic neurological deficit
APUD	Amine precursor uptake decarboxylase	DIPJ	Distal interphalangeal joint
		DMSA	Dimercaptosuccinic acid
ARDS	Acute respirator distress syndrome	DVT	Deep vein thrombosis
ARF	Acute renal failure		
ASA	American Society of Anesthesiologists	ECG	Electrocardiogram
		EGF	Epidermal growth factor
ASD	Atrial septal defect	EMQ	Extended matching question
ASI	Acute serum conversion illness	EPSP	Excitatory post synaptic potential
AST	Aspartate transaminase	ERCP	Endoscopic retrograde cholangiopancreatography
BE	Base excess	ERV	Expiratory reserve volume
BIPP	Bismuth iodoform paraffin paste	ELISA	Enzyme-linked immunosorbent assay
BMI	Body mass index		
BP	Blood pressure	ESR	Erythrocyte sedimentation rate
BSA	Body surface area	ESWL	Extracorporeal shockwave lithotripsy
CABG	Coronary artery bypass graft	EWS	Early warning scoring system
CAPD	Continuous ambulatory peritoneal dialysis		
		FAP	Familial adenomatous polyposis
CBD	Common bile duct	FAST	Focused assessment with sonography for trauma
CEA	Carcino-embryonic antigen		
CHD	Congenital heart disease	FBC	Full blood count
CI	Cardiac index	FEV	Forced expiratory volume
CLI	Chronic limb ischaemia	FISH	Fluorescence in situ hybridisation

FNAC	Fine need aspiration cytology	MAC	Minimal alveolar concentration
FOB	Faecal occult blood	MCH	Mean corpuscular haemoglobin
FRC	Functional residual capacity	MCHC	Mean corpuscular haemoglobin concentration
FVC	Forced vital capacity		
		MCPJ	Metacarpophalangeal joint
GCS	Glasgow coma score	MCQ	Multiple choice question
GIST	Gastrointestinal stromal tumour	MCV	Mean corpuscular volume
GFR	Glomerular filtration rate	MEN	Multiple endocrine neoplasia
GMC	General Medical Council	MI	Myocardial infarction
GORD	Gastroesophageal reflux	MIBG	Metaiodobenzylguanidine
GnRH	Gonadotrophin-releasing hormone	MODS	Multiple organ dysfunction syndrome
HCC	Hepatocellular carcinoma	MRA	Magnetic resonance angiography
HCV	Hepatitis C virus	MRCS	Membership of the Royal College of Surgeons
HDU	High dependency unit		
HIAA	Hydroxyindolacetic acid	MRSA	Methicillin-resistant *Staphylococcus aureus*
HIV	Human immunodeficiency virus		
HNPCC	Hereditary non-polyposis colorectal cancer	MRI	Magnetic resonance imaging
		MSH	Melanocyte-stimulating hormone
HRT	Hormone replacement therapy	MSU	Mid-stream urine
		MTPJ	Metatarsophalangeal joint
IC	Inspiratory capacity	MUGA	Multiple-gated apposition
ICP	Intracranial pressure		
IGF	Insulin-like growth factor	NCEPOD	National Clinical Enquiry into Perioperative Deaths
IMA	Inferior mesenteric artery		
ILP	Isolated limb perfusion	NICE	National Institute for Clinical Excellence
IPSP	Inhibitory postsynaptic potential		
IRV	Inspiratory reserve volume	NPI	Nottingham Prognostic Index
ISCP	Intercollegiate Surgical Curriculum Programme	NPV	Negative predictive value
		NSAID	Non-steroidal anti-inflammatory drugs
ISS	Injury Severity Score		
ITU	Intensive therapy unit		
IUCD	Intrauterine contraceptive devise	OCP	Oral contraceptive pill
IVC	Inferior vena cava	OSCE	Objective structured clinical examination
IVU	Intravenous urogram		
KPPT	Kaolin partial thromboplastic time	PAF	Platelet activating factor
		PCA	Patient controlled analgesia
LCIS	Lobular carcinoma in situ	PCI	Percutaneous coronary intervention
LDL	Low density lipoproteins		
LFTs	Liver function tests	PCR	Polymerase chain reaction
LMA	Laryngeal mask airway	PCV	Packed cell volume
LMWH	Low molecular weight heparin	PCWP	Pulmonary capillary wedge pressure
LSV	Long saphenous vein		

PDA	Patent ductus arteriosus	SPJ	Saphenopopliteal junction
PDGF	Platelet-derived growth factor	SSV	Short saphenous vein
PE	Pulmonary embolus	SV	Stroke volume
PEG	Percutaneous endoscopic gastroenterostomy	SVR	Systemic vascular resistance
PEEP	Positive end expiratory pressure	TENS	Transcutaneous electrical nerve stimulation
PGI	Persistent generalised lymphadenopathy	TGF	Transforming growth factor
PID	Pelvic inflammatory disease	TIA	Transient ischaemic attack
PIPJ	Proximal interphalangeal joint	TIPPS	Transjugular intrahepatic portal systemic shunt
PONV	Postoperative nausea and vomiting		
POSSUM	Physiological and Operative Severity Score for the enUmeration of Mortality and Morbidity	TLC	Total lung capacity
		TNF-α	Tumour necrosis factor-α
		TOF	Trachea-oesophageal fistula
PPD	Purified protein derivative	TPN	Total parenteral nutrition
PPV	Positive predictive value	tPA	Tissue plasminogen activator
PT	Prothrombin time	TRH	Thyrotrophin-releasing hormone
PTFE	Polytetrafluoroethylene	TSH	Thyroid-stimulating hormone
PTH	Parathyroid hormone	TV	Tidal volume
PUJ	Pelviureteric junction		
		U&E	Urea and electrolytes
QoL	Quality of life	UTI	Urinary tract infection
RBC	Red blood cell	VF	Ventricular fibrillation
RCT	Randomised controlled trial	VIP	Vasoactive intestinal polypeptide
RES	Reticulo-endothelial system	VMA	Vanillyl mandelic acid
RTS	Revised Trauma Score	VRE	Vancomycin-resistant enterococcus
RV	Residual volume	VUR	Vesicoureteric reflux
		vWF	von Willebrand factor
SBE	Standard base excess		
SFJ	Saphenofemoral junction	WCC	White cell count
SIRS	Systemic inflammatory response syndrome	WHO	World Health Organization
SLE	Systemic lupus erythematosus	VC	Vital capacity
SMA	Superior mesenteric artery	VSD	Ventricular septal defect

Chapter 1

Professional skills in clinical practice

Duties of a doctor

Patients must be able to trust doctors with their lives and wellbeing. To justify that trust, the profession has a duty to maintain a good standard of practice and care and to show respect for human life. In particular a doctor must:

- Make the care of his or her patient their first concern
- Treat every patient politely and considerately
- Respect patients' dignity and privacy
- Listen to patients and respect their views
- Give patients information in a way that the patient can understand
- Respect the rights of patients to be fully involved in decisions about their care
- Keep his or her professional knowledge and skills up to date
- Recognise the limits of his or her own professional confidence
- Be honest and trustworthy
- Respect and protect confidential information
- Make sure that his or her personal beliefs do not prejudice patient care
- Act quickly to protect patients from risk if there are concerns to believe that he, she or a colleague may not be fit to practice
- Avoid abusing their position as a doctor
- Work with colleagues in ways that best serve patients' interests

In all of these matters, doctors must never discriminate unfairly against their patients or colleagues. They must always be prepared to justify their actions.

Communication skills

Good communication is integral to medical practice. Communication is important not only in professional–patient interactions, but also to share information within the healthcare team. The benefits of effective communication include good working relationships and increased patient satisfaction. Effective communication may also increase patient understanding of treatment, improve compliance and, in some cases, lead to improved health. It engenders meaningful and trusting relationships between healthcare professionals and their patients.

Benefits for patients

The doctor–patient relationship is improved. The doctor is better able to seek the relevant information and recognise the problems of the patient by way of interaction and attentive listening. As a result, the patient's problems may be identified more accurately. Good communication helps the patient to recall information and comply with treatment instructions. It may improve patient health and outcomes. Better communication and dialogue, by means of reiteration and repetition between doctor and patient, has a beneficial effect in terms of promoting better emotional health, resolution of symptoms and pain control. The overall quality of care may be improved by ensuring that patients' views and wishes are taken into account. Good communication is likely to reduce the incidence of clinical errors.

Benefits for doctors

Effective communication skills may relieve doctors of some of the pressures of dealing with the difficult situations. Problematic communication with patients is thought to contribute to emotional burn-out and low personal accomplishment in doctors, as well as high psychological morbidity. Being able to communicate competently may also enhance job satisfaction. Patients are less likely to complain if doctors communicate well.

Good communication skills expected of healthcare professional include the ability to:

- Talk to patients, carers and colleagues effectively and clearly, conveying and receiving the intended message
- Enable patients and their carers to communicate effectively
- Listen effectively, especially when time is pressured
- Identify potential communication difficulties and work through solutions
- Understand the differing methods of communication used by individuals
- Understand that there are differences in communication signals between cultures
- Cope in specific difficult circumstances
- Understand how to use and receive non-verbal messages given by body language
- Utilise spoken, written and electronic methods of communication
- Know when the information received needs to be passed on to another person or professional for action
- Know and interpret the information needed to be recorded on patients records, writing discharge letters, copying letters to patients and gaining informed consent
- Recognise the need for further development to acquire specialist skills

Key tasks in communication with patients include:

- Eliciting the patient's main problems, the patients perception of these and the physical, emotional and social impact on the patient and family
- Tailoring the information to what the patient wants to know and checking their understanding
- Eliciting the patient's reactions and their main concerns
- Determining how much the patient wants to participate in decision making
- Discussing the treatment options so that the patient understand the implications
- Maximising the chance that the patient will follow the agreed treatment plan

Documentation and record keeping

Accurate documentation and record keeping is important for both clinical and legal reasons. Records provide a means of communication and record of events. Patient records should be:

- Factual, consistent and accurate
- Written as soon as possible after the event
- All entries should be dated and signed
- The signature should clearly identify the author
- Personal slur and value-judgment should be avoided

Clinical governance
Definition

Clinical governance is a framework through which healthcare organisations are accountable for maintaining and improving the quality of their services, by creating an environment in which excellence is allowed to flourish. It embodies three key attributes:

- Recognising high standards of care
- Transparent responsibility and accountability for standards
- A constant dynamic of improvement

Clinical governance addresses those structures, systems and processes that assure the quality and accountability. It ensures proper management of an organisation's operation and delivery of service. Clinical governance is composed of the following elements:

- Education and training
- Clinical effectiveness
- Research and development
- Openness
- Risk management
- Clinical audit

Education and training

It is no longer acceptable for any clinician to abstain from continuing education after qualification. The continuing professional development of clinicians is the responsibility of the individual and his employer. It is the professional duty of clinicians to remain up-to-date.

Clinical effectiveness

Clinical effectiveness is a measure of the extent to which a particular intervention works. The measure on its own is useful, but it is enhanced by considering whether the intervention is appropriate and whether it represents value for money. In the modern health service, clinical practice needs to be refined in the light of emerging evidence of effectiveness. It also has to consider aspects of efficiency and safety from the perspective of the patient.

Research and development

Good professional practice has always sought to change in the light of evidence from research. The time lag for introducing such change can be very long. Reducing the time lag and associated morbidity requires emphasis not only on carrying out and implementing research. Techniques such as critical appraisal of the literature, project management and the development of guidelines, protocols and implementation strategies are all tools for promoting the implementation of research practice.

Openness

Poor performance and practice can too often thrive behind closed doors. Processes which are open to public scrutiny, while respecting individual patient and practitioner confidentiality are an essential part of quality assurance. Open proceedings and discussion about clinical governance issues should occur. Any organisation providing high quality care has to show that it is meeting the needs of the population it serves. Health needs assessment and understanding the problems and aspirations of the community require the cooperation between healthcare organisations, public health departments, local authorities and community health councils. The system of clinical governance brings together all the elements which seek to promote quality of care.

Risk management

Risk management can be defined as a proactive approach that addresses the various activities of an organisation. It identifies the risks that exist and assesses each risk for the potential frequency and severity. It eliminates the risks that can be eliminated and reduces the effect of those that cannot be eliminated. It establishes financial mechanisms to absorb the consequences of the risks that remain. Risk management involves consideration of:

- Risks to patients
- Risks to practitioners
- Risks to the organisation

Compliance with statutory regulations can help to minimise risks to patients. This can be further reduced by ensuring that systems are regularly reviewed and questioned. Maintenance of medical ethical standards is also a key factor in maintaining patient and public safety and wellbeing. It is vital to ensure that clinicians work in a safe environment. Poor quality is a threat to any organisation. They need to reduce their own risks by ensuring high quality employment practice, a safe environment and well-designed policies on public involvement.

Risk management is essential to:

- Providing a safe working environment
- Meeting the personal and professional responsibility to patients
- Complying with health and safety legislation
- Reducing the risk of litigation

Risks can be clinical or non-clinical. Once a risk is identified it must be analysed:

- How often it is likely to occur?
- What are the potential effects of managing the risk?
- What are the potential effects if the risk is ignored?
- How much is it likely to cost?

Consideration needs to be given to measures to control the risk. It may be possible to totally eliminate the risk. If it can not be eliminated, the risk should be minimised. Funding for risk management is part of every hospital's budget through the Clinical Negligence Scheme for Trusts and existing liabilities schemes.

Clinical audit

Clinical audit is the review of clinical performance and the refining of clinical practice as a result and the measurement of performance against agreed standards. It is a systematic, critical analysis of the quality of medical care, including the procedures used for diagnosis and treatment, to help to provide reassurance that the best quality of service is being achieved, having regard to the available resources. Clinical audit is an assessment of total care and can assess:

- Structure – type of resources
- Process – what is done to patients
- Outcome – the result of clinical interventions

Medical audit

Medical audit involves a systematic approach that highlights opportunities for improvement and provides a mechanism for change. It is not simply case presentations at morbidity and mortality meetings. The audit cycle (**Figure 1.1**) involves:

- Observation of existing practice
- The setting of standards
- Comparison between observed and set standards

- Implementation of change
- Re-audit of clinical practice

Audit techniques include:

- Basic clinical audit – throughput, morbidity, mortality
- Incident review – critical incident reporting
- Clinical record review
- Criterion audit – retrospective analysis judged against chosen criteria
- Adverse occurrence screening
- Focused audit studies – specific outcome
- Global audit – comparison between units
- National studies – e.g. National Confidential Enquiry into Patient Outcome and Death (NCEPOD)

Comparative audit requires:

- High quality data collection
- Relevant and valid measure of outcome
- Appropriate and valid measures of case mix
- A representative population
- Appropriate statistical analysis

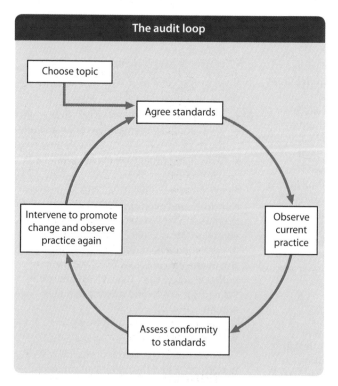

The audit loop

- Choose topic
- Agree standards
- Observe current practice
- Assess conformity to standards
- Intervene to promote change and observe practice again

Figure 1.1 The audit loop

Ethics and the law

The Coroner

There are approximately 600,000 deaths per year in England and Wales. The cause of death is certified by the attending doctor in 75% cases. Of the 150,000 deaths referred to the coroner, 60% are referred by doctors, 38% by the police and 2% by the Registrar of Births, Marriages and Deaths. Initial investigations are conducted by coroner's officers. They are often retired policemen. A death certificate may be issued after discussion with a coroner's officers. Coroners hold inquests for about 10% of deaths that they certify.

Referral to the coroner

A death should be referred to the coroner if:

- The cause of death is unknown
- The deceased had not been seen by the certifying doctor either after death or within 14 days of death
- The death was violent, unnatural or suspicious
- The death may be due to an accident
- The death may be due to self-neglect or neglect by others
- The death may be due to an industrial disease or related to the deceased's employment
- The death may be due to an abortion
- The death occurred during an operation or before recovery from the effects of an anaesthetic
- The death may be due to suicide
- The death occurred during or shortly after detention in police or prison custody

Role of the coroner

The Coroner's Act 1988 defines when an inquest should be held. Inquests are held in public and may involve a jury. The purpose of an inquest is to determine:

- Who is the deceased
- How, when and where he died
- Details of the cause of death

The coroner is not concerned with civil or criminal liability. A coroner may record the cause of death as:

- Natural causes
- Accident/misadventure
- Industrial disease
- Sentence of death
- Dependence on drugs or non-dependent abuse of drugs
- Lawful killing
- Open verdict
- Want of attention at birth
- Unlawful killing
- Suicide
- Still birth
- Attempted or self-induced abortion

Medical litigation

Definition of negligence

For an allegation of negligence to succeed claimant must prove:

- The defendant had a duty of care to the claimant
- There was a breach of the duty of care
- The claimant suffered actionable harm or damage
- The damage was caused by the breach of the duty of care

Duty of care

All healthcare professional have a duty to become and remain competent. The level of skill will depend on experience and seniority of the professional. If a senior delegates responsibility to a junior he must be sure the junior is competent. Otherwise he remains responsible for any resulting error – vicarious liability. A breach of duty of care occurs if the healthcare professional fails to reach the proficiency of his peers. This is known as the Bolam test. It applies equally in treatment, diagnosis and advice. The breach can be something done (commission) or something not done (omission). A doctor can not be negligent if he acted in accordance with relevant professional opinion and this principle applies even if another doctor would have adopted a different practice. Ignorance is not a defence for negligence. Errors of clinical judgment (e.g. wrong diagnosis) often do not amount to negligence.

Actionable harm or damage

Actionable harm or damage is the disability, loss or injury suffered by the claimant.

However negligent the defendant has been, the claimant must have suffered quantifiable harm. Quantifiable harm includes:

- Loss of earnings
- Reduced quality or quantity of life
- Disfigurement
- Disability
- Mental anguish

There may also be an element of contributory negligence. This occurs if the actions of the claimant is judged to have made the situation worse and can reduce the amount of damages awarded.

Causation

Causation is the link between actionable harm and breach of duty of care. The harm has to have occurred as a result of the actions of the defendant.

Legal process

The burden of proof lies with the claimant. The standard of proof is the civil standard of balance of probabilities. Actions must be brought within 3 years. Different rules apply for children and mentally ill. If a claim is brought, the solicitor issues a Letter of Claim. A Letter of Response should be provided within 3 months. If the case continues, claim forms are raised by the solicitor and submitted to the court.

Civil Procedure Rules 1998

The Woolf report in 1994 noted that in medical negligence cases there was a disproportionate relationship between the costs and the amounts awarded. There were long delays in the settling of claims and unmeritorious cases were often pursued. Clear-cut cases were defended longer than should have been and success rate was lower than for any other personal injury litigation. There was less co-operation between opposing parties and 90% of litigants were legally aided. Woolf has proposed case management by the courts, alternative means of dispute resolution, court-based experts and judges with specialist medical knowledge. The future may include no-fault compensation, early settlement using fixed tariffs depending on the injury caused and greater use of mediation to settle disputes.

Preoperative assessment

Preoperative assessment aims to reduce the morbidity and mortality associated with surgery. It may prevent unnecessary cancellations and reduce hospital stay. Evidence-based guidelines reduce the time and cost associated with unnecessary investigations. An effective preoperative assessment process should inform the patient of the proposed procedure and allow informed consent for surgery to be obtained. It should assess pre-existing medical conditions and plan both the preoperative and postoperative management of these conditions. The issues that should be addressed include:

- Time of admission and starving instructions
- Management of usual medication
- Any specific preoperative preparation that may be required
- Transport to theatre
- Any specific anaesthetic issues
- Anticipated duration of surgery
- Likely recovery period
- Need for drains and catheter
- Likely discharge date
- Need for dressing change or specific postoperative care
- Follow-up requirements
- Likely date of return to work or full activity

Important medical diseases that increase the morbidity and mortality following surgery include:

- Ischaemic heart disease
- Congestive cardiac failure
- Hypertension
- Cardiac arrhythmias
- Chronic respiratory disease
- Diabetes mellitus
- Endocrine dysfunction
- Chronic renal failure
- Nephrotic syndrome
- Obstructive jaundice
- Obesity

Assessment of fitness for surgery

ASA Grading

Medical co-morbidity increases the risk associated with anaesthesia and surgery. The America Society of Anesthesiologists (ASA) grade is the most commonly used system to grade co-morbidity. The ASA grade is as follows:

- 1 = Normal healthy individual
- 2 = Mild systemic disease that does not limit activity
- 3 = Severe systemic disease that limits activity but is not incapacitating
- 4 = Incapacitating systemic disease which is constantly life-threatening
- 5 = Moribund, not expected to survive 24 hours with or without surgery

ASA grade accurately predicts morbidity and mortality. Over 50% of patients undergoing elective surgery are ASA grade 1. Operative mortality for these patients is less than 1 in 10,000.

POSSUM Scoring

POSSUM stands for Physiologic and Operative Severity Score for the enUmeration of Mortality and Morbidity. It was developed in a general surgical population and has since been adapted for use in vascular, colorectal, and oesophago-gastric patients. It is being increasingly ultilised in other specialties. It uses 12 physiological and biochemical variables, and six operative variables to give an estimation of mortality risk.

Elective surgery grades

The type of surgery is graded according to the degree of stress it will cause. Different types of surgery carry different risks and need differing levels of preoperative assessment. Elective surgery can be graded as follows:

- Minor – e.g. excision of a skin lesion
- Intermediate – e.g. inguinal hernia repair
- Major – e.g. hysterectomy
- Major plus – e.g. colonic resection

Preoperative investigations

The main purpose of preoperative investigations is to provide additional diagnostic and prognostic information with the aim of:

- Providing information that may confirm the appropriateness of the current course of clinical management
- Using the information to reduce the possible harm to patients by altering their clinical management
- Using the information to help assess the risk to the patient and opening up the possibility of discussing potential increases of risk with the patient
- Predicting postoperative complications
- Establishing a baseline measurement for later reference

The request for preoperative investigations should be based on factors apparent from the clinical assessment and the likelihood of asymptomatic abnormalities. It should also take into consideration the severity of the surgery contemplated. Preoperative investigations rarely uncover unsuspected medical conditions. It is inefficient as a means of screening for asymptomatic disease. Only 5% of patients have abnormalities on investigations not predicted by a clinical assessment. Only 0.1% of these investigations ever change the patient's management. Over 70% of preoperative investigations could be eliminated without adverse effect. The National Institute for Clinical Excellence (NICE) has produced guidelines on preoperative tests. These tests include:

- Chest x-ray
- ECG
- Echocardiography
- Full blood count
- Renal function
- Coagulation screen
- Glycosylated haemoglobin (HbA1c)
- Liver function
- Lung function tests

The tests recommended are based on the age of the patient, ASA grade and grade of the proposed surgery. Recommendations are graded:

- Red – not required
- Amber – test to be considered
- Green – recommended

Indications for preoperative investigations

Chest x-ray

- All patients for major vascular surgery
- Suspected malignancy
- Patients with cardiac or pulmonary disease for grade 4 (major+) surgery
- Patients who have severe (ASA 3) cardiac or pulmonary disease
- Anticipated ICU admission

ECG

- All patients aged 60 and over
- All patients with cardiovascular disease, including hypertension
- All patients with severe (ASA 3) respiratory or renal disease aged 40 and over

Echocardiography

- Severe aortic or mitral stenosis
- Severe left ventricular dysfunction
- Cardiomyopathy
- Pulmonary hypertension

Full blood count

- All patients undergoing major (grade 3 or 4) surgery
- Patients with severe (ASA 3) cardiac or respiratory disease
- Severe renal disease (creatinine > 200)
- Patients with a history of anaemia
- Patients who require a cross match or group and save
- Patients with a bleeding disorder
- Patients with chronic inflammatory conditions such as rheumatoid arthritis.

Renal function

- All patients with known or suspected renal dysfunction
- All patients with cardiac disease (including hypertension on treatment)
- All patients on diuretic treatment
- Patients with severe respiratory disease on steroid or theophylline therapy
- All patients with diabetes
- All patients for major (grade 3 or 4) surgery

Coagulation screen

- Personal or family history of abnormal bleeding
- Suspected liver dysfunction (cirrhosis, alcohol abuse, metastatic cancer)
- Current anticoagulant therapy
- Patients on haemodialysis

Glycosylated haemoglobin (HbA1c)

- Result within past 3 months for all diabetic patients
- Current random blood glucose in known or suspected diabetes

Liver function

- Hepato-biliary or pancreatic disease
- Known alcohol abuse
- Major gastrointestinal surgery

Lung function

- Patients with severe (ASA 3) respiratory disease undergoing major surgery
- Patients having scoliosis surgery
- Asthmatics need a peak flow recorded

Tests of respiratory, cardiac and renal disease

Respiratory function

Lung function tests should be able to predict the type and severity of any lung disease and correlate with the risk of complications and postoperative mortality. Tests fall in to three categories:

- Lung mechanics
- Gas exchange
- Control of breathing

Useful radiological investigations include a chest x-ray and high-resolution thoracic CT. Arterial blood gases may provide additional helpful information. Lung function tests allow assessment of lung volumes, airway caliber and gas transfer.

Spirometry

Lung volumes are assessed with spirometry (**Figure 2.1**). The total amount of air moved in and out of the lungs each minute depends upon the tidal volume (TV) and respiratory rate (RR). Pulmonary ventilation is the product of RR and TV. The extra inspiration available is called the inspiratory reserve volume (IRV). The extra expiration available is called the expiratory reserve volume (ERV). After maximum expiration, some air is still present in the lungs and is known as the residual volume (RV). The maximum volume available for breathing is the vital capacity (VC). Vital capacity is the sum of IRV, TV and ERV.

Peak flow rates

Airway calibre can be assessed by peak flow measurements (**Figure 2.2**). Accurate assessment requires co-operation and maximum voluntary effort of the patient. The flow rates measured include:

- FVC = Forced vital capacity
- FEV1 = Forced expiratory volume in one second

Absolute values depend on the height, weight, age, sex and race of the patient. The FEV_1/FVC ratio is a useful derived measurement. Lung function can be classified as:

- Normal
- Restrictive
- Obstructive

In restrictive lung disease, the FVC is reduced but FEV_1/FVC is normal. In obstructive lung disease, the FVC is normal or reduced and FEV_1/FVC is reduced.

Gas transfer

Arterial blood gases are the best measure available for the measurement of gas transfer. They also allow the assessment of ventilation/perfusion mismatch. Important parameters to measure are:

- pH
- Partial pressure of oxygen
- Partial pressure of carbon dioxide

Pulse oximetry gives an indirect estimate of gas transfer. This technique may be unreliable in the presence of other medical problems (e.g. anaemia).

Cardiac function

Simple non-invasive and more complicated invasive tests of cardiac function exist. Non-invasive tests include:

- Chest x-ray
- ECG
- Echocardiography
- Exercise test

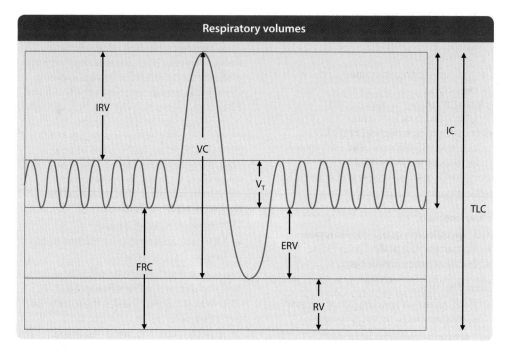

Figure 2.1 Respiratory volumes. IC = Inspiratory capacity. IRV = Inspiratory reserve volume. TV = Tidal volume. VC = Vital capacity. FRC = Functional residual capacity. RV = Residual volume. ERV = Expiratory reserve volume. TLC = Total lung capacity. (Reproduced from Thillai M and Hattotuwa K. Pocket Tutor Understanding ABGs and Lung Function Tests. London: JP Medical Ltd, 2012.)

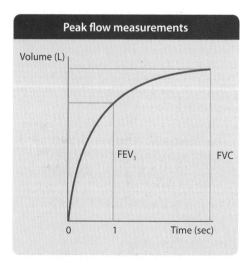

Figure 2.2. Peak flow measurements. FVC = Forced vital capacity. FEV_1 = forced expiratory volume in one second

Invasive tests include:

- Coronary angiography
- Thallium scanning

Chest x-ray

Routine preoperative chest x-ray is not recommended for all patients, but it is indicated in the presence of cardiorespiratory symptoms or signs. Important signs associated with increased cardiac morbidity are cardiomegaly, pulmonary oedema or a change in the cardiac outline characteristic of specific diseases.

ECG

A resting ECG is normal in 25–50% of patients with ischaemic heart disease. Characteristic features of ischaemia or previous infarction may be present. An exercise ECG provides a good indication of the degree of cardiac reserve.

24-hour ECG monitoring is useful in the detection and assessment of arrhythmias.

Echocardiography

Can be performed percutaneously or via the transoesophageal route. Two-dimensional echocardiography allows assessment of muscle mass, ventricular function, ejection fraction, end-diastolic and end-systolic volumes, valvular function and segmental defects. Doppler ultrasound allows assessment of valvular flow and pressure gradients.

Nuclear medicine

Myocardial scintigraphy allows assessment of myocardial perfusion. Radiolabelled thallium is the commonest isotope used. Areas of ischaemia or infarction appear as 'cold' spots on the scan. Vasodilators can be used to evaluate reversibility of ischaemia. Radiolabelled albumin or red cells can be used to assess ejection fraction. Such dynamic studies are performed 'gated' to the ECG.

Renal function

Glomerular filtration rate is the gold standard test of renal function. It can be calculated by measuring creatinine clearance rate but this requires 24-hour urine collection. Serum creatinine allows a good estimate of renal function. However the use of serum creatinine may be inaccurate in patients with obesity, oedema, pregnancy or ascites.

Management of associated medical conditions

Some medical conditions increase the risk associated with surgery. These need to be assessed preoperatively and where possible, the patient's condition optimised.

Cardiovascular disease

Several scoring systems exist for stratifying cardiac risk prior to non-cardiac surgery. They are simple to use and identify patients in need of further investigation.

Eagle index

One point is allocated for each of:

- History of myocardial infarction of angina
- Q wave on preoperative ECG
- Non-diet controlled diabetes mellitus
- Age more than 70 years
- History of ventricular arrhythmia

Patients scoring zero are at low-risk, patients scoring one are intermediate risk and those scoring two or more are at high-risk. Low-risk patients require no further investigation. Intermediate risk patients require an exercise ECG and thallium scan. High-risk patient should be considered for coronary angiography prior to major non-cardiac surgery.

Revised cardiac risk index

One point is allocated for each of:

- High-risk surgery
- Ischaemic heart disease
- History of congestive heart failure
- History of cerebrovascular disease
- Insulin therapy for diabetes mellitus
- Renal impairment

The risk of a major cardiac event during surgery increases with the number of points from 0.5% for zero points to 10% for more than two points.

Myocardial infarction

Elective surgery should be deferred for 6 months after a myocardial infarct. Risk factors for postoperative myocardial re-infarction include:

- Short time since previous infarct
- Residual major coronary vessel disease
- Prolonged or major surgery
- Impaired myocardial function

The risk of postoperative re-infarction after a previous myocardial infarct is 35% between 0 and 3 months, 15% between 3 and 6 months and 4% more than 6 months. Approximately 60% of postoperative myocardial infarcts are silent. The mortality of re-infarction is approximately 40%.

Hypertension

In patients with hypertension, an assessment is needed of the severity of hypertension and the presence of end organ damage. The risk of cardiovascular morbidity is increased in poorly controlled hypertension. Increased risk is present if the diastolic pressure is greater than 95 mmHg. Elective surgery should be cancelled if diastolic pressure is greater than 120 mmHg.

Respiratory disease

Patients with lung disease are at increased risk of respiratory complications. The complications include:

- Bronchospasm
- Atelectasis
- Bronchopneumonia
- Hypoxaemia
- Respiratory failure
- Pulmonary embolism

In addition to routine preoperative investigations, in patients with respiratory disease it is necessary to consider a chest x-ray, spirometry and arterial blood gases. A recent upper respiratory tract infection increases the risk postoperative chest complications. Elective surgery should be deferred for 2–4 weeks.

Smoking

Smoking doubles the risk of postoperative pulmonary complications. The increased risk persists for 3–4 months after stopping smoking. Smoking increases blood carboxyhaemoglobin. Increased carboxyhaemoglobin persists for 12 hours after the last cigarette.

Obesity

Morbidity and mortality after all surgery is increased in the obese. The risk is increased even in the absence of other disease. The Body Mass Index (BMI) is the best available measure of the degree of obesity. A patient's BMI = Weight (kg)/height (m)^2. The normal BMI is 22–28. A BMI greater than 30 equates to being significantly overweight. A BMI greater than 40 equals morbid obesity. Patients are at risk of numerous complications shown in **Table 2.1**.

Diabetes mellitus

Pre- and perioperative management of diabetic patients depends on the severity of the disease. Diet-controlled diabetics require no specific precautions. The blood sugar should be checked prior to surgery and consideration given to a glucose–potassium–insulin (GKI) infusion if more than 12 mmol/L. Those patients on long acting sulphonylureas should stop them 48 hours prior to surgery. Short acting agents should be omitted on the morning of operation. All oral hypoglycaemics can be recommenced when the patient is eating normally. A GKI infusion should be considered for non-insulin dependent diabetics undergoing major surgery. Insulin dependent diabetics should be placed early on an operating list and give a GKI infusion until eating normally. A GKI infusion is made up with 15 units of insulin, 10 mmol potassium chloride and 500 mL 10% dextrose and infused at a rate dependent on the blood sugar level.

Chronic renal failure

Chronic renal failure affects multiple organ systems. Effects that need to be considered by both surgeons and anesthetists include:

Complications associated with obesity		
Cardiovascular	**Respiratory**	**Other**
Hypertension	Difficult airway	Gastro-oesophageal reflux
Ischaemic heart disease	Difficult mechanical ventilation	Abnormal liver function
Cerebrovascular disease	Chronic hypoxaemia	Insulin resistance and type 2 diabetes
Deep venous thrombosis	Obstructive sleep apnoea	Poor postoperative pain control
Difficult vascular access	Pulmonary hypertension	Unpredictable pharmacological response
	Postoperative hypoxaemia	

Table 2.1 Complications associated with obesity

- Electrolyte disturbances
- Impaired acid–base balance
- Anaemia
- Coagulopathy
- Impaired autonomic regulation
- Protection of veins, shunts and fistula

Preparation for surgery

Drugs

Most medication can be continued in the perioperative period. A few drugs need to be discontinued as they present either anaesthetic or surgical risks. Oral anticoagulation with warfarin is managed according to the indication for its use. Patients with prosthetic heart valves need to continue anticoagulation with therapeutic doses of low molecular weight heparin. Patients on warfarin for atrial fibrillation can have their anticoagulation stopped prior to surgery. Warfarin should be discontinued for 5 days prior to surgery but can be restarted the night following the operation.

For minor surgery, there is no need to stop either the oral contraceptive pill or hormone replacement therapy. The oral contraceptive pill increases the risk of venous thromboembolism four-fold and for major surgery patients should be informed of the increased risk and an appropriate decision made.

Preoperative fasting

General anaesthesia increases the risk of aspiration of gastric contents. Traditionally patients have been starved since midnight prior to elective surgery the following morning. It is now known that clear fluids leave the stomach within 2 hours and that they do not increase the volume or acidity of gastric contents. For elective surgery, patients can be allowed food and clear fluids until 6 and 2 hours prior to their surgery, respectively. For emergency surgery, oral intake should be restricted as many surgical emergencies are associated with delayed gastric emptying.

Informed consent

Patient autonomy must be respected at all times. They should be given sufficient information to determine what treatment that they are or are not willing to receive. They have the right to decide not to undergo a treatment even if this could adversely affect the outcome or result in their death. Patients must be given sufficient information to make these decisions. Obtaining informed consent is not an isolated event. It involves a continuing dialogue between the doctor and patient.

Types of consent

Expressed consent can be oral or written. It is needed for most investigations or treatments with risks attached. Implied consent is non-written and occurs when a patient co-operates with a particular action, such as a physical examination or simple practical procedure. When obtaining consent, patients should be informed of:

- Details of the diagnosis and prognosis with and without treatment
- Uncertainties about the diagnosis
- Options available for treatment
- The purpose of a proposed investigation or treatment
- The likely benefits and probability of success
- Any possible side effects
- A reminder that the patients can change their mind at any stage
- A reminder that the patients have the right to a second opinion

All questions should be answered honestly. Information should not be withheld that might influence the decision making process. Patients should not be coerced. The person who obtains consent must be suitably trained and qualified. They must have sufficient knowledge of the proposed treatment and its risks. It is good practice for this to be the clinician providing the treatment.

Specific problems

No-one else can make a decision on behalf of a competent adult. In an emergency, a life-saving procedure can be performed without consent. All actions must, however, be justifiable to one's peers. Advanced care directives and living wills are legally binding and should be followed.

Consent in children

At the age of 16 years a child can be presumed to have the capacity to decide on treatment. Below the age of 16 years, a child may have the capacity to decide depending on their ability to understand what the treatment involves (Gillick competence). If a competent child refuses treatment, a person with parental responsibility may authorise treatment which is in the child's best interests.

Mental Capacity Act

In the UK, the Mental Capacity Act is designed to protect people who can't make decisions for themselves or lack the mental capacity to do so. This could be due to a mental health condition, a severe learning difficulty, a brain injury, a stroke or unconsciousness due to an anaesthetic or sudden accident. The Act's purpose is:

- To allow adults to make as many decisions as they can for themselves
- To enable adults to make advance decisions about whether they would like future medical treatment
- To allow adults to appoint, in advance of losing mental capacity, another person to make decisions about personal welfare on their behalf at a future date
- To allow decisions concerning personal welfare and affairs to be made in the best interests of adults when they have not made any future plans and cannot make a decision at the time
- To ensure an NHS body or local authority will appoint an independent mental capacity advocate to support someone who cannot make a decision about serious medical treatment when there are no family or friends to be consulted
- To provide protection against legal liability for carers who have honestly and reasonably sought to act in the person's best interests
- To provide clarity and safeguards around research in relation to those who lack capacity.

Under the Mental Capacity Act, a person is presumed to make their own decisions 'unless all practical steps to help him (or her) to make a decision have been taken without success'. Every person should be presumed to be able to make their own decisions. One can only take a decision for someone else if all practical steps to help them to make a decision have been taken without success. Incapacity is not based on the ability to make a wise or sensible decision. To determine incapacity, it is necessary to consider whether the person one is looking after is able to understand the particular issue that they are making a decision about. It is necessary to consider if they have:

- An impairment or disturbance in the functioning of their mind or brain, and
- An inability to make decisions

A person is unable to make a decision if they cannot:

- Understand the information relevant to the decision
- Retain that information
- Use or weigh that information as part of the process of making the decision, or communicate the decision

If, having taken all practical steps to assist someone, it is concluded that a decision should be made for them, that decision must be made in that person's best interests. It is essential to consider whether there is another way of making the decision which might not affect the person's rights. The Mental Capacity Act sets out a checklist of things to consider when deciding what is in a person's best interests including:

- Do not make assumptions on the basis of age, appearance, condition or behaviour
- Consider all the relevant circumstances
- Consider whether or when the person will have capacity to make the decision
- Support the person's participation in any acts or decisions made for them
- Do not make a decision about life-sustaining treatment 'motivated by a desire to bring about death'
- Consider the person's expressed wishes and feelings, beliefs and values
- Take into account the views of others with an interest in the person's welfare, their carers and those appointed to act on their behalf

Perioperative risk management

We all take risks in everyday life. The degree of risk taken depends on the perceived benefit. Most decisions are made on previous experiences. Risk assessment forms an integral part of patient care. An assessment needs to be made of the risks versus benefits for an procedure performed. These will then influence decisions made by the surgeon or the patient

Risk assessment models

Assessment of risk in surgery depends on many factors. These involve knowledge of the:

- Patient
- Disease
- Co-morbidities
- Proposed surgery
- Physiological status

Risk assessment tools

Decision making is rarely simple and straight forward. Risk assessment tools have been developed and are in common use to help assess risk. They include:

- Goldman Cardiac Risk Index
- Parsonnet Score
- POSSUM
- Injury Severity Score
- Revised Trauma score
- APACHE I, II and III

WHO Safe Surgery Check List

In Western industrialised countries, major complications are reported to occur following about 15% of inpatient surgical procedures with permanent disability or death occurring following 0.5% of operations. Some of this morbidity and mortality results from human error and is preventable. The WHO Safe Surgery Check List recommends a series of checks – Sign In, Time Out and Sign Out, be performed prior to, during and after any surgical procedure. The aim of the use of the checklist is to strengthen the commitment of clinical staff to address safety issues within the surgical setting. This includes improving anaesthetic safety practices, ensuring correct site surgery, avoiding surgical site infections and improving communication within the team. Its routine use has been shown to reduce the risk of complications and death.

Principles of anaesthesia
Pharmacokinetics and pharmacodynamics

Definitions

Pharmacokinetics is the study of the bodily absorption, distribution, metabolism, and excretion of drugs. Pharmacodynamics is the study of the biochemical and physiological effects of drugs and their mechanisms of action. Pharmacokinetics of a drug are dependent on:

- Absorption into the body
- Distribution throughout the fluids and tissues of the body
- Metabolism and its daughter metabolites
- Excretion or elimination from the body

First order kinetics

With first order kinetics, a constant fraction of the drug in the body is eliminated per unit time. The rate of elimination is proportional to the amount of drug in the body. The majority of drugs are eliminated in this way. With drugs displaying first order kinetics various properties can be defined:

- The clearance is defined as the apparent volume of plasma from which a drug is entirely removed per unit time. It is usually expressed in proportion to body weight or surface area.
- The volume of distribution is the volume into which a drug appears to be uniformly distributed at the concentration measured in plasma. It is usually a steady state volume of distribution equal to the amount of drug in the body. Drugs that are lipid soluble have a high volume of distribution. Drugs that are lipid insoluble have a low volume of distribution.
- The half life is the time taken for the plasma concentration of a drug to fall by 50% when first-order kinetics are observed. Many drugs have an initial redistribution phase with a short half-life followed by an elimination phase with a longer half-life.

- The bioavailability is the proportion of a dose of a specified drug preparation entering the systemic circulation after administration by a specified route.

Multicompartment models

First order kinetics is often only displayed in drugs that are distributed around a single compartment. The human body is more complex. It has several compartments – muscle, blood, brain fat etc. Some drugs (induction anaesthetic agents) are initially transported to organs with a rich blood supply. After a few minute the agent redistributes to other parts of the body. Initially, the blood concentration rapidly falls due to redistribution. Later, the blood concentration decreases more slowly due to metabolism or elimination of the drug.

General anaesthesia

General anaesthesia is a drug-induced state of unresponsiveness and is usually achieved by the use of a combination of agents. It has three phases:

- Induction
- Maintenance
- Reversal and recovery

Premedication

Is the administration of drugs prior to a general anaesthetic. It has three potentially useful effects:

- Anxiolysis
- Reduced bronchial secretions
- Analgesia

Anxiolysis, if needed, can be achieved with either benzodiazepines or phenothiazines. Opiate analgesics also have useful sedative properties. Reduction of sections is not as important today with modern inhalational agents. Ether was notorious for stimulating bronchial secretions. If required, secretions can be reduced with hyoscine. It also reduces salivation and prevents bradycardia. Analgesia is best achieved with strong opiates.

Drugs used in premedication include:

- Anxiolysis – benzodiazepines, phenothiazines
- Analgesia – opiates, non-steroids anti-inflammatories
- Amnesia – benzodiazepines, anticholinergics
- Antiemetic – anticholinergics, antihistamines, 5HT antagonists
- Antacid – alginates, proton pump inhibitors
- Anti-autonomic – anticholinergics, β-blockers
- Adjuncts – bronchodilators, steroids

Induction of anaesthesia

Induction agents are usually administered intravenously. They are highly lipid soluble and rapidly cross the blood–brain barrier. They are distributed to organs with a high blood flow such as the brain. With falling blood levels they are rapidly redistributed. As a result they have rapid onset and, without maintenance, have a rapid recovery.

Thiopentone is a short-acting barbiturate that was first used at Pearl Harbour in 1942. It depresses the myocardium and in hypovolaemic patient can induce profound hypotension. Propofol is now one of the most commonly used induction agents. It has very short half-life and can also cause hypotension. It can also be used as an infusion for the maintenance of anaesthesia. Chemically, it is unrelated to barbiturates and has largely replaced thiopentone for the induction of anaesthesia. Propofol has no analgesic properties, so when used in the maintenance of anaesthesia, opioids such as fentanyl may be need to administered.

Rapid-sequence induction

Rapid-sequence induction involves the rapid induction of anaesthesia. Cricoid pressure is used to reduce the risk of aspiration. Pressure is released once tracheal intubation with a cuffed tube has been achieved. It is achieved by the use of thiopentone and suxamethonium and is used for patients who are not fasted, have a history of gastro-oesophageal reflux, have intestinal obstruction, pregnancy or intra-abdominal pathology that will delay gastric emptying.

Endotracheal intubation

Endotracheal intubation is the placement of a tube into the trachea to maintain a patient airway. Following insertion, air entry is confirmed by listening with a stethoscope for breath sounds over each side of the chest and by monitoring end tidal carbon dioxide levels. The benefits of an endotracheal airway include:

- Protection against aspiration and gastric insufflation
- More effective ventilation and oxygenation
- Facilitation of suctioning
- Delivery of anaesthetic and other drugs via the endotracheal tube

Potential complications include:

- Failed intubation and hypoxaemia
- Aspiration and post-intubation pneumonia
- Pneumothorax
- Trauma from the laryngoscope – teeth and soft tissues
- Right mainstem intubation
- Oesophageal intubation
- Hypotension and arrhythmias
- Vocal cord damage

Laryngeal mask airway

The laryngeal mask airway (LMA) is an alternative to the use of an endotracheal tube. It consists of a tube with an inflatable cuff that is inserted blindly into the pharynx, forming a low-pressure seal around the laryngeal inlet and permitting gentle positive pressure ventilation. The apex of the mask, with its open end pointing downwards toward the tongue, is pushed backwards towards the uvula. The cuff follows the natural bend of the oropharynx and is seated over the pyriform fossae. The advantages of an LMA is that it does not require the use of a laryngoscope or muscle relaxants and it provides an airway for spontaneous or controlled ventilation that is well tolerated. An LMA does not protect the lungs from aspiration, making it unsuitable for patients at risk of this complication.

Maintenance of anaesthesia

Balanced anaesthesia has three aspects:

- Hypnosis – suppression of consciousness
- Analgesia – suppression of physiological responses to stimuli
- Relaxation – suppression of muscle tone and relaxation

The ideal inhalational anaesthetic agent

The ideal inhalational anaesthetic agent should have several properties. In its preparation it should:

- Be easily administered
- Have a boiling point above ambient temperature
- Have a low latent heat of vaporisation
- Be chemically stable with long shelf-life
- Be compatible with soda-lime, metals and plastics
- Be non-flammable
- Be cheap

Its pharmacokinetic should be:

- Low solubility
- Rapid onset, rapid offset, adjustable depth
- Minimal metabolism
- Predictable in all age groups

Its pharmacodynamic should be:

- High potency – allows high FiO_2
- High therapeutic index
- Analgesic

The agent should have few adverse actions and have minimal toxicity. There should be no toxicity with chronic low-level exposure to staff.

Anaesthesia is normally maintained with inhaled volatile gases. They are lipid soluble hydrocarbons. They have high saturated vapour pressures. Modern inhalational agents are potent, non-inflammable and non-explosive. The minimum alveolar concentration (MAC) is the alveolar concentration required to keep 50% of population unresponsive. The adverse effects of inhalational anaesthetics are shown in **Table 2.2.**

Halothane

Halothane is a potent anaesthetic but poor analgesic agent (MAC = 0.75). It can be used for gaseous induction in children. About 20% is metabolised in the liver and it can cause hepatic dysfunction. Occasionally it causes severe hepatitis that can progress to liver necrosis. It depresses myocardial contractility and can induce arrhythmias.

Isoflurane

Isoflurane is a potent anaesthetic but poor analgesic agent (MAC = 1.05). It is less

Adverse effects of inhalational anaesthetic			
Cardiovascular	Respiratory	Central nervous system	Other
Decrease myocardial contractility	Depress ventilation	Increase cerebral blood flow	Decrease renal blood flow
Reduce cardiac output	Laryngospasm and airway obstruction	Reduce cerebral metabolic rate	Stimulate nausea and vomiting
Hypotension	Decrease ventilatory response to hypoxia and hypercapnia	Increase risk of epilepsy	Precipitate hepatitis
Arrhythmias			
Increase myocardial sensitivity to catecholamines	Bronchodilatation	Increase intracranial pressure	

Table 2.2 Adverse effects of inhalational anaesthetics

cardiotoxic than halothane but causes greater respiratory depression. It reduces peripheral resistance and can cause a 'coronary steal'. Few adverse effects have been reported.

Nitrous oxide

Nitrous oxide is a weak anaesthetic agent (MAC = 103). It can not be used as an anaesthetic agent alone without causing hypoxia. It is however a very potent analgesic agent. It is often used as a 50% N_2O/50% O_2 mixture known as Entonox. It is used in anaesthesia mainly for its analgesic properties.

Muscle relaxants

Muscle relaxants are either depolarising or non-depolarising agents. Depolarising agents (e.g. suxamethonium) act rapidly within seconds and their effects last for approximately 5 minutes. They are used during induction of anaesthesia. Side effects include:

- Histamine release producing a 'scoline rash'
- Bradycardia
- Somatic pain resulting from fasciculation
- Hyperkalaemia
- Increased intraocular pressure
- Increased gastric pressure

Persistent neuromuscular blockade can result in 'scoline apnoea'. This affects

approximately 1:7000 of population and is due to pseudocholinesterase deficiency. Malignant hyperpyrexia affects approximately 1:100,000 of population. It is due to increased calcium influx and uncontrolled metabolism and results in a rapid increase in body temperature with increased $PaCO_2$.

Non-depolarising agents (e.g. vecuronium) act over 2–3 minutes and the effects last for 30 minutes to 1 hour. They act as competitive antagonists of acetylcholine receptor and are used for intraoperative muscle relaxation.

Perioperative monitoring

General anaesthesia removes the ability of a patient to protect themselves. The safety and physiological control of the patient becomes the responsibility of the anaesthetist. The anaesthetist needs to:

- Maintain airway and oxygenation
- Preserve circulation
- Prevent hypothermia
- Prevent injury
- Monitor during anaesthesia

Airway management

General anaesthesia removes muscle tone. Without assistance the airway will be compromised. Methods of maintaining airway include:

- Manual methods (e.g. jaw thrust)
- Guedel airway
- Laryngeal mask
- Endotracheal tube
- Tracheostomy tube

Monitoring during anaesthesia

The continuous presence of an adequately trained anaesthetist is essential. Accurate monitoring of vital signs is obligatory. Facilities for cardiopulmonary resuscitation should be immediately available. Monitoring of the following is considered essential for all patients:

- Temperature
- Heart rate
- Blood pressure
- ECG
- Oxygen content of inspiratory gas mix
- End-tidal carbon dioxide
- Pulse oximetry

The following may be considered for major surgery:

- Invasive blood pressure monitoring
- Central venous pressure
- Urine output

Alarms should indicate oxygen supply failure and ventilator disconnection.

Invasive and non-invasive monitoring

Cardiac output is the 'gold standard' measure of cardiovascular function. Measurement normally requires invasive pressure monitoring. Cardiovascular function can however be assessed non-invasively with:

- Electrocardiogram
- Blood pressure
- Central venous pressure
- Urine output

Blood pressure can be monitored with a cuff (intermittent) or arterial line (continuous) and in the absence of vasoconstriction provides a good estimate of cardiac output.

The ECG

An electrocardiogram (ECG) provides information on both heart rate and rhythm. It also serves as a valuable monitor of electrolyte abnormalities. A 12-lead ECG provides information on myocardial ischaemia or infarction. ECG monitoring is essential for all patients and is of particular use in:

- All patients in ITU or HDU
- Patients with poor cardiac reserve
- Patients receiving vasoactive drugs
- Patients with drug toxicity
- Monitoring of electrolyte disturbances

Arterial pressure monitoring

Invasive arterial pressure monitoring requires:

- An arterial cannula
- A monitoring line
- A transducer
- A monitoring system

It provides information on systolic and diastolic pressure and arterial waveform. Complications and problems associated with invasive monitoring include:

- Over and under dampening
- Incorrect zeroing
- Haematoma
- Distal ischaemia
- Inadvertent drug injection
- Disconnection and haemorrhage
- Infection

Central venous pressure

Clinical assessment of jugular venous pressure is unreliable. The central venous system can be cannulated by the internal jugular or subclavian routes to provide more accurate information about central venous pressure and intravascular volume. It also allows assessment of the cardiac pre-load. Complications of CVP lines include:

- Pneumothorax
- Arterial puncture
- Air embolism
- Infection

The site at which transducers are zeroed are very variable. They also change with patient movement. Therefore changes in pressure rather than absolute values are important. The pressure response to a fluid bolus (e.g. 200 mL of colloid given as quickly as possible) give a good estimate of intravascular volume status. A low CVP with a transient increase with a fluid bolus indicates hypovolaemia. A high CVP with a persistent increase with a fluid bolus indicates hypervolaemia.

Cardiac output and left-sided pressures

If both ventricle are functioning normally, cardiac pre-load will allow an assessment of cardiac output. However, in ischaemic heart disease or sepsis, left ventricular function can be reduced. Pulmonary hypertension reduces right ventricular function. In these situations, assessment of left heart pressures may be important. Also a more direct measure of cardiac output may be needed. Cardiac output can be measured either invasively with a pulmonary artery catheter or non-invasively using an oesophageal Doppler.

Swan–Ganz catheter

A Swan–Ganz catheter is a balloon-tipped catheter inserted through a central vein. It is floated through the right side of heart into the pulmonary artery. The balloon allows 'wedging' in a branch of the pulmonary artery. The pressure recorded is known as the pulmonary capillary wedge pressure. It is a good estimate of left atrial pressure. The tip of the catheter contains a thermistor. The cardiac output can be measured using thermodilution principal. If blood pressure and cardiac output are known then vascular resistance can be calculated. Complications of a Swan–Ganz catheter include:

- Arrhythmias
- Knotting and misplacement
- Cardiac valve trauma
- Pulmonary infarction
- Pulmonary artery rupture
- Balloon rupture
- Catheter thrombosis or embolism

The primary haemodynamic data obtained from a Swan–Ganz catheter includes:

- Heart rate
- Mean arterial pressure
- Central venous pressure
- Mean pulmonary artery pressure
- Mean pulmonary artery occlusion pressure
- Cardiac output
- Ventricular ejection fraction

The derived haemodynamic data obtained from a Swan–Ganz catheter includes:

- Cardiac index
- Stroke volume
- Stroke volume index
- Systemic vascular resistance
- Systemic vascular resistance index
- Pulmonary vascular resistance index
- Left ventricular stroke work index
- Right ventricular stroke work index
- Oxygen delivery
- Oxygen consumption

Recovery from anaesthesia

Recovery from anaesthesia should be monitored by a suitably trained nurse and it should occur in a properly equipped recovery area. An anaesthetist should be immediately available. Causes of failure to breath after general anaesthesia include:

- Obstruction of the airway
- Central sedation due to opiates or anaesthetic agent
- Hypoxia
- Hypercarbia
- Hypocarbia due to overventilation
- Persistent neuromuscular blockade
- Pneumothorax
- Circulatory failure leading to respiratory arrest

Care of the patient under anaesthesia
Thermoregulation

Mammals maintain a constant body temperature. They are known as homeotherms. Their body temperature is usually above the environmental temperature. Homeotherms have many advantages but do need a higher metabolic rate.

Body temperature results from a balance between production and heat loss. In a balanced state, production and loss of heat will be equal and the body temperature will be constant. Tight control of temperature is essential for normal physiological functions. The core temperature is invariably higher then the skin temperature.

Control of body temperature

Temperature is controlled by the hypothalamus. Control requires sensors, a control centre and effectors. Temperature sensors are found throughout the body in the skin, brain and other organs. There are two types of sensors that respond to hot and cold. The hypothalamus acts as a thermostat and has a temperature set point. Effectors produce more heat (increased metabolic rate, shivering, brown fat metabolism) or change heat loss (blood vessel dilation or constriction, erection of hair, curling up, sweating).

The skin

The skin is the primary organ for removal of metabolic heat. About 90% of heat is lost through the skin. The remaining 10% is lost in urine and exhaled air. If the body temperature is too high, blood vessels in the skin can dilate and increase blood flow by 150 times to lose excess heat. In cold weather, blood vessels in the skin will contract and reduce heat loss. Heat loss is by:

- Radiation
- Conduction
- Convection
- Sweating

Newton's law of cooling governs heat loss by radiation and conduction. Heat loss = heat conductance x temperature difference. The temperature difference = body temperature – ambient temperature. Sweating can be used to lose enormous amounts of heat. The heat of vaporisation of water is about 580 calories/litre. If the ambient temperature is higher than the body temperature, sweating is the only way heat can be lost. Sweat glands are activated by nerves from the sympathetic nervous system.

Mechanisms of pyrexia

Fevers are caused by in increase in the temperature set point – the thermostat has been set higher. Often caused by bacterial toxins or inflammatory mediators, they act directly on the hypothalamus. Fevers result from either increased metabolism, reduced heat conduction, or both. The benefits of a fever are uncertain.

Perioperative hypothermia

Surgical patients are at risk of developing hypothermia at any stage of the perioperative pathway. Inadvertent perioperative hypothermia is a common but preventable complication of surgical procedures. It is associated with increased morbidity. Hypothermia is defined as a patient core temperature of below 36.0°C. During the early phase of anaesthesia, a patient's temperature can easily fall. Reasons for this include:

- Loss of the behavioural response to cold
- Impairment of thermoregulatory heat-preserving mechanisms under general anaesthesia
- Anaesthesia-induced peripheral vasodilatation
- Patient getting cold while waiting for surgery on the ward

It is important to prevent inadvertent perioperative hypothermia.

Perioperative care

Patients should be informed that the hospital environment may be colder than their own home and that staying warm before surgery will reduce the risk of postoperative complications. They should bring additional clothing, such as a dressing gown, a vest and warm clothing. They should tell staff if they feel cold at any time during their hospital stay. When using any device to measure patient temperature, healthcare professionals should be aware of, and carry out, any adjustments that need to be made in order to obtain an estimate of core temperature.

Preoperative phase

Each patient should be assessed for their risk of inadvertent perioperative hypothermia. Patients should be managed as higher risk if any two of the following apply:

- ASA grade II to V
- Preoperative temperature below 36.0°C
- Undergoing combined general and regional anaesthesia
- Undergoing major or intermediate grade surgery
- At risk of cardiovascular complications

If the patient's temperature is below 36.0°C, forced air warming should be started preoperatively on the ward and it should be maintained throughout the intraoperative phase.

Intraoperative phase

The patient's temperature should be measured and documented before induction of anaesthesia. It should be repeated every 30 minutes until the end of surgery. Induction of anaesthesia should not begin unless the patient's temperature is 36.0°C or above. Intravenous fluids (500 mL or more) and blood products should be warmed to 37°C using a fluid warming device. Patients who are at higher risk of inadvertent perioperative hypothermia and who are having anaesthesia for less than 30 minutes should be warmed intraoperatively from induction of anaesthesia using a forced air warming device. All patients who are having anaesthesia for longer than 30 minutes should be warmed intraoperatively from induction of anaesthesia using a forced air warming device.

Postoperative phase

The patient's temperature should be measured and documented on admission to the recovery room and then every 15 minutes. Ward transfer should not be arranged unless the patient's temperature is 36.0°C or above. If the patient's temperature is below 36.0°C, they should be actively warmed using forced air warming until they are discharged from the recovery room or until they are comfortably warm.

Prevention of injuries

General anesthesia removes many of the bodies natural protective mechanisms. If care is not taken, iatrogenic injuries are possible. Many of these injuries can produce lasting disability and can lead to litigation. Recognition of risks and prevention is essential. Tissues at risk include nerves, eyes, teeth and skin.

Nerve injuries

The incidence of nerve injuries during anaesthesia is unknown. However, in the USA, they account for 15% of postoperative litigation claims. Most are due to careless positioning of the patient. The commonest nerves affected are the ulnar and common peroneal nerves and the brachial plexus. Predisposing factors include:

- Medical conditions associated with a neuropathy (e.g. diabetes mellitus)
- Nerve ischaemia due to hypotension
- Local injections or direct nerve injury
- The use of a tourniquets

Most nerve injuries are due to a neuraproxia. About 90% undergo complete recovery. However about 10% are left with some residual weakness or sensory loss.

Ulnar nerve injuries are caused by positioning the arms along side the patient in pronation. The nerve is compressed at the elbow between the operating table and medial epicondyle. Injury can be prevented by positioning arms in supination. Brachial plexus injuries are caused by excessive arm abduction or external rotation and can be prevented by avoiding more than 60° of abduction. Common peroneal nerve injuries are caused by direct pressure on the nerve, often with the legs in lithotomy position. The nerve can be compressed against the neck of the fibula. Injury can be prevented by adequate padding of lithotomy poles. The radial nerve can damaged by a tourniquet or misplaced injection in the deltoid muscle. Injury can be prevented by adequate padding of any tourniquet used.

Haematological problems in surgery

Function and components of blood

Blood has both cellular and fluid components. The cellular components make up 45% of the volume. The fluid component makes up 55% of the volume.

Plasma

Plasma is the fluid component. Its normal pH is 7.35–7.45. About 90% is water and 10% is solutes. Solutes include albumin (60%), globulins (35%), fibrinogen, thrombin, hormones, cholesterol, nitrogenous wastes, nutrients and electrolytes.

Erythrocytes

Erythrocytes or red blood cells are biconcave discs. They are approximately 7.5 μm in diameter. They are formed in the bone marrow and removed from circulation in the spleen and liver. They have no nuclei or mitochondria. They have a life span of about 120 days. Normal red cell production requires iron, amino acids, vitamins and hormones – erythropoietin. Reticulocytes are immature red blood cells. They account for 1–2% of circulating red blood cells. Red cell production is stimulated by haemorrhage, anaemia, hypoxia and increased oxygen requirement.

Leukocytes

Leukocytes or white blood cells account for 1% of blood volume. They have both nuclei and mitochondria. There are five types of while blood cells as follows:

- Neutrophils (40–70%)
- Lymphocytes (20–40%)
- Monocytes (4–8%)
- Basophils (1%)
- Eosinophils

Neutrophils are responsible for phagocytosis of bacteria. Eosinophils are involved in defence against parasites and in immune complex destruction. Basophils release histamine and produce chemotactic agents. Monocytes are the precursors of tissue macrophages. Lymphocytes are produce in both lymph nodes and the spleen. B lymphocytes produce antibodies. T lymphocytes are involved in cell-mediated immunity. NK cells are lymphocytes that are involved in immune surveillance.

Platelets

Platelets are not true cells. They are fragments of cells known as megakaryocytes and are formed in the bone marrow and have a life span of about 10 days. They have granules that contain calcium, ADP, serotonin and platelet derived growth factor. They have an important role in blood coagulation.

Iron metabolism

The body contains about 5 g of iron. About 65% of the body's iron is found in haemoglobin, 30% is in ferritin and haemosiderin and 3% is in myoglobin. Daily dietary requirements are about 1 mg in a man and 3 mg in a woman. An average diet contains about 15 mg of iron daily, only 5–10% of which is absorbed. Absorption occurs in the ferrous (2+) form in the upper part of small intestine. Erythropoiesis occurs in the bone marrow. Iron is carried to the bone marrow by plasma transferrin. Iron is stored bound to ferritin and as haemosiderin.

Ferritin

Ferritin is a water-soluble protein-iron complex. It is made up of apoferritin and a iron-phosphate-hydroxide core. About 20% of its weight is iron. Synthesis is stimulated by the presence of iron. Iron is in the ferric (3+) form.

Haemosiderin

Haemosiderin is an insoluble protein–iron complex. About 40% of its weight is iron. It is formed by lysosomal digestion of ferritin.

Transferrin

Transferrin is a β-globulin that is synthesised in the liver. It has a half-life of 8–10 days. Each molecule binds two iron atoms and is normally only about 30% saturated. Erythroblasts have transferrin receptors.

Dietary iron

Iron is present in food as ferric hydroxide and ferric–protein complexes. Meat and liver are good sources of dietary iron. The average Western diet contains 10–15 mg of iron and 5–10% is absorbed in the duodenum and jejunum. Absorption is increased in pregnancy and iron-deficiency states. In a normal individual, the daily iron requirement is 1–2 mg per day.

Iron absorption

Iron absorption is favoured by acid and reducing agents and it is better absorbed in the ferrous form. The amount of iron absorbed is controlled in the epithelial cells. Excess iron forms ferritin and is shed with the cells into the gut lumen. Iron enters the plasma in the ferric form.

Iron transport

Most iron is transported to the bone marrow and is used mainly for erythropoiesis. It binds to transferrin in the portal blood. About 6 g of haemoglobin are produced each day and this requires about 20 mg of iron. Total plasma iron turns over about seven times per day.

Iron deficiency anaemia

As the body has a limited ability to absorb iron and excess loss of iron through bleeding is common, then iron deficiency is the commonest cause of anaemia worldwide. It results in hypochromic and microcytic red blood cells. The diagnosis of iron deficiency is usually straightforward. Determining the cause can be difficult.

Clinical features

The clinical features of iron deficiency anaemia depend of the rate of onset. If the onset is insidious, then symptoms are often few. The commonest symptoms are lethargy and dyspnoea. Skin atrophy occurs in about 30% of patients. Nail changes include koilonychia (spoon-shaped nails). Patients may also develop angular stomatitis and glossitis. Oesophageal and pharyngeal webs may be seen. Examination should be directed to identifying possible underlying causes.

Causes of iron deficiency

The causes of iron deficiency anaemia include:

- Increased blood loss – uterine, GI tract, urine
- Increased demands – prematurity, growth, child-bearing
- Malabsorption – post-gastrectomy, coeliac disease
- Poor diet

Investigation

The following investigations may be required:

- Full blood count and blood film examination
- Haematinic assays (serum ferritin, vitamin B12 and folate)
- Faecal occult bloods
- Mid-stream urine
- Endoscopic or radiological studies of the gastrointestinal tract

The diagnosis of iron deficiency can be based on:

- Reduced haemoglobin (men < 13.5 g/dL, women < 11.5 g/dL)
- Reduced mean cell volume (< 76 fL)
- Reduced mean cell haemoglobin (< 27 pg)
- Reduced mean cell haemoglobin concentration (< 300 g/L)
- Blood film – microcytic, hypochromic red cells
- Reduced serum ferritin (< 10 mg/L)
- Reduced serum iron (men < 14 mmol/L, women < 11 mmol/L)
- Increased serum iron binding capacity (> 75 mmol/L)

A diagnostic bone marrow examination is rarely required.

Other causes of a hypochromic microcytic anaemia include:

- Anaemia of chronic disease
- Thalassaemia trait
- Sideroblastic anaemia

Management

The management of iron deficiency anaemia relies on identification and management of the underlying cause and iron replacement therapy. Oral replacement with ferrous salts is the preferred option. Preparations include ferrous sulphate, fumarate and gluconate. They provide approximately 200 mg of iron per day. The side effects of iron supplements include epigastric pain, constipation and diarrhoea. Effective treatment should increase the haemoglobin concentration by 1 g/L/day and treatment should continue for 3 months after a normal haemoglobin level is achieved. Intravenous iron preparations are available on a named patient basis but severe side effects (e.g. anaphylaxis) may occur. Injections can result in skin staining and arthralgia and should only be used when patients can not tolerate oral preparations.

Sickle cell anaemia

Pathology

Sickle cell anaemia is an autosomal recessive disease. Normal haemoglobin has two α and 2 β chains. In sickle cell disease a single amino acid substitution occurs on the β chain. Valine is substituted for glutamic acid at position 6. Patients who are homozygous have sickle cell anaemia. Patients who are heterozygous have sickle cell trait. It is commonly seen in patients of Afro-Caribbean descent. The resulting Hb S is less soluble than Hb A. When deoxygenated, haemoglobin undergoes polymerisation and forms characteristic sickle cells. The abnormal cells result in blockage of small vessels and causes vaso-occlusive events. Sickling may be precipitated by infection, fever, dehydration, cold or hypoxia.

Clinical features

Patients with sickle cell anaemia have a chronic haemolytic anaemia with a high reticulocyte count. They are at increased risk of infection by encapsulated bacteria. Acute complications include:

- Painful crises
- Worsening anaemia
- Acute chest symptoms
- Symptoms and signs of neurological or ocular events
- Priapism

Investigation

The diagnosis can be confirmed by:

- Sickle solubility test
- High performance liquid chromatography

Prevention of complications

Patient and parent education of the risks associated with sickle cell anaemia is important. Patients need to avoid the cold and dehydration. Antibiotic prophylaxis should be considered in children less than 5 years of age. Usually phenoxymethylpenicillin is the antibiotic of choice. Children should be vaccinated with the pneumococcal vaccine.

Patients with sickle cell anaemia are at high-risk of acute sickling complications during general anaesthesia. They require careful pre and perioperative management. Preoperative transfusion may be required to ensure a haemoglobin of 9–10 g/dL. During surgery it is essential to avoid dehydration and hypoxia. Adequate intraoperative and postoperative pain relief is essential.

Management of complications

Patients with suspected complications require:

- Intravenous fluids
- Adequate pain relief often with opiates
- Oxygen
- Early antibiotic therapy if suspected infection

Painful crises

Approximately 60% of patients with sickle cell anaemia will have one episode per year. Bony crises result from localised ischaemia. Avascular necrosis may occur. Treatment of crises involves rest and analgesia. Abdominal crises present with pain, vomiting, distension and features of peritonism. About 40% of adolescents with sickle cell anaemia will have gallstones.

Anaemia

Worsening anaemia often presents with tiredness and cardiac failure. It results from acute splenic sequestration or an aplastic crisis. In both situations urgent transfusion may be required.

Acute chest syndrome

Patients present with chest pain, cough, fever and tachypnoea accompanied by clinical and radiological features of consolidation. *Chlamydia* and *Mycoplasma* are important causes of chest infections. Management requires parenteral antibiotic therapy.

Acute neurological events

A stroke occurs in approximately 10% of patients before the age of 20 years. All acute neurological symptoms require investigation. Acute stroke requires urgent exchange transfusion.

Priapism

Priapism occurs in about 20% of males before the age of 20 years. If it lasts for more than a few hours it can result in impotence. Blood should be aspirated from the corpora cavernosa. Intra-cavernosal injection of an α agonist (e.g. phenylephrine) may be of benefit.

Haemostasis

The haemostatic response has three elements:

- Vasoconstriction
- Platelet aggregation
- Clotting cascade

Vasoconstriction

Vasoconstriction occurs as a direct result of vessel injury. It is enhanced by vasoconstricting elements released from platelets. Pain can also result in reflex sympathetic vasoconstriction.

Platelet aggregation

Platelets are formed in the bone marrow from megakaryocytes. They contain the contractile proteins actin and myosin. They have no nucleus but contain endoplasmic reticulum and a Golgi apparatus that can produce proteins. They contain mitochondria that can produce ATP and ADP. They can also synthesis prostaglandins and thromboxane A2. They have a half-life in the blood of 8 to 12 days.

In response to tissue damage, platelets undergo a number of changes. Platelet aggregation can result in a 'platelet plug'. Platelets adhere to damaged endothelium (via von Willebrand factor). Aggregating platelets release arachadonic acid which is converted to thromboxane A2 and calcium mediated contraction of actin and myosin results in degranulation. Release of ADP can induce further aggregation and release in a positive feedback fashion.

Clotting cascade

The clotting cascade has two semi-independent pathways (**Figure 2.3**). The intrinsic pathway has all of its components within blood. The extrinsic pathway is triggered by extravascular tissue damage and is activated by exposure to a tissue factor. Both pathways result in activation of prothrombin (Factor II). The final common pathway converts fibrinogen to fibrin monomers. Polymerisation of fibrin monomers results in the formation of long fine strands held together by H-bonds. These are then converted into covalent bonds with stabilisation of the fibrin polymer. The intrinsic pathway is relatively slow (2–6 minutes). The extrinsic pathway is quite fast (15 seconds).

Disorders of bleeding and coagulation

Coagulation tests

Prothrombin time

The prothrombin time (PT) tests both the extrinsic and common pathways. Thromboplastin and calcium are added to the patient's plasma. The PT is expressed as a ratio known as the International Normalised Ratio (INR). It is prolonged in:

- Warfarin treatment
- Liver disease
- Vitamin K deficiency
- Disseminated intravascular coagulation

Activated partial thromboplastin time

The activated partial thromboplastin time (APPT) tests both the intrinsic and common pathways. Kaolin is added to the patient plasma. It is prolonged in:

- Heparin treatment
- Haemophilia and factor deficiencies
- Liver disease
- Disseminated intravascular coagulation
- Massive transfusion
- Lupus anticoagulant

Thrombin time

The thrombin time tests the common pathway. Thrombin is added to patient plasma. This converts fibrinogen into fibrin it is prolonged in:

- Heparin treatment
- Disseminated intravascular coagulation
- Dysfibrinogenaemia

Bleeding time

The bleeding time measures capillary bleeding. It is prolonged in:

- Platelet disorders
- Vessel wall disorders

Classification of bleeding disorders

Bleeding diatheses can arise from disorders of the:

- Vessel wall

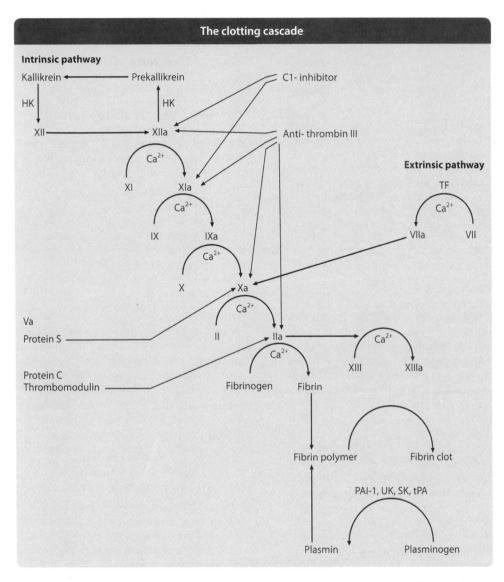

The clotting cascade

Intrinsic pathway

Kallikrein ← Prekallikrein C1- inhibitor

HK HK

XII — XIIa ← Anti- thrombin III

Ca^{2+}

Extrinsic pathway

XI XIa TF

Ca^{2+} Ca^{2+}

IX IXa VIIa VII

Ca^{2+}

X Xa

Ca^{2+}

Va

Protein S II IIa Ca^{2+}

Ca^{2+} XIII XIIIa

Protein C
Thrombomodulin Fibrinogen Fibrin

Fibrin polymer Fibrin clot

PAI-1, UK, SK, tPA

Plasmin Plasminogen

Figure 2.3 The clotting cascade (HK = High molecular weight kininogen. TF = Tissue factor. PAI-1 = Plasminogen activator inhibitor-1. UK = Urokinase. SK = Streptokinase. tPA = Tisse plasminogen activator.)

- Platelets
- Coagulation system

A classification of bleeding disorders is shown in **Table 2.3**.

Haemophilia

Haemophilia A is due to factor VIII deficiency. Haemophilia B (Christmas disease) is due to factor IX deficiency. Haemophilia A affects about 1 in 10,000 population. It is a sex-linked

clotting disorder but one-third of patients have no family history.

Clinical features

Haemophilia usually presents in childhood with prolonged haemorrhage after dental extraction, recurrent haemarthroses or muscle haematomas. Sub-periosteal haematomas can result in haemophilic pseudo-tumours. The clinical severity

Classification of bleeding disorders		
Vessel wall	**Platelets**	**Coagulation system**
Hereditary haemorrhagic telangiectasia	Congenital platelet disorders	von Willebrand's disease
	Thrombocytopenia	Factor VIII, IX deficiency
Ehlers–Danlos syndrome	Myeloproliferative disorders	Liver disease
Drugs (e.g. steroids)	Drugs (e.g. aspirin)	Anticoagulants
Sepsis		Disseminated intravascular coagulation
Trauma		
Vasculitis		

Table 2.3 Classification of bleeding disorders

depends on the extent of the clotting factor deficiency. Patients with less than 1% clotting factor activity have severe disease with life-threatening bleeding. Those with 1–5% activity have moderate disease with post-traumatic bleeding. Those with 5–20% activity have mild disease.

Investigation
Investigation will show the APPT to be prolonged. The PT is normal. The whole blood coagulation time is prolonged and Factor VIII levels are reduced.

Treatment
Bleeding episodes are treated with factor VIII replacement given as either factor VIII concentrate or cryoprecipitate. Bleeding is usually well-controlled if the factor VIII levels are raised to above 20% of normal. Desmopressin will increase intrinsic factor VIII levels. About 5-10% of patients develop antibodies to factor VIII which renders patients refractory to factor replacement therapy.

von Willebrand's disease
In 1926, Erik von Willebrand described an inherited bleeding disorder in a family from the Aland Islands off the coast of Finland. It is due to deficiency or dysfunction of a protein termed the von Willebrand factor

(vWF). Haemostasis is impaired because of defective interaction between platelets and the vessel wall. vWF mediates the adhesion of platelets to sites of vascular injury and binds and stabilises the procoagulant protein factor VIII. Like haemophilia, it usually presents with skin bruising, nose-bleeds, haematomas and prolonged bleeding from trivial wounds. Diagnosis is based on demonstrating a deficiency of vWF. Treatment is usually with desmopressin.

Recombinant factor VIIa
Factor VIIa is a trypsin-like serine protease. It is an initiator of thrombin generation. It acts via two pathways to activate Factor Xa. One pathway is at the site of tissue injury complexed with Tissue Factor. The other pathway is on the platelet surface independent of Tissue Factor. Tissue Factor is found in the subendothelial layer of the vascular wall and is not normally available to complex with Factor VIIa. Following injury, the subendothelial layer is exposed and Tissue Factor can bind to Factor VIIa. Theoretically both mechanisms localise the action of Factor VIIa to the site of trauma.

Clinical uses
Recombinant Factor VIIa is licensed for use in haemophiliacs with antibodies to Factor VIII.

It may also be useful in trauma patients with massive blood loss. It significantly reduces blood transfusion requirements in patients with blunt trauma and may also reduce the incidence of multi-organ failure.

Disseminated intravascular coagulation

Disseminated intravascular coagulation (DIC) is due to widespread intravascular activation of the clotting cascade. It causes a bleeding tendency due to consumption of clotting factors. Patients present with bruising, purpura and oozing from surgical wounds and venepuncture sites. Causes include:

- Severe (usually Gram-negative or meningococcal) infection
- Widespread mucin-secreting metastatic adenocarcinoma
- Hypovolaemic shock
- Burns
- Transfusion reactions
- Eclampsia
- Amniotic fluid embolus
- Promyelocytic leukaemia

Investigation

Investigation will show the APPT and PT to be increased. Serum fibrinogen levels will be reduced and fibrin degradation products will be increased. There will be a thrombocytopenia and Factor V and VIII activities will be reduced.

Management

Management of DIC involves fluid resuscitation and treatment of the underlying cause. The clotting abnormalities can be corrected with fresh frozen plasma, cryoprecipitate and platelet transfusion.

Blood transfusion

Blood products

Blood products available include:

- Whole blood
- Packed red cells
- Granulocyte concentrates
- Platelet concentrates
- Human plasma – fresh frozen plasma
- Plasma protein fraction

- Human albumin 25%
- Cryoprecipitate
- Clotting factors – Factor VIII/IX
- Immunoglobulins

Blood groups

ABO system

The ABO blood groups system consists of three allelic genes – A, B and O. The A and B genes control synthesis of enzymes that add carbohydrate residues to cell surface glycoproteins. The O gene is an amorph and does not transform the glycoprotein. Six possible genotypes and four phenotypes exist. Naturally occurring antibodies are found in the serum of those lacking the corresponding antigen. Blood group O is the universal donor. Blood group AB is the universal recipient. A summary of the ABO blood group system is shown in **Table 2.4**.

Rhesus system

Rhesus antibodies are immune antibodies requiring prior exposure during transfusion or pregnancy. About 85% of the population are rhesus positive and 90% of rhesus-negative patients transfused with rhesus-positive blood will develop anti-D antibodies.

Cross matching

Cross matching of blood requires three stages. First, blood grouping is performed when the patient's red cells are grouped for ABO and Rhesus antigens. A serum test is performed to confirm the patient's ABO group. Second, antibody screening is carried out to detect atypical red cell antibodies in the recipient's serum. Third, cross matching is performed to test the donor red cells against the patient's serum.

Complications of blood transfusion

Complications of blood transfusion are rare. However, when they do occur they can be life-threatening. They can be classified as early or late (**Table 2.5**).

Acute haemolytic or bacterial transfusion reactions

Acute haemolysis or a reaction to bacterial contamination of blood can be difficult to

The ABO blood group system				
Phenotype	Genotype	Antigens	Antibodies	Frequency (%)
O	OO	O	Anti-A & B	46
A	AA or AO	A	Anti-B	42
B	BB or BO	B	Anti-A	9
AB	AB	AB	None	3

Table 2.4 The ABO blood group system

Complications of blood transfusion
Early
Haemolytic reactions (immediate or delayed)
Bacterial infections from contamination
Allergic reactions to white cells or platelets
Acute lung injury
Pyogenic reactions
Circulatory overload
Air embolism
Thrombophlebitis
Citrate toxicity
Hyperkalaemia
Clotting abnormalities
Late
Infections – hepatitis or CMV
Iron overload
Immune sensitisation

Table 2.5 Complications of blood transfusion

differentiate on clinical grounds alone. It may occur after infusion of a small volume of incompatible or infected blood and is associated with high morbidity and mortality. In the unconscious patient, bleeding due to DIC may be the only sign. Most ABO mismatched transfusions are due to human error. The patient feels unwell and agitated. Symptoms include back pain and pain at the site of infusion. These may be associated with shortness of breath and rigors. Examination will show hypotension, oliguria and bleeding from venepuncture sites. Urinalysis may show haemoglobinuria.

If acute haemolysis is suspected then the transfusion should be immediately stopped and the giving set removed. The unit of blood should be rechecked against the patient's identity. Intravenous crystalloid should be given. Blood should be taken for a full blood count, plasma haemoglobin, clotting, blood cultures and repeat grouping. Broad spectrum antibiotics should be given and the urine output monitored.

Anaphylaxis

Anaphylaxis usually occurs soon after the start of a transfusion and may be seen in IgA deficient patients reacting to transfused IgA. The patient presents with circulatory collapse and bronchospasm. The transfusion should be discontinued and the giving set removed. The airway should be maintained and oxygen given. Adrenaline, chlorpheniramine, and salbutamol should be administered. If the patient is IgA deficient, any further transfusion must be carefully planned.

Non-haemolytic transfusion febrile reaction

Non-haemolytic transfusion febrile reactions usually occur more than 30 minutes after the start of a transfusion. Patient feels generally well but may be shivering. Temperature is usually less than 38.5°C and the blood pressure is often normal. The transfusion should be stopped and the possibility that this may be a more significant reaction considered. The transfusion should be restarted at a slower rate. Consideration should be given to the use of paracetamol. Hydrocortisone should not be routinely be used during a transfusion.

Transfusion-related acute lung injury

Transfusion-related acute lung injury occurs following administration of plasma-containing blood components. It is due to interaction of donor antibodies with recipient white cells. The clinical picture is similar to the acute respiratory distress syndrome (ARDS) and occurs 30 minutes to several days after transfusion. Clinical features include fever, cough and shortness of breath. A chest x-ray shows perihilar shadowing and it should be treated as ARDS.

Delayed haemolytic transfusion reaction

Delayed haemolytic transfusion reaction occurs 5–10 days after transfusion. The clinical features are usually minimal. The possibility should be considered if there is unexplained pyrexia, jaundice or a drop in haemoglobin. Urinalysis may show urobilinogenuria.

Autologous transfusion

Autologous blood transfusion is the use of the patient's own blood. It is particularly useful in elective surgery and accounts for about 5% of all transfusions performed in the USA. It is less commonly performed in the UK. It reduces both the need for allogeneic blood transfusion and the risks of postoperative complications (e.g. infection, tumour recurrence). The three main techniques are:

- Predeposit transfusion
- Intraoperative acute normovolaemic haemodilution
- Intraoperative cell salvage

Predeposit transfusion

For predeposit transfusion, blood collection begins 3–5 weeks preoperatively. Between 2 and 4 units are often stored. The last unit is should be collected more than 72 hours before surgery. Predeposit transfusion eliminates the risk of viral transmission and reduces the risk of immunological transfusion reactions. It also reduces the risk of postoperative immunosuppression seen with allogeneic transfusion. Collection is expensive and time-consuming and it is only suitable for elective surgery.

Intraoperative acute normovolaemic haemodilution

With intraoperative acute normovolaemic haemodilution, whole blood is removed at start of the operative procedure. Up to 1.5 litres of blood can be collected and replaced with crystalloid or colloid solution. Few detrimental effects of acute anaemia have been demonstrated. The blood is stored in theatre at room temperature and it is re-infused during or immediately following surgery. It is cheaper than predeposit transfusion. There is little risk of administrative or clerical error. It is suitable for elective or emergency surgery at which considerable blood loss is anticipated.

Intraoperative cell salvage

With intraoperative cell salvage, shed blood is collected from the operative field. The blood is anticoagulated with citrate or heparin and filtered to remove debris and clots. Cells are then washed with saline and concentrated by centrifugation. The concentrate is then reinfused. Large volumes of blood can be salvaged. Salvaged blood is not haemostatically intact as both platelets and clotting factors are consumed. It is suitable for use in cardiac, trauma, vascular and obstetric surgery. Its use is contraindicated in contaminated operative fields and in the presence of malignancy.

Preoperative anaemia

Tissue oxygenation is dependent on arterial oxygen content, capillary blood flow and the position on the oxygen dissociation curve. The haemoglobin concentration affects all of these factors. Anaemia reduces arterial oxygen content. Reduced plasma viscosity increases capillary blood flow. Increased levels of 2,3 bisphosphoglycerate shifts the oxygen dissociation curve to the right.

Both anaemia and polycythaemia increase postoperative mortality. A perioperative haemoglobin concentration of approximately 10 g/dL is ideal. Preoperative transfusion may induce immunosuppression, increase the risk of infection and increase the risk of tumour recurrence. If a blood transfusion is required, it should be given at least 2 days preoperatively as blood transfused immediately prior to operation has reduced O_2 carrying capacity.

Chapter 3

Postoperative management and critical care

Autonomic nervous system

The autonomic nervous system (ANS) controls the body's internal environment and is important in the process of homeostasis. It controls the heart rate, blood pressure, digestion, respiration, blood pH and other bodily functions. The functions of the autonomic nervous system are summarised in **Table 3.1**. The control of the ANS is done automatically below the conscious level. The hypothalamus has an important role in coordinating autonomic function. In the ANS there are two nerves between the central nervous system (CNS) and the end organ. The nerve cell bodies for the second nerve are organised into ganglia. The ANS effects its function via neural transmission as follows:

- Central nervous system
- Preganglionic nerve
- Ganglion
- Postganglionic nerve
- End organ

At each junction neurotransmitters are released. The ANS has two divisions that differ in anatomy and function.

Sympathetic nervous system

The sympathetic nerves arise from the thoracic and lumbar regions of the spinal cord. The preganglionic nerves are short and synapse in paired ganglia adjacent to the spinal cord. The adrenal medulla, technically an endocrine gland, is functionally a part of the sympathetic nervous system. Acetylcholine is the neurotransmitter released from the preganglionic neurones. Noradrenaline is the neurotransmitter released from the postganglionic neurones.

The sympathetic nervous system is the 'fight or flight' branch of the ANS. Emergency situations are handled by the sympathetic system. The sympathetic system increases cardiac output and pulmonary ventilation, diverts blood to the muscles, raises blood glucose and slows down digestion, kidney

Functions of the autonomic nervous system		
	Sympathetic	**Parasympathetic**
Eye	Iris dilates	Iris constricts
Heart	Increased heart rate	Decreased heart rate
Bronchioles	Bronchodilatation	Bronchoconstriction
Bladder	Sphincter constricts	Sphincter dilates
	Detrusor muscle relaxes	Detrusor muscle constricts
Intestine	Secretions decrease	Secretions increase
	Motility decreases	Motility increases
Rectum	Sphincter relaxes	Sphincter constricts
	Muscle wall contracts	Muscle wall relaxes

Table 3.1 Functions of the autonomic nervous system

filtration and other functions not needed during emergencies. The adrenal medulla behaves like a combined autonomic ganglion and postsynaptic sympathetic nerve, It releases both adrenaline (80%) and noradrenaline (20%).

Parasympathetic nervous system

The parasympathetic nerves arise from the cranial and sacral regions of the CNS. The cranial nerves involved are III, VII, IX, X. They have long preganglionic nerves which synapse at ganglia near or on the organs innervated. Acetylcholine is the neurotransmitter released from both the pre- and postganglionic neurones.

The parasympathetic nervous system is the 'rest and digest' branch of the ANS. The parasympathetic system promotes normal maintenance of the body. It increases secretions and mobility of different parts of the digestive tract. It is also involved in urination and defecation.

Autonomic receptors

There are multiple types of receptors in the autonomic nervous system. For the sympathetic system the major receptor types are α and β receptors. These are subdivided into α-1, α-2, β-1 and β-2. The parasympathetic system has nicotinic and muscarinic receptors.

Receptors subtypes are not evenly distributed throughout the body. The sympathetic and parasympathetic systems often have opposing actions on the same organ.

Adrenergic receptors are usually stimulated by noradrenaline or adrenaline. The α-1 receptor is found in the smooth muscle of arterioles and in the sphincter muscles of the gastrointestinal tract and bladder. The α -2 receptor is found in presynaptic nerves and other parts of the gastrointestinal tract. The β-1 receptor is the dominant type in the heart. The β-2 receptor is found in the bronchioles of the lung and the muscles of the bladder.

Cholinergic receptors are usually stimulated by acetylcholine. Nicotinic types are found in autonomic ganglia. These receptors are different to the nicotinic receptor found in neuromuscular junctions. Muscarinic types are found on all organs with parasympathetic innervation.

Pain

Pain is an unpleasant sensory and emotional experience associated with potential or actual tissue damage. It is a complex interaction of sensory, emotional and behavioural factors. Stimuli activate the nociceptive system which then conveys the information to the brain by an adaptable pathway. Pain is only experienced in the conscious brain.

Types and physiology of pain

Somatic pain

First pain

First or 'fast' pain is a protective response which allows rapid withdrawal from a painful stimulus. It occurs due to stimulation of high threshold thermo/mechanical receptors. The information is transmitted by fast myelinated A fibres. They enter the dorsal horn of the spinal cord. Secondary fibres in the spinothalamic tract transmit the stimulus to the posterior thalamic nuclei. Tertiary fibres transmit the stimuli to somatosensory post-central gyrus.

Secondary pain

Secondary or 'slow' pain is responsible for the delayed sensation of pain. It elicits behaviour to protect damaged tissue. It initiates reflex responses such as tachycardia, hypertension and increased respiratory rate. It is due to stimulation of high threshold polymodal receptors. They respond to mechanical, thermal and chemical stimuli. The information is transmitted by slow unmyelinated C fibres which enter the dorsal horn. Secondary fibres in the palaeo-spinothalamic tract transmit the stimuli to the medial thalamic nuclei. Collateral fibres transmit the stimulus to the midbrain, medullary reticular formation and hypothalamus. Further information is transmitted to the forebrain limbic system.

Visceral pain

There are fewer visceral nociceptors than somatic receptors and cortical mapping is less concentrated. Therefore, visceral pain is poorly localised. Visceral pain is also qualitatively different due to progressive stimulation and summation. It may also be referred to a site away from the source of stimulation.

Physiology

Peripheral activation

Most pain originates following tissue damage. It is due to the local release of inflammatory mediators. The mediators involved include:

- Leukotrienes D4 and B4
- Bradykinin
- Histamine
- 5HT

They activate or sensitise high threshold nociceptors and results in primary hyperalgesia.

Spinal level activation

Spinal level activation occurs in the dorsal horn of spinal cord. It is a complex interaction between excitatory and inhibitory interneurones. It also involves descending inhibitory tracts in the spinal cord. The gate control theory (**Figure 3.1**) explains the non-linear relation between injury and response. It suggests that pain can be 'gated-out' in the dorsal horn by other stimuli. The neurotransmitters involved are excitatory amino acids and neuropeptides. Some neuropeptides increase nociception (e.g. Substance P, bombesin, VIP). Other neuropeptides reduce nociception (e.g. galanin, somatostatin, GABA).

Supraspinal level activation

Perception of pain is associated with activity in the thalamus and the primary and secondary cortex. Various regions of the brain are involved with descending inhibition. The stimuli originate at level of cortex and thalamus and are mediated via relays in the brainstem and dorsal columns to the dorsal horns. The mediators involved include noradrenaline, 5HT and endogenous opioids.

Postoperative pain control

Pain is a complex process influenced by both physiological and psychological factors. Management of postoperative pain has generally been shown to be inadequate. Adverse effects of postoperative pain include:

- Respiratory – reduced cough, atelectasis, sputum retention and hypoxaemia
- Cardiovascular – increased myocardial oxygen consumption and ischaemia
- Gastrointestinal – decreased gastric emptying, reduced gut motility and constipation
- Genitourinary – urinary retention
- Neuroendocrine – hyperglycaemia, protein catabolism and sodium retention
- Musculoskeletal – reduced mobility, pressure sores and increased risk of venous thrombosis
- Psychological – anxiety and fatigue

Assessment of pain

Pain is a subjective experience. Observer assessment of patient behaviour is unreliable. Pain should be assessed and recorded by visual analogue scales, verbal numerical reporting scale and categorical rating scales.

Management of pain

Non-pharmacological methods of pain relief include:

- Preoperative explanation and education
- Relaxation therapy
- Hypnosis
- Cold or heat
- Splinting of wounds, etc.
- Transcutaneous electrical nerve stimulation (TENS)

Pharmacological methods of pain relief include:

- Simple analgesia
- Non-steroidal anti-inflammatory agents
- Opiates
- Local anaesthetic agents

Simple analgesia

Paracetamol is a weak anti-inflammatory agent. It modulates prostaglandin production in the central nervous system. It can be administered orally, intravenously or rectally. It is best taken on a regular rather than 'as

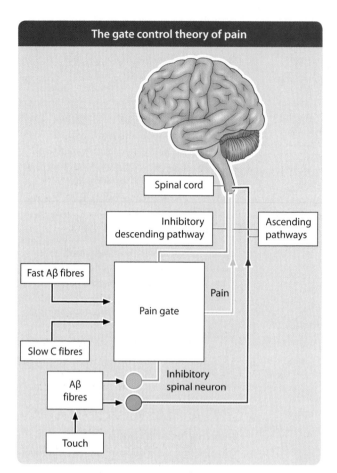

The gate control theory of pain

Figure 3.1 The gate control theory of pain

required' basis. Overdose results in hepatic necrosis. It is often used in combination with weak opiates (e.g. dihydrocodeine).

Non-steroidal anti-inflammatory agents

Non-steroidal anti-inflammatory agents inhibit the enzyme cyclo-oxygenase. They reduce prostaglandin, prostacyclin and thromboxane production. They also have a weak central analgesic effect. They are often used for their 'opiate sparing' effects. Side effects include gastric irritation and peptic ulceration, precipitation of bronchospasm in asthmatics, impairment of renal function and platelet dysfunction and bleeding.

Opiates

The most commonly used opiates are diamorphine and morphine. Diamorphine is a prodrug rapidly hydrolysed to morphine and 6-monoacetyl-morphine. It is more lipid soluble than morphine with greater central effects. Both act on μ receptors in the brain and spinal cord. μ 1 receptors are responsible for analgesia. μ 2 receptors are responsible for respiratory depression. The side effects of opiates include sedation, nausea and vomiting, vasodilatation and myocardial depression, pruritus, delayed gastric emptying, constipation and urinary retention.

Morphine can be administered by several routes. Intramuscular administration produces peaks and troughs in both plasma levels and pain relief. Subcutaneous infusion is useful for chronic pain relief, particularly in chronic pain and palliative care. Intravenous injection is reliable but can produce both sedation and respiratory depression. With patient-controlled analgesia (PCA), morphine is administered intravenously but the patient determines their own analgesic requirement. A 'lock-out' period prevents accidental overdose. It is a safe means of administration as sedation occurs before respiratory depression.

Lipid soluble opiates (e.g. fentanyl) can be used for spinal or epidural injection/infusion. They produces good analgesia with reduced risk of side effects. Intrathecal morphine administration is an attractive analgesic technique since the opioid is injected directly into the cerebrospinal fluid, close to the structures of the central nervous system where the opioid acts. The procedure is simple, quick, and relatively low-risk. Respiratory depression is however a major safety concern.

Local and regional anaesthesia

Local anaesthetic agents act by reducing membrane permeability to sodium. They act on the small unmyelinated C fibre before large A fibres. Therefore, they reduce pain and temperature sensation before touch and power.

Lignocaine

Lignocaine is a weak base. At physiological pH, it is mainly ionised. It has a rapid onset but short duration of action. With the addition of adrenaline, the duration of action can be increased to 2 hours. The main toxicity is on central nervous and cardiovascular systems. Plain lignocaine should be used for local anaesthesia in digits and appendages as adrenaline containing solutions can cause tissue ischaemia.

Bupivacaine

Bupivacaine is chemically related to lignocaine but has a more prolonged onset and longer duration of action. It acts for 6–8 hours. Like lignocaine its main toxicity is on the central nervous and cardiovascular systems. Its duration of action can also be prolonged by the addition of adrenaline

Spinal and epidural anaesthesia

Spinal anaesthesia is the administration of local anaesthetic or opiate into the cerebrospinal fluid (CSF) below the termination of the spinal cord at L1. Epidural anaesthesia is the use of local anaesthetic or opiate administration into the fatty epidural space. A single bolus dose, can produce good anaesthesia for several hours. The use of both requires an experienced anaesthetist as complications are common and can be life-threatening (**Table 3.2**). The quality of the block is often better with a spinal anaesthetic. Contraindications to spinal or epidural anaesthesia are pre-existing neurological disease, known coagulopathy and sepsis.

	Characteristic	Spinal	Epidural
Complications of spinal and epidural anaesthesia			
Immediate	Hypotension	Common	Less common
	local anaesthetic toxicity	Rare	Occasional
	High blockade	Occasional	Occasional
Early	Urinary retention	Common	Less common
	Headache	1–5%	Never unless dural puncture
	Local infection	Almost never	Uncommon
	Meningism	Uncommon	Very rare
	Epidural haematoma	Almost never	Very rare
	Backache	Common	Common

Table 3.2 Complications of spinal and epidural anaesthesia

Postoperative epidural infusions

Postoperative epidural analgesia attenuates the postoperative stress response, improves postoperative pain control, reduces the incidence of postoperative pulmonary complications and allows the more rapid return of gastrointestinal function. When used as part of an enhanced recovery programme it can shorten hospital stay.

Opioid alone epidurals allow opioid analgesia without sedation. There is no motor or sympathetic blockade. However the quality of analgesia can be variable. Itch is a common side effect. Serious respiratory depression can occur after stopping the infusion.

Local anaesthetic alone epidural infusions have the potential for complete anaesthesia. They have no sedative effects or respiratory depression. However, sympathetic and motor blockade are common. Cardiovascular side effects can occur and the block occasionally is patchy or unilateral. A combination of local anaesthetic and opioid allows for synergy between the two mechanisms of action and the doses of both drugs can be reduced.

Hypotension

The sympathetic outflow from the spinal cord occurs between T1 and L2. It is blocked to varying degrees in both spinal and epidural anaesthesia. The higher the block the greater the degree of sympathetic blockade. In hypovolaemic patients, there is a greater risk of hypotension. Hypotension during spinal and epidural anaesthesia usually requires fluid resuscitation.

Post spinal headache

A headache follows about 2% of spinal anaesthetics and is usually due to a CSF leak. In most patients is settles after about 3 days. The headache is characteristically occipital and is worse on standing and relieved by lying down. Initial treatment is with bed rest, simple analgesia and fluids. If it persists, a 'blood-patch' may be required when the patient's own blood is injected into epidural space to seal the leak.

Postoperative nausea and vomiting

Postoperative nausea and vomiting (PONV) may be the most unpleasant memory associated with a patient's surgical experience. PONV is common and in adults its incidence has been estimated to be approximately 25%. Prolonged vomiting can result in electrolyte imbalance, dehydration and may prolong hospital stay. PONV can be induced by many physiological and pathological factors, including drugs.

Nausea and vomiting is primarily controlled by the vomiting centre. It is located in the dorso-lateral reticular formation of the medulla. This is an area in the brainstem that integrates neural responses. Afferent stimuli arrive from chemoreceptors and pressure receptors in the gut, from the CNS and from peripheral pain receptors. Other sites of input include the cerebral cortex, vestibular and cerebellar nuclei. Efferent impulses from this area influence other related brainstem nuclei including the chemoreceptor trigger zone (CTZ). This is located in the area postrema of the 4th ventricle and is outside the blood–brain barrier. The afferent and efferent connections to the vomiting centre and CTZ are summarised in **Figure 3.2**.

Dopamine and 5-HT play an important role in the activity of the CTZ. 5-HT has an important role in drug-induced emesis and 5-HT3 receptors appear to be an important part in the mediation of nausea and vomiting induced by high doses of cytotoxic agents. Other neurotransmitters implicated in the control of nausea and vomiting include acetylcholine and dopamine. Hence anti-emetics act as antagonists to one or more of these neurotransmitters. These include domperidone, metoclopramide, prochlorperazine, cyclizine, hyoscine and ondansetron. There is now great interest in the use of combinations of anti-emetics to increase efficacy. There is increasing evidence that combinations of different classes of antiemetics show improvements over monotherapy.

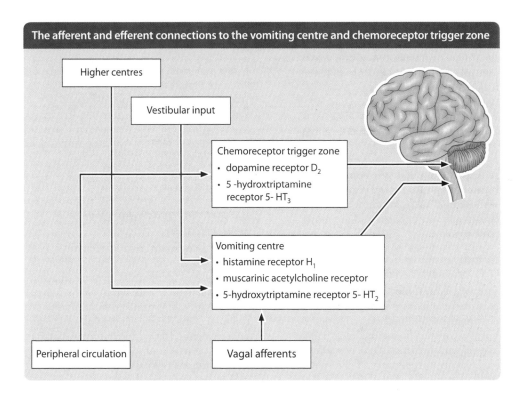

The afferent and efferent connections to the vomiting centre and chemoreceptor trigger zone

Figure 3.2 The afferent and efferent connections to the vomiting centre and chemoreceptor trigger zone

Metabolic and nutritional support
Fluid and electrolyte management

For the 'average' 70 kg man, the total body water is 42 litres. This represents about 60% of the body weight. This is made up of 28 litres in the intracellular and 14 litres in the extracellular compartments. The plasma volume is 3 litres and the extravascular volume is 11 litres. The total body sodium is 4200 mmol of which 50% is in the extracellular fluid compartment. The total body potassium is 3500 mmol of which only about 50 mmol is in the extracellular fluid compartment. The normal osmolality of extracellular fluid is 280–295 mosmol/kg. When calculating fluid replacement for a patient, it is necessary to consider:

- Maintenance requirements
- Pre-existing and ongoing losses
- Insensible losses

Maintenance requirements

Daily maintenance fluid requirements vary between individuals. For a 70 kg male it is about 3 litres of water, 120 mmol sodium and 70 mmol potassium. For a 40 kg woman it is 90 mmol sodium and 40 mmol potassium. The daily maintenance fluid requirements for children can be estimated as follows:

- 0–10 kg is 100 mL/kg
- 10–20 kg is 1000 mL + 50 mL/kg for each kg more than 10
- More than 20 kg is 1500 mL + 25 mL/kg for each kg more than 20

Pre-existing and on-going losses

Pre-existing and ongoing losses can be rich in electrolytes. Most 'surgical' pre-existing and ongoing losses are rich in sodium and should be replaced with 0.9% saline. They include:

- Vomit and diarrhoea
- Nasogastric aspirate
- Stoma, drain and fistula output

Insensible losses

Insensible losses occur via faeces (100 mL/day), the lungs (400 mL/day) and skin (600 mL/day). Total insensible losses are usually about 1 litre per day.

Fluid replacement therapy

Fluids can be replaced with crystalloid or colloid solutions. There is no evidence from RCTs that resuscitation with colloids reduces the risk of death, compared to resuscitation with crystalloids, in patients with trauma, burns or following surgery. Crystalloids are cheaper and are more widely used.

Crystalloids

The composition of different crystalloid solutions vary (**Table 3.3**). Normal saline contains only sodium and chloride. Hartmann's solution has less chloride but also contains potassium, bicarbonate and calcium. Dextrose saline contains significantly less sodium and chloride in relation to its volume than normal saline.

Colloids

Colloids can be either monodispersed with all molecules of similar molecular weight or polydispersed with molecules having a spread of molecular weights. The properties of commonly used colloid solutions is shown in **Table 3.4**. Albumin is monodispersed, has a long half life and accounts for 60–80% of normal plasma oncotic pressure. It has no adverse effect on coagulation. Dextrans are polydispersed polysaccharides with a molecular weight in the range of 10 to 90 kDa.

They reduce plasma viscosity, reduce platelet aggregation and have a risk of anaphylaxis. Gelatins are polydispersed polypeptides with a molecular weight of about 35 kDa. They are rapidly lost from vascular space. Hydroxyethyl starch is a polydispersed synthetic polysaccharide polymer derived from amylopectin with a molecular weight in the range 50 to 450 kDa. The large molecules are engulfed by the reticuloendothelial system and their use may be associated with a bleeding diathesis.

Assessment of adequacy of resuscitation

Clinical assessment and observations will provide a rough guide to the need for resuscitation. Tachycardia, hypotension and reduced skin turgor are signs of dehydration. In most situations, urine output is a good estimate of the degree of hypovolaemia with oliguria defined as a urine output of less than 0.5 mL/kg/hr. If doubt remains, then invasive monitoring with an assessment of central venous pressure may be required.

The response of the urine output or central venous pressure to a fluid challenge can be used to assess the adequacy of resuscitation. A fluid challenge should be regarded as a 200–250 mL bolus of colloid, administered as quickly as possible. A response in the central pressure or urine output should be seen within minutes. A rapid rise followed by a prompt fall suggests hypovolaemia. A rapid rise that is maintained suggests good intravascular volume replacement. The size and duration of the response rather the actual values recorded are more important.

The composition of crystalloid solutions			
	Hartmann's	Normal saline	Dextrose saline
Sodium (mmol/L)	131	150	30
Chloride (mmol/L)	111	150	30
Potassium (mmol/L)	5	Nil	Nil
Bicarbonate (mmol/L)	29	Nil	Nil
Calcium (mmol/L)	2	Nil	Nil

Table 3.3 The composition of crystalloid solutions

The properties of colloid solutions			
	Volume effect (%)	Molecular weight (kDa)	Half-life
Gelatins (Haemaccel)	80	35	2–3 hours
4% Albumin	100	69	15 days
Dextran 70	120	41	2–12 hours
6% Hydroxyethyl starch	100	70	17 days

Table 3.4 The properties of colloid solutions

Techniques of venous access

Peripheral venous access is required for administration of fluids and drugs. Central venous access is required for parenteral nutrition, monitoring of central venous pressure, cardiac pacing and in patients with difficult peripheral access.

Anatomy of venous access

Central venous access can be via either the internal jugular or subclavian veins. The internal jugular vein is used more often and right-sided access is preferred as the apical pleura does not rise as high on the right and it also avoids the thoracic duct found on the left. The patient is positioned head down. In the low approach, the triangle formed by the two heads of sternomastoid and clavicle is identified and the cannula is aimed down and lateral towards ipsilateral nipple. The subclavian vein is usually approached from below clavicle. The patient is positioned head down. The needle is inserted below the junction of medial two-third and lateral one-third of the clavicle. The needle is aimed towards the suprasternal notch, passing immediately behind clavicle. The vein is encountered after 4–5 cm.

Techniques

Aseptic techniques should be used for all cannulations. Local anaesthetic should be used for central catheters. Both success and safety may be improved by using ultrasound guidance. Techniques of gaining access include:

- Catheter over needle
- Catheter through needle
- Seldinger technique
- Surgical cutdown

Seldinger technique

There are four steps to the Seldinger technique:

- Venepuncture is performed with an introducer needle
- A soft tipped guide wire is passed through the needle and the needle removed
- A dilator is passed over the guide wire
- The dilator is removed and the catheter is passed over wire which is then removed

After insertion, a chest x-ray should be performed to check the position of catheter. Early complications of central venous catherisation include:

- Haemorrhage
- Air embolus
- Pneumothorax
- Cardiac arrhythmias
- Pericardial tamponade
- Failed cannulation

Late complications of central venous catherisation include:

- Venous thrombosis
- Infection

Approximately 10% of central lines become colonised with bacteria. About 2% of patients in intensive care develop catheter-related sepsis. Central line infections are usually due to coagulase-negative staphylococcus infection. They are occasionally due to *Candida* and *Staphylococcus aureus*. The incidence of infection can be significantly reduced by aseptic techniques and adequate care of lines. Closed systems should be used at all times. Dedicated lines should be used for parenteral nutrition. Antimicrobial coating of lines may reduce the risk of infection.

Venous cutdown

Venous cutdown is useful for gaining access in shocked, hypovolaemic patients. The commonest sites used are the long saphenous vein at the ankle – 2 cm anterior to medial malleolus or the basilic vein and at the elbow – 2.5 cm lateral to the medial epicondyle. At both sites, the vein is dissected and ligated distally. A small transverse venotomy is made. The cannula is passed through the venotomy and secured.

Surgical nutrition

Malnutrition is common in surgical patients and results in:

- Delayed wound healing
- Reduced ventilatory capacity
- Reduced immunity
- Increased risk of infection

Nutritional assessment

Weight loss of 10% and 30% should be regarded as mild and severe malnutrition, respectively. Useful anthropometric measurements in the assessment of nutritional status include triceps skin fold thickness, mid-arm circumference and hand-grip strength.

Methods of nutritional support

Enteral nutrition

The gastrointestinal tract should be used for nutritional support if it is available. Prolonged postoperative starvation is not required. Early enteral nutrition is associated with reduced postoperative morbidity. Enteral feeding prevents intestinal mucosal atrophy and supports the gut-associated immunological shield. It attenuates the hypermetabolic response to injury and surgery. It is cheaper than parenteral nutrition and has fewer complications.

Polymeric liquid diet is made up of short peptides, medium chain triglycerides, polysaccharides, vitamins and trace elements. Enteral feed can be taken orally or administered via a nasogastric tube. Long-term feeding can

be by a surgical gastrostomy or jejunostomy, percutaneous endoscopic gastrostomy or needle catheter jejunostomy. Enteral feeding is often started at a low rate of infusion and then increased. Complications of enteral feeding include malposition and blockage of the tube, gastro-oesophageal reflux and feed intolerance.

Parenteral nutrition

Intestinal failure can be defined as a reduction in the functioning gut mass to below the minimum necessary for adequate digestion and absorption of nutrients. It is a useful concept for assessing the need for parenteral nutrition which can be given by either a peripheral or central line. Indications for parenteral nutrition include:

- Enterocutaneous fistulae
- Moderate or severe malnutrition
- Acute pancreatitis
- Abdominal sepsis
- Prolonged ileus
- Major trauma and burns
- Severe inflammatory bowel disease

Central parenteral nutrition is hyperosmolar and has a low pH. It is irritant to vessel walls. Typical feed contains the following in 2.5 L:

- 14 g nitrogen as L amino acids
- 250 g glucose
- 500 mL 20% lipid emulsion
- 100 mmol sodium
- 100 mmol potassium
- 150 mmol chloride
- 15 mmol magnesium
- 13 mmol calcium
- 30 mmol phosphate
- 0.4 mmol zinc
- Water and fat soluble vitamins
- Trace elements

Monitoring of parenteral nutrition

Feeding lines should only be used for that purpose. Drugs and blood products should be given via a separate peripheral line or other channels on a multiple lumen central line. About 5% of patients on total parenteral nutrition develop metabolic derangement. Parenteral nutrition should be monitored:

- Clinically – weight
- Biochemically twice weekly
- FBC, U+E, LFT

- Magnesium, calcium, zinc, phosphate
- Nitrogen balance
- Blood cultures on any sign of sepsis

Metabolic complications of parenteral nutrition include:

- Hyponatraemia
- Hypokalaemia
- Hyperchloraemia
- Trace element and folate deficiency
- Deranged LFTs
- Linoleic acid deficiency

Postoperative complications
Postoperative pyrexia

Pyrexia is a common problem seen after surgery. The underlying cause can often be identified clinically depending on the time since operation, the type of surgery undertaken and associated clinical features. Specific complications often occur at certain times after an operation (**Table 3.5**). However, the time scales should be regarded as a rough guide and not absolute rules.

Assessment

Adequate assessment requires a full history and examination, supplemented by investigations as required. Respiratory complications are often associated with breathlessness, cough and chest pain. Wound infections may show erythema, purulent discharge or wound dehiscence. Abdominal pain, distension and ileus may suggest a collection or anastomotic leak. Calf pain and tenderness may suggest a DVT. Useful investigations may include:

- Chest x-ray
- ECG
- Arterial blood gases
- Ventilation/perfusion scan
- Abdominal ultrasound or CT scan

Wound dehiscence

Wound dehiscence affects about 2% of mid-line laparotomy wounds. It is a serious complication with a mortality of up to 30%. It is due to failure of the wound closure technique such as a broken suture, slipped knot or inadequate muscle bites often in the presence of infection. It usually occurs between 7 and 10 days after surgery and is often heralded by a serosanguinous discharge from the wound. Even if the dehiscence only seems to affect part of the wound, it should be assumed that the underlying defect involves the whole of the closure.

Management

Opiate analgesia should be given and a sterile dressing applied to the wound. Fluid resuscitation may be required. An early return to theatre is necessary and the wound should be resutured under general anaesthesia. The optimal technique is controversial. Interrupted or mass closure with non-absorbable sutures is often used. The use of 'deep tension' sutures is controversial and is regarded by many as being almost obsolete as it is believed to strangulate muscle and weaken the closure. It is also painful and associated with increased risk of infection.

Timing of common postoperative complications			
First 24 hours	**24–72 hours**	**3–7 days**	**7–10 days**
Systemic response trauma	Pulmonary atelectasis	Chest infection	Deep venous thrombosis
	Chest infection	Wound infection	
Pre-existing infection		Intraperitoneal sepsis	Pulmonary embolus
		Urinary tract infection	
		Anastomotic leak	

Table 3.5 Timing of common postoperative complications

Postoperative pulmonary complications

Postoperative hypoxia

Postoperative hypoxia occurs due to a lack of alveolar ventilation or perfusion. Poor alveolar ventilation can occur as a result of:

- Hypoventilation (airway obstruction, opiates)
- Bronchospasm
- Pneumothorax
- Arteriovenous shunting (collapse, atelectasis)

Poor alveolar perfusion can occur as a result of:

- Ventilation–perfusion mismatch (pulmonary embolism)
- Impaired cardiac output
- Decreased alveolar diffusion
- Pneumonia
- Pulmonary oedema

Atelectasis

Hypoxaemia is often seen during the first 48 hours after most major surgery. It occurs as a result of a reduction in functional residual capacity. Significant atelectasis is more often seen in those with pre-existing lung disease, in those with upper rather than lower abdominal incisions, obese patients and cigarette smokers. The basic mechanisms leading to atelectasis are an increase in the volume of bronchial secretions, an increase in viscosity of secretions and a reduction in tidal volume and ability to cough.

Clinical features

Atelectasis usually presents as a postoperative pyrexia starting at about 48 hours after surgery. It is often accompanied by tachycardia and tachypnoea. Examination will show reduced air entry, dullness on percussion and reduced breath sounds. A chest x-ray may show consolidation and collapse.

Treatment

The management of atelectasis involves intensive chest physiotherapy, nebulised bronchodilators and appropriate antibiotics for a possible associated infection.

Pneumonia

Nosocomial pneumonia occurs in about 1% of all patients admitted to hospital. It occurs in 15–20% of non-ventilated and 40–60% of ventilated ITU patients. The organisms responsible for hospital-acquired chest infections include:

- Gram-negative bacteria (*Pseudomonas aeruginosa, Enterobacter*)
- *Staphylococcus aureus*
- Anaerobes
- *Haemophilus influenzae*

There is no evidence that prophylactic antibiotics reduce the risk of pneumonia.

Aspiration pneumonitis

Aspiration of gastric contents results in a chemical pneumonitis. It is most commonly seen in the apical segments of the right lower lobe. If it is unrecognised or inadequately treated, it can result in a secondary bacterial infection. Secondary infection is usually with Gram-negative and anaerobic organisms. A chest x-ray of a patient with aspiration pneumonitis is shown in **Figure 3.3**.

Treatment

Immediate treatment of aspiration should involve tilting the head of the operating table down and sucking out the pharynx. Consideration should be given to intubation and endotracheal suction. Prophylactic antibiotics should be given. There is no evidence that steroids reduce the inflammatory response.

Other postoperative complications

Cardiovascular complications

Postoperative cardiovascular complications include:

- Hypotension
- Hypovolaemia
- Ventricular failure
- Cardiogenic shock
- Arrhythmias
- Conduction defects
- Hypertension

Perioperative arrhythmias can occur as result of:

- Physiological disturbances – acidosis, hypercapnoea and hypoxaemia
- Electrolyte imbalance
- Vagal manoeuvres

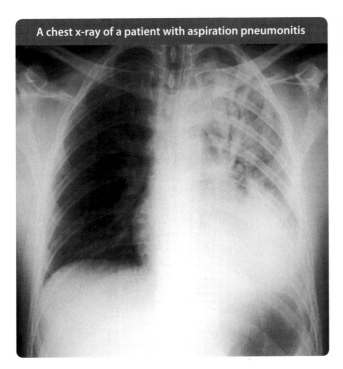
A chest x-ray of a patient with aspiration pneumonitis

Figure 3.3 A chest x-ray of a patient with aspiration pneumonitis

- Hypovolaemia
- Pathological disturbances – myocardial ischaemia, pulmonary embolus
- Pharmacological agents

Postoperative renal failure

Acute renal failure is commonly seen in the perioperative period and is associated with a high morbidity and mortality. It is therefore important to either prevent its occurrence or recognise its presence and treat it early. Causes of postoperative renal failure can be classified as prerenal, renal or postrenal (**Table 3.6**).

Renal hypoperfusion from any cause makes the kidney concentrate urine, and decreases the urine output. Therefore, prerenal failure is not a failure per se but a normal response to inadequate renal perfusion. Treating the precipitating cause may reverse the renal dysfunction. Direct renal injury may occur if there is a superimposed insult such as exposure to a nephrotoxic agent. Postrenal renal failure occurs when there is obstruction to urine flow anywhere distal to the renal pelvis.

Obstruction is the most likely diagnosis when there is anuria.

Urinary tract infections

Approximately 10% of patients admitted to hospital have a urinary catheter inserted. The risk of catheter-related infection depends on the age and sex of the patient, the duration of catheterisation and the indication for its use. Bacterial colonisation of catheters is common. If a catheter is required for more than 2 weeks, 90% of patients will develop bacteriuria. The commonest organisms identified are enterobacter and enterococci. Colonisation does not require treatment unless the patient is systemically unwell. Infection can be prevented by maintaining a closed drainage system, good infection control standards and preventing the backflow of urine from the cather bag.

Postoperative confusion

Postoperative confusion occurs in about 10% of postoperative patients. It is associated with increased morbidity and morality and

Causes of postoperative renal failure		
Prerenal	**Renal**	**Postrenal**
Shock (hypovolaemia, cardiogenic, septic)	Acute tubular necrosis	Bladder outflow obstruction
	Glomerulonephritis	Single ureter (calculus, tumour)
Renal artery disease	Interstitial nephritis	Both ureters (bladder malignancy)

Table 3.6 Causes of postoperative renal failure

leads to increased duration of hospitalisation. Clinical features include a reduced level of consciousness, impaired thinking and memory, perceptional abnormalities and disturbances of emotion. Causes of postoperative confusion include:

- Hypoxia – respiratory disease, cardiac failure, arrhythmia
- Trauma – head injury
- Infection – intracranial, extracranial
- Neoplasia – primary and secondary cerebral tumours
- Vitamin deficiency – thiamine (Wernicke encephalopathy), B_{12} deficiency
- Endocrine – hypothyroidism, hyperthyroidism, Addison's disease
- Degenerative
- Vascular – CVA, TIAs
- Drugs
- Metabolic derangement

Principles of intensive care
High-risk surgical patients

There is growing concern that high-risk surgical patients receive sub-optimal care which has important implications for both the patient and the health economy. In the UK, 170,000 patients undergo high-risk non-cardiac surgery each year. Of these, 100,000 will develop significant complications resulting in 25,000 deaths. Each year, emergency general surgical patients account for 14,000 admissions to intensive care in England and Wales and this group of patients has a mortality rate of 25%.

It is important that hospitals formalise pathways for unscheduled surgical care.

All patients should have a clear diagnostic and monitoring plan documented on admission. Prompt recognition of complications is essential. Patients often require complex management and delay worsens outcome. Adequate and prompt access to emergency operating theatres is essential.

The seniority of the staff involved a the patients management should be guided by a risk assessment. High-risk surgical patients, with a predicted hospital mortality of more than 5% should have direct diagnostic, surgical, anaesthetic and critical care consultant input. Surgical procedures with a predicted mortality of more than 10% should be performed under the direct supervision of both a consultant surgeon and anaesthetist. Each patient should have their risk of death re-assessed at the end of surgery and the optimum location for postoperative care determined. All high-risk patients should be admitted to critical care.

Outreach services

Outreach services are an essential component of critical care services and have three essential objectives:

- To assess potential admissions
- To enable discharges
- To share critical care skills

They often use Early Warning Scoring (EWS) systems to identify sick patients, based on assessment of physiological dysfunction which trigger a clinical response. Various validated early warning systems have been developed based on:

- Heart rate
- Blood pressure

- Respiratory rate
- Temperature
- Conscious level

Each observation is given a score. A normal observation is scored zero. The greater the physiological derangement the higher the score (**Table 3.7**). The sum of all parameters scored gives a global ESW which should be acted on as follows:

- Low score – increased frequency of observation
- Medium score – request appropriate medical review
- High score – request critical care assessment

Criteria for intensive care assessment include:

- Threatened airway
- Respiratory arrest
- Respiratory rate more than 40 or less than 8 breaths/min
- Oxygen saturation less than 90% on more than 50% oxygen
- Cardiac arrest
- Pulse rate less than 40 or more than 140 beats/min
- Systolic blood pressure less than 90 mmHg
- Sudden fall in level of consciousness
- Repeated or prolonged seizures
- Rising arterial carbon dioxide tension with respiratory acidosis

The indication for admission to ICU is support of organ function including:

- Respiratory – ventilation/CPAP
- Renal – haemofiltration/haemodialysis

- Cardiac – ECG and inotropic drugs
- Hepatic – blood transfusion
- Neurological – intracranial pressure monitoring

Factors to be considered when assessing admission to ICU include:

- Diagnosis
- Severity of illness
- Age
- Coexisting disease
- Physiological reserve
- Prognosis
- Availability of suitable treatment
- Response of treatment to date
- Recent cardiopulmonary arrest
- Anticipated quality of life
- The patient's wishes

Sepsis and SIRS

Sepsis is a clinical syndrome that complicates severe infection. It is characterised by the cardinal signs of inflammation occurring in tissues that are remote from the site of infection. The systemic inflammatory response syndrome (SIRS) is an identical clinical syndrome that can arise from a number of aetiological triggers including:

- Sepsis – bacterial, viral, fungal
- Hypovolaemic shock
- Trauma
- Burns
- Tissue ischaemia
- Pancreatitis

Both sepsis and SIRS response can lead to the multiple organ dysfunction syndrome

Physiological variables and scores of an early warning system							
	3	2	1	0	1	2	3
Heart rate (beats/min)		< 40	41–50	51–100	101–110	111–130	> 130
Mean BP (mmHg)	< 70	71–80	81–100	101–199		> 200	
Respiration rate (breaths/min)		< 8		9–14	15–20	21–29	> 30
Temperature		< 35	35.1–36.5		36.6–37.4	> 37.5	
Consciousness level				Awake	Respond to voice	Respond to pain	No response

Table 3.7 Physiological variables and scores of an early warning system

(MODS), which is the cause of the high mortality associated with these syndromes. The definitions of bacteraemia, SIRS, sepsis and septic shock are shown in **Table 3.8**.

Bacterial infection is the commonest cause of sepsis with 50% and 40% of cases due to Gram-negative and Gram-positive organisms, respectively. The incidence of both sepsis and SIRS is increasing as a result of advancing age, immunosuppression and multidrug-resistant infection. Despite improvements in critical care, the mortality from SIRS, sepsis, severe sepsis, and septic shock is 5%, 15%, 20%, and 50% respectively.

Pathophysiology

Sepsis and SIRS usually arises as a result of failure of control of the inflammatory response. The over-production of inflammatory mediators, the under-production of anti-inflammatory mediators and receptor abnormalities appear to be important in both initiation and propagation of the response. There is decreased destruction of inflammatory mediators and the production of abnormal leukocytes. The major inflammatory mediators involved in SIRS are:

- Platelet activating factor
- Tumour necrosis factor-α
- Interleukin-1
- Interleukin-6
- Interleukin-8
- Interleukin-10

Clinical features

The cardiorespiratory effects include:

- Increased cardiac output
- Decreased vascular resistance
- Increased oxygen consumption
- Fever or hypothermia
- Tachycardia
- Tachypnoea

The metabolic or haematological effects include:

- Respiratory alkalosis
- Deranged liver function
- Deranged renal function
- Altered white cell count and platelets
- Disseminated intravascular coagulation

Severe sepsis

Severe sepsis refers to sepsis plus at least one of the following signs of hypoperfusion or organ dysfunction:

- Areas of mottled skin
- Capillary refilling requires 3 seconds or longer
- Urine output < 0.5 mL/kg for at least one hour
- Lactate > 2 mmol/L

	The definitions of SIRS, sepsis and septic shock	
	Definition
Bacteraemia	The presence of viable bacteria in the bloodstream
SIRS	The systemic inflammatory response to a variety of clinical insult manifest by two or more of the following:
	Temperature > 38°C or < 36°
	Heart rate > 90 bpm
	Respiratory rate > 20 breaths per minute or P_aCO_2 > 4.3 kPa
	White cell count > 12,000 or < 4000 per mm³
Sepsis	SIRS with documented infection
Severe SIRS	SIRS with documented infection and hypoperfusion, hypotension and organ dysfunction
Septic shock	Sepsis with hypotension despite adequate fluid resuscitation

Table 3.8 The definitions of systemic inflammatory response syndrome (SIRS), sepsis and septic shock

- Abrupt change in mental status
- Abnormal electroencephalographic findings
- Platelet count < 100,000 platelets/mL
- Disseminated intravascular coagulation
- Acute lung injury or acute respiratory distress syndrome (ARDS)
- Cardiac dysfunction as defined by echocardiography or direct measurement of the cardiac index

MODS refers to progressive organ dysfunction in an acutely ill patient, such that homeostasis cannot be maintained without intervention. It is at the severe end of the severity of illness spectrum of both SIRS and sepsis. MODS can be classified as primary or secondary. Primary MODS is the result of a well-defined insult in which organ dysfunction occurs early and can be directly attributable to the insult itself. Secondary MODS is organ failure that is not in direct response to the insult itself, but is a consequence of the host's response.

Management

In the management of severe sepsis there are two priorities:

- Prompt assessment and resuscitation
- Early control the source of sepsis

Prompt assessment has been aided by the development and uses of EWS systems. Blood should be taken for culture and measurement of the serum lactate. Oxygen, intravenous fluids and broad-spectrum antibiotics should be administered. The effect of resuscitation should be closely monitored. These actions can be summarised in the 'sepsis six':

- High flow oxygen
- Blood cultures
- Intravenous antibiotics within 1 hour
- Fluid resuscitation
- Measurement of lactate and haemoglobin
- Catheterise and monitor urine output

The control of sepsis in surgical patients often requires radiological or surgical intervention. This can be determined by the appropriate use of radiological procedures. There is a progressive deterioration in outcome associated with increasing delay to source control. A delay of more than 12 hours after

the onset of hypotension increases the mortality associated with sepsis three-fold.

Respiratory support

Oxygen delivery depends on:

- Cardiac output
- Haemoglobin concentration
- Arterial oxygen saturation (S_aO_2)
- Arterial oxygen tension (P_aO_2)

Pulse oximetry

Arterial oxygen saturation can be measured non-invasively using pulse oximetry. It consists of two light emitting diodes of two different wavelengths. The frequencies are in the red (660 nm) and infrared (940 nm) spectrum. The monitor has one photodetector. The absorption spectrum of haemoglobin at the two frequencies depends on the degree of oxygenation and this allows calculation of the oxygen saturation. The arterial component of the circulation is targeted by restricting analysis to the signal that is pulsatile. Pulse oximetry readings can be unreliable if there is:

- Intense vasoconstriction
- Jaundice
- Methaemoglobinaemia

Respiratory failure

Respiratory failure is used to describe inadequate gas exchange with the result that arterial oxygen and/or carbon dioxide levels cannot be maintained within their normal ranges. A fall in blood oxygenation is known as hypoxaemia. A rise in arterial carbon dioxide levels is called hypercapnia. Patients with hypoxaemic respiratory failure (type 1) have reduced P_aCO_2 and reduced P_aO_2 and those with ventilatory respiratory failure (type 2) have increased P_aCO_2 and reduced P_aO_2.

Hypoxaemic failure can result from:

- Low inspired oxygen partial pressure
- Alveolar hypoventilation
- Diffusion impairment
- Ventilation to perfusion mismatch
- Right-to-left shunt

Ventilatory failure can result from:

- Abnormalities of central respiratory drive
- Neuromuscular dysfunction
- Abnormalities of the chest wall

- Abnormalities of the airway
- Abnormalities of the lung

Artificial ventilation

Artificial ventilation eliminates carbon dioxide and improves oxygenation by reducing respiratory work and oxygen consumption, administering a higher inspired oxygen content (F_iO_2) and preventing or reversing atelectasis.

Indications for tracheal intubation include:

- Facilitation of mechanical ventilation
- Protection from aspiration
- Facilitation of tracheobronchial suction
- Relief of upper airway obstruction

Indications for mechanical ventilation include:

- Support in respiratory failure
- Coma (head injury, drug overdose)
- Control of intracranial pressure
- Reduction of metabolic demands
- Allow muscle relaxation and facilitate surgery
- Postoperative ventilation

Most ventilators are volume/time-cycled with a pressure limit. They deliver a preset tidal volume irrespective of lung compliance. The pressure limit reduces the risk of over-inflation. Possible modes in which they can be used are:

- Controlled mechanical ventilation
- Assisted controlled or triggered ventilation
- Intermittent mandatory ventilation
- Pressure support

Variables on a ventilator that can be preset or altered include:

- Tidal volume
- Ventilation rate
- Inspiratory to expiratory ratio
- Flow waveform
- Partial pressure of inspired oxygen
- Pressure limit
- Positive end expiratory pressure (PEEP)
- Positive airway pressure (CPAP)

Complications of mechanical ventilation include:

- Problems associated with endotracheal tube – obstruction, misplacement
- Disconnection
- Barotrauma

- Impaired venous return
- Sodium and water retention
- Bronchopneumonia

Acute respiratory distress syndrome

Acute respiratory distress syndrome (ARDS) was first recognised in the 1960s. It was initially termed 'adult' respiratory distress syndrome but it is seen in both children and adults. It occurs following many different inflammatory insults to the lungs. The causes of ARDS are shown in **Table 3.9**.

Pathology

Irrespective of the aetiology, the main pathological feature is diffuse alveolar damage. Endothelial injury results in increased permeability. Protein-rich exudate is found in the alveoli. Neutrophils appear to be important in the inflammatory process. Cytokines and enzymes may be responsible for many of the features. Resolution of inflammation can occur but is usually associated with some degree of pulmonary fibrosis.

Clinical features

ARDS is usually a progressive clinical problem presenting with acute respiratory failure. The hypoxaemia is often refractory to increasing respiratory support. Lung compliance is reduced and hypoxaemia persists. Resolution can occur and lung function can return to normal. Overall mortality is approximately 50%.

Diagnosis

Two conditions are now recognised, acute lung injury (ALI) and ARDS. Both consist of an acute lung injury with bilateral pulmonary infiltrates on chest x-ray, a pulmonary capillary wedge pressure of less than 18 mmHg and no evidence of left atrial hypertension. In ALI the P_aO_2/F_iO_2 is less than 200 and in ARDS the P_aO_2/F_iO_2 is more than 300.

Management

Supportive intensive care therapy is important. Sepsis should be treated with appropriate antibiotics. Careful fluid balance

The causes of ARDS	
Direct lung injury	**Indirect lung injury**
Pneumonia	Sepsis
Aspiration pneumonitis	Trauma
Pulmonary contusion	Cardiopulmonary bypass
Fat embolism	Acute pancreatitis
Inhalational injury	

Table 3.9 The causes of ARDS

is important and over hydration should be avoided. The nutritional status should be addressed. Mechanical ventilation is important but the exact strategy is controversial. It is generally believed that ventilation with low tidal volumes is beneficial. High tidal volumes can exacerbate the lung injury. The role of positive end-expiratory pressure is unclear. Inhaled nitric oxide or surfactant are of no proven benefit. Steroids may have some clinical effect.

Acid–base balance

pH is a logarithmic scale and the blood pH is normally maintained at 7.36–7.44. A change in pH of 0.3 units is equivalent to a doubling of the hydrogen ion concentration. Blood pH is maintained by biological buffering mechanisms involving proteins, bicarbonate and haemoglobin. The relationship between serum pH and bicarbonate concentration is described by the Henderson–Hasselbach equation. Compensatory mechanisms exist to compensate for changes in pH. Important definitions include:

- Acidosis = a rise serum in hydrogen iron concentration or fall in pH
- Alkalosis = a reduction in hydrogen iron concentration or rise in pH
- Respiratory acidosis = a fall in pH due to a rise in partial pressure of carbon dioxide
- Respiratory alkalosis = a rise in pH due to a fall in partial pressure of carbon dioxide
- Metabolic acidosis = a fall in pH due to a metabolic cause
- Metabolic alkalosis = a rise in pH due to a metabolic cause

The anion gap is the sum of the positive and negative charges in the plasma. The cations are sodium and potassium. The anions are chloride, bicarbonate. The difference between the two is the anion gap. If a metabolic acidosis is due to anion excess the anion gap is increased. If metabolic acidosis is due to bicarbonate loss the anion gap is normal. Lactic acidosis and renal failure are associated with an increased anion gap.

Blood gas analysis
A blood gas analyser measures:

- Partial pressure oxygen
- Partial pressure carbon dioxide
- pH

Other variables are derived using Henderson-Hasselbach equation and are summarised in **Table 3.10**.

Interpretation of results
Blood gas results should be interpreted with knowledge of the patient's clinical condition. It is important to check for the consistency within the blood gas sample. To fully interpret results it is important to:

- Look at the pH for the primary acid–base disorder
- Assess a respiratory component by looking at the partial pressure of carbon dioxide
- Assess the metabolic component by looking at the base excess
- Calculate the anion gap

Lactic acidosis
Metabolic acidosis is defined as a state of decreased systemic pH resulting from either

a primary increase in hydrogen ion or a reduction in bicarbonate concentrations. In the acute state, respiratory compensation of acidosis occurs by hyperventilation resulting in a relative reduction in $PaCO_2$. Chronically, renal compensation occurs by means of reabsorption of bicarbonate. The underlying aetiology of metabolic acidosis is classically categorised into those that cause an elevated anion gap and those that do not. Lactic acidosis, identified by a state of acidosis and an elevated plasma lactate concentration is one type of anion gap metabolic acidosis.

The normal blood lactate concentration is 0.5–1.0 mmol/L. Patients with a critical illness can be considered to have normal lactate concentrations of less than 2 mmol/L. Hyperlactataemia is defined as a mild to moderate persistent increase in blood lactate concentration without metabolic acidosis. Lactic acidosis is characterised by a persistently increased blood lactate levels in association with a metabolic acidosis. Elevated lactate levels are a marker of inadequate tissue perfusion and should be considered in relation the patient's clinical presentation. An elevated serum lactate alone cannot provide definitive confirmation of disease presence, severity or prognosis.

Shock

Shock is a pathological condition characterised by inadequate tissue perfusion reducing the delivery of oxygen and other essential nutrients to a level below that required for normal cellular activities. Cellular injury and destruction may follow and tissue and organ function deteriorate. There is progressive cardiovascular collapse resulting in:

- Hypotension
- Hyperventilation
- Reduced level of consciousness
- Oliguria

The causes of shock include:

- Hypovolaemia
- Cardiogenic
- Septic shock
- Anaphylaxis

Physiology of shock

Compensation

Loss of effective circulating blood volume initiates reactive changes. Re-distribution of the circulating blood volume occurs. Perfusion to the coronary and cerebral circulations is maintained by autoregulation. Acute hypovolaemia results in reduced central

Variables derived from a blood gas analyser	
	Normal value
Temperature	37°C
pH	7.36–7.44
Partial pressure CO_2 (pCO_2)	4.6–5.6 kPa
Partial pressure O_2 (pO_2)	10.0–13.3 kPa
Bicarbonate	22 –26 mmol/L
Total carbon dioxide	24–28 mmol/L
Standard bicarbonate (SBC)	22–26 mmol/L
Base excess (BE)	–2 to +2 mmol/L
Standard base excess (SBE)	–3 to +3 mmol/L
Oxygen saturation	>95%
Haemoglobin	11.5–16.5 g/dL

Table 3.10 Variables derived from a blood gas analyser

venous pressure, cardiac filling and cardiac output. Sympathetic stimulation causes reduced splanchnic perfusion, cutaneous vasoconstriction and reduced renal perfusion. The venous return is increased and myocardial contractility is maintained. The renin/angiotensin system is stimulated, antidiuretic hormone is released and the urine output is reduced. If compensation is adequate, blood pressure is maintained and oxygen delivery to the essential tissues remains adequate.

Progression

If compensatory mechanisms are inadequate, ischaemia and hypoxia occur. Anaerobic metabolism results in increased lactate production. Capillary permeability increases and pulmonary oedema may occur resulting in ARDS. Renal hypoperfusion can result in acute tubular necrosis.

Irreversibility

If compensatory mechanisms fail, then vasodilatation occurs and capillary permeability is increased. Progressive tissue hypoxia occurs. When the systolic blood pressure falls below about 50–60 mmHg, reduced coronary circulation results in myocardial ischaemia. Cerebral ischaemia causes vasomotor depression and visceral vasodilatation. Disseminated intravascular coagulation occurs and water and electrolyte disturbances develop.

Acute blood loss

Following acute blood loss, the haemoglobin and packed cell volume (PCV) remain normal for the first 3–4 hours. Plasma volume then expands and the haemoglobin and PCV fall, associated with an increase in neutrophils and platelets. The reticulocyte count increases on day 2 or 3 and this reaches a maximum of 10–15% by day 8 to 10. Without treatment haemoglobin begins to rise by day 7.

Cardiovascular support

In all forms of shock, there is a need to re-establish adequate cardiac output and tissue perfusion. The aim is to achieve a mean arterial pressure of at least 80 mmHg. For this to occur it requires preload optimisation with volume replacement and patients may need inotropic support. Some patients require inotropes and vasopressor. Others require inodilators to redistribute the blood flow. The choice of inotrope depends on their relative actions on the sympathetic nervous system.

Cardiogenic shock

For patients who have low cardiac output with high filling pressure and vascular resistance, dobutamine is an inotrope that reduces vascular resistance. Inodilators such as dopexamine are also useful. Pure vasodilators such as nitrates or nitroprusside also have a role.

High output states

In severe cases of sepsis, vasodilatation is often resistant to the use of vasoconstrictors. The perfusion pressure can be restored with noradrenaline. Dobutamine can be added to increase cardiac output. Adrenaline aggravates splanchnic ischaemia.

Acute renal failure

Acute renal failure is a reduction in renal excretory or regulatory function resulting in the retention of waste products normally excreted by the kidney. A normal adult urine output is about 0.5 mL/kg/hr. Renal failure can be anuric, oliguric or polyuric. Biochemical changes of acute renal failure include:

- Hyponatraemia
- Hyperkalaemia
- Hypocalcaemia
- Metabolic acidosis

Management

The management of acute renal failure is to correct the precipitating cause. Most surgical patients are hypovolaemic and require volume resuscitation. If there is inadequate renal perfusion pressure then consideration needs to be given to inotropic support. Oxygen should be administered. Consideration should be given to the use of bicarbonate if the base excess is more than 10 or the arterial pH less than 7. Hyperkalaemia requires urgent treatment if the patient is:

- Symptomatic
- ECG changes – increased PT interval, tented T waves, ventricular tachycardia
- Serum potassium more than 6 mmol/L

Treatment options are:

- 10 mL 10% calcium gluconate intravenously
- 10 units actrapid in 50 mL 50% dextrose
- Salbutamol nebuliser
- Calcium resonium 15–30 mg as required up to twice daily

Physiological scoring systems

Patients admitted to intensive care form a heterogeneous population. They differ in many respects including age, previous health status, reason for admission and severity of illness. All these factors influence prognosis. Scoring system have been developed to quantity this case mix. Scoring systems can be generic or specific and can be used for audit, research and clinical management. Limitations and errors associated with their use include missing data, observer error, inter-observer variability and lead time bias.

APACHE II score

The APACHE II score is a general measure of disease severity based on current physiologic measurements, age and previous health condition. Scores range from 0 to 71 and with an increasing score there is an increasing risk of hospital death. The APACHE II score is made up of:

- Acute physiology score
- Age points
- Chronic health points

POSSUM system

The outcome of surgery depends on several factors including the physiological status of the patient and the disease process that requires surgical intervention. Raw morbidity and mortality data can provide a biased picture. POSSUM stand for the Physiological and Operative Severity Score for the enUmeration of Mortality. It allows risk-adjusted assessment of surgical quality and accurately predicts 30-day morbidity and mortality. It is two-part scoring system including a physiological assessment and operative severity measure.

Chapter 4

Surgical technique and technology

Surgical wounds

Pathophysiology of wound healing

Wound healing starts with an initial vascular response. Vasoconstriction occurs as a direct response to trauma. Exposed subendothelial tissue activates the coagulation and complement cascades. Platelet adhesion and aggregation causes clot formation. Degranulation of platelets releases growth factors and chemotactic factors. An inflammatory response occurs due to histamine and 5HT release which produces vasodilatation, increased capillary permeability and margination of neutrophils.

This is followed by a cellular response with migration of neutrophils, macrophages and lymphocytes. Macrophages produce growth factors leading to migration of fibroblast and epithelial cells. This causes cellular proliferation with three components:

- Epithelialisation
- Contraction
- Fibroplasia

The formation of an epithelial barrier is important to prevent infection and maintain fluid balance. This is achieved by both migration and proliferation of epithelial cells. Migration requires the presence of granulation tissue. When epithelial cover is complete contact inhibition prevents further epithelial growth. Wound contraction can account for up to 80% reduction in wound size. This occurs due to myofibroblasts in the granulation tissue. Fibroplasia occurs due to procollagen production by fibroblasts. The extracellular matrix contains fibronectin and glycosaminoglycans. These regulate collagen synthesis and cellular differentiation. Fibroplasia is accompanied by simultaneous angiogenesis. Fibrous proliferation is followed by remodeling. Maximum collagen production occurs at 20 days after injury and wound strength increases up to 3 to 6 months. Initial collagen production is disorganised. Remodelling lines it up with stresses in skin. The physiology of wound healing is summarised in **Figure 4.1**.

Important growth factors in wound healing include:

- Platelet derived growth factors (PDGF)
- Insulin like growth factor (IGF-1)
- Epidermal growth factor (EGF)
- Transforming growth factor (TGF-β)

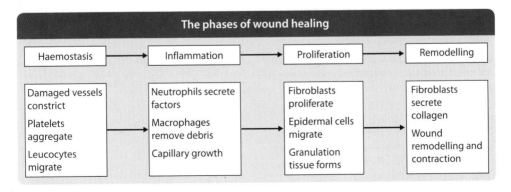

Figure 4.1 The phases of wound healing

Factors that influence wound healing can be both systemic and local.

Systemic factors include:

- Age and sex
- Nutrition
- Vitamin and trace element deficiencies – vitamin C, vitamin A, zinc
- Drugs – steroids, chemotherapy, immunosuppression
- Systemic disease – diabetes, jaundice, malignancy
- Hypoxia

Local factors include:

- Blood supply
- Infection
- Foreign bodies
- Surgical technique

Scars and contractures

Factors that influence scar formation include:

- Individual genetic make up
- Race
- Anatomical site
- Wound tension
- Age
- Placement of incision
- Surgical technique

To minimise the degree of postoperative scarring:

- Incisions should run along Langer lines
- The finest suture possible should be used
- Tension should be avoided
- Sutures should be removed as soon as possible
- Traumatic wounds should be clean and edges excised
- Exposure to sunlight should be avoided in the early postoperative period

Contractures result if scars shorten. They are particularly seen in badly aligned scars not corresponding to Langer lines. They can reduce joint mobility and may require surgery such as a Z-plasty or skin graft to correct the deformity. Depressed scars occur if skin becomes attached to deep tissue. They can be treated by the release of normal skin from margins of scar. The scar can then de-epithelialised and skin edges closed over the top.

Keloid and hypertrophic scars

All scars become red and thickened during the normal healing process. After several months maturation results in flattening of the wound. In some scars collagen formation is excessive resulting in elevated and red scar. If this process is confined to the area of the wound the scar is described as hypertrophic. If it extends beyond the wound into normal tissue the scar is described as keloid scar. Keloid scars are seen particularly in patients of Afro-Caribbean origin and often affect the presternal and deltoid areas. Treatment can be difficult. Treatment options include:

- Intra-lesional steroid injections (e.g. triamcinolone)
- Compression dressings with elasticated compression garments
- Silastic gel therapy
- Excision and radiotherapy
- Laser therapy

Principles of anastomoses

Gastrointestinal anastomoses

An anastomosis is a surgically created join between two hollow viscera or vessels in order to create a confluent channel. Anastomoses can be fashioned in various ways including:

- End-to-end
- End-to-side
- Side-to-side

Any anastomotic technique is required to maintain apposition of the two sides of the anastomosis until collagen is laid down. Gastrointestinal anastomoses show serosal healing and require a good blood supply and minimal tension. Anastomotic leak or failure my occur if there is:

- Distal obstruction
- Peri-anastomotic sepsis
- Peri-anastomotic haematoma
- Hypotension
- Hypoxia
- Jaundice
- Corticosteroids
- Uraemia

An anastomosis should promote primary healing by accurate alignment and minimal disruption of the local vasculature. It should incorporate a minimum amount of foreign material. It should avoid implantation of malignant cells and should not enhance the risk of metachronous tumours.

Conventional methods of fashioning an anastomosis is with sutures or staples. There is no evidence to suggest that hand-sewn are superior to stapled anastomoses. A 'two layered' technique is the classic method of gastrointestinal anastomosis. It requires the use of an inner continuous all layer suture and interrupted outer seromuscular suture. It produces serosal apposition and mucosal inversion. The inner layer was believed to be haemostatic but may strangulates mucosa. A 'single layered' technique is the modern teaching of gastrointestinal anastomoses. It requires an interrupted seromuscular absorbable suture that incorporates a strong submucosal layer. There should be minimal damage to the submucosal vascular plexus.

Stapled anastomoses can be fashioned side-to-side anastomosis with linear staplers or end-to-end with circular devices. Stapled anastomoses may reduce radiologically detected anastomotic leaks but may be associated with increased rate of anastomotic strictures.

The use of drains around anastomoses is controversial. There is no evidence that the use of a drain reduces the risk of anastomotic leakage above pelvic brim. The presence of a drain may actually increase the risk of leakage.

Surgical technique

Incisions

Incisions should allow access to the surgical site and should:

- Be capable of extension if required
- Be secure when closed
- Have a low complication rate
- Be associated with minimal pain
- Have a good cosmetic appearance when healed

Various profiles of surgical blades are available to optimise incisions (**Figure 4.2**).

Wound closure

Wound closure is a matter of personal preference influenced by experience. Mass closure of midline abdominal incision is the preferred technique using an '0' or '1' non-absorbable monofilament suture. About 1 cm bite should be placed 1 cm apart. Applying 'Jenkin's Rule', the suture length:wound length should be about 4:1. A no touch technique of needles should be used. The use of deep tension sutures is controversial. Deep tension sutures offer no extra security and often produce a painful and cosmetically unacceptable scar. The use of a 'fat stitch' reduces dead space but adds no strength to wound repair. There is no evidence that the use of fat sutures reduces the risk of wound infection. The use of silk sutures for skin closure should be avoided as they increase risk of stitch abscesses. If there

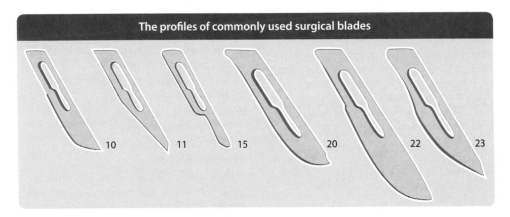

The profiles of commonly used surgical blades

10   11   15   20   22   23

Figure 4.2 The profiles of commonly used surgical blades

is concern about possible wound infection, consideration should be given to leaving the skin wound open.

Sutures should be removed as early as possible. On the head and face, limbs and abdomen they should be removed at 5, 7 and 10 days respectively.

Suture materials and needles

The purpose of a suture is to hold a wound together, in good apposition, until such time as the natural healing process is sufficiently well established to make the support from the suture material unnecessary and redundant.

The ideal suture material should:

- Have good handling characteristics
- Not induce a significant tissue reaction
- Allow secure knots
- Have adequate tensile strength
- Not cut through tissue
- Be sterile
- Be non-allergenic
- Be cheap

The choice of suture will depend on:

- Properties of the suture material
- Absorption rate
- Handling and knotting properties
- Size of suture
- Type of needle

Suture characteristics

Suture materials vary in their physical characteristics. Monofilament sutures (e.g. polypropylene) are smooth. They slide well in tissues but if handled inappropriately they can fracture. Multifilament sutures (e.g. polyglactin) are braided. They have a greater surface area. They are easier to handle and knot well. Some suture materials have a 'memory' and return to former shape when tension is removed. Absorbable suture are broken down by either proteolysis or hydrolysis. The rate of breakdown varies between individual suture materials.

Suture sizes

Sutures are sized by the USP (United States Pharmacopoeia) scale. The available sizes and diameters are:

- 6–0 = 0.07 mm
- 5–0 = 0.10 mm
- 4–0 = 0.15 mm
- 3–0 = 0.20 mm
- 2–0 = 0.30 mm
- 0 = 0.35 mm
- 1 = 0.40 mm
- 2 = 0.5 mm

Needle points

Five types of needle points are in common use and are shown in **Figure 4.3**:

- Cutting needle
- Reverse cutting needle
- Round-body needle
- Taper cutting needle
- Blunt point needle

Needles vary in their diameter and the circumference of the curve as shown in **Figure 4.4**.

Other techniques of wound closure

SteriStrips are self adhesive tapes. They can be used to reduce tension on a wound and are particularly useful for superficial lacerations. Tension from the tapes can cause skin blisters. Tissue adhesive is based on cyanoacrylate monomer. It is simple and pain free to use but wounds does need to be clean and tension free.

Wound dressings

The 'ideal wound dressing' should:

- Maintain a moist environment at the wound interface
- Remove excess exudate without allowing 'strike through' to the surface of dressing
- Provide thermal insulation and mechanical protection
- Act as a barrier to micro-organisms
- Allow gaseous exchange
- Be non-adherent and easily removed without trauma
- Leave no foreign material in the wound
- Be non-toxic, non-allergenic and non-sensitising

Hydrocolloids

Hydrocolloids are a matrix of cellulose and other gel forming agents such as gelatin and pectin. They form an occlusive dressing and should be avoided if infection is a risk. This

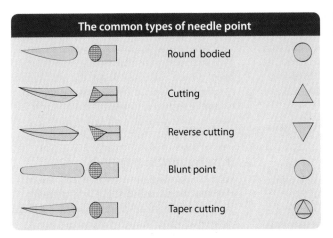

Figure 4.3 The common types of needle point

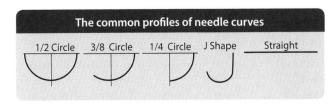

Figure 4.4 The common profiles of needle curves

type of dressing promotes autolysis and aids granulation. It can remain in place for up to a week. Over-granulation can occur.

Alginates

Alginates are made from calcium and sodium salts of alginic acid obtained form seaweed. They are highly absorbent. They are useful in medium to heavily exudating wounds and form a gel in contact with wound exudates.

Foam dressings

Foam dressings are useful for moderately exudating wounds. They prevents 'strike through' of exudate to wound surface. They deslough wounds by maintaining a moist environment.

Hydrogels

Hydrogels have a high water content which creates a moist wound surface. They debride wounds by a combination of hydration and promotion of autolysis. They will absorb light exudates but are not appropriate for heavily exudating wounds.

Debriding agents

Debriding agents remove eschar and necrotic tissue. They do not maintain a moist environment and need frequent changes. They damage granulation tissue and can potentially delay healing.

Negative pressure topical dressings

Negative pressure topical dressings apply pressure via a foam dressing. They remove wound exudate and reduce extravascular and interstitial fluid. They improve blood supply to the wound during the phase of inflammation. The mechanical effect appears to stimulate cellular proliferation. A polyurethane or polyvinyl-alcohol foam dressing is cut to the shape of the wound. The foam is then covered with an adhesive dressing with a small hole. A therapeutic regulated accurate care (TRAC) pad is applied over the hole and is connected to a negative pressure generator. The pressures achieved at the TRAC pad–foam interface are regulated. A pressure of approximately 125 mmHg is often used. Intermittent application of pressure may be advantageous.

The dressings should be changed every 48–72 hours. Wounds suitable for negative pressure topical dressings include those resulting from trauma, burns, pressure sores, leg ulcers and infection. Contraindications include grossly infected and bleeding wounds, malignancy and exposed vessels and bowel.

Diathermy

Diathermy is the use of high frequency electrical current to produce heat. It is used to either cut and destroy tissue or to produce coagulation. Mains electricity is 50 Hz and produces intense muscle and nerve activation. The electrical frequency used by diathermy is in the range of 300 kHz to 3 MHz. The patient's body forms part of the electrical circuit but the current has little effect on muscles and the myocardium.

Monopolar diathermy

With monopolar diathermy (**Figure 4.5**), an electrical plate is placed on the patient and acts as an indifferent electrode. The current passes between the instrument and the indifferent electrode. As the surface area of the instrument is an order of magnitude less than that of the plate, localised heating is produced at the tip of instrument and minimal heating effect is produced at the indifferent electrode. The effects of diathermy depend on the current intensity and wave-form used. Coagulation is produced by interrupted pulses of current (50–100/second) and the use of a square wave-form. Cutting is produced by continuous current in a sinus wave-form.

Diathermy can interfere with pacemaker function. Arcing can occur with metal instruments and implants. Superficial burn can occur if a spirit-based skin preparation is used. A burn can occur under the indifferent electrode if the plate is not properly applied. Channeling effects can occur if diathermy is used on a viscus with a narrow pedicle (e.g. penis or testis).

Bipolar diathermy

With bipolar diathermy (**Figure 4.6**), the two electrodes are combined in the instrument (e.g. forceps) and the current passes between the tips and not through the patient. The advantage of bipolar diathermy is that the electrical current does not pass through parts of the body which are not being treated. It is possible to be much more precise with the quantity of tissue being coagulated.

Lasers

Laser is an acronym for Light Amplification by the Stimulated Emission of Radiation. Laser emissions vary and are:

- Collimated – parallel output beam results in little energy loss
- Coherent – waves are all in phase resulting in little loss of energy
- Monochromic – all of the same wave length

The effects of a laser depends on its photochemical, photomechanical and photothermal effects. Tissue penetration increases with wavelength. Pulsing of output can reduce thermal damage.

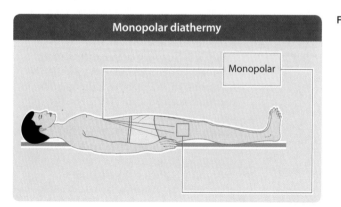

Figure 4.5 Monopolar diathermy

Monopolar diathermy

Monopolar

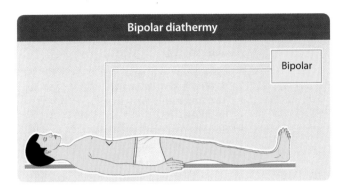

Bipolar diathermy

Bipolar

Figure 4.6 Bipolar diathermy

Lasers are classified according to the amount of damage they can cause:

- Class 1 – generally safe
- Class 2 – safe within the time of the blink reflex
- Class 3 – cause blindness after short exposure from mirrored surfaces
- Class 4 – unsafe even with reflection from non-mirrored surfaces

All medical lasers belong to class 4 and both patients and operators are required to wear goggles. The properties and uses of different types of laser are shown in **Table 4.1.** Risks associated with the use of lasers include excessive burning, scar formation, accidental skin exposure and corneal or retinal burns.

Surgical procedures
Day care surgery

During recent years, the duration of hospital stay has been reduced. This has been associated with an expansion in the use of day case surgery. Approximately 50% of elective operations are now performed as day cases. Potential benefits of day surgery include:

- Reduced disruption to patients' normal lives
- Psychological benefit of avoiding prolonged hospital stay
- Reduced morbidity including nosocomial infections
- Reduced inpatient waiting lists
- Increased availability of inpatient beds
- Reduced costs

Properties and uses of different types of laser			
Laser	Wavelength (nm)	Pulse length	Uses
Carbon dioxide	10,600	Continuous	Tissue cutting
Neodymium-YAG	1064	Continuous	Coagulation
Neodymium-YAG	1064	10 ns	Posterior capsulotomy
Ruby	694	100 µs	Tattoo removal
Argon	488–514	Continuous	Coagulation
Excimer	308	10 ns	Photorefractive keratotomy

Table 4.1 The properties and uses of different types of laser

Safe day case surgery requires appropriate:

- Patient selection
- Operative procedures
- Anaesthetic techniques

Patient selection

For day surgery patients should generally fulfill the following criteria:

- Age less than 70 years
- ASA Grade 1 or 2
- BMI less than 30
- Availability of a responsible adult
- Access to a telephone
- Live within an hour's travelling time from the hospital

Appropriate patient selection requires close co-operation between surgeon, anaesthetist and day unit. Preoperative screening should be performed. It can be carried out by a questionnaire and/or in a nurse-led assessment clinic. Patients requiring extensive preoperative investigation are not suitable for day case surgery.

Operation selection

Operations suitable for day case surgery vary between specialties. The appropriateness can be expanded by the facility for an overnight stay. Generally operations should be:

- Short duration
- Low incidence of postoperative complications
- Not require blood transfusion
- Not require major postoperative analgesia

Laparoscopic surgery can be performed, usually with an overnight stay. Surgery should be performed by an experienced surgeon. There should be access to inpatient beds should they be required.

Day case anaesthesia

The principles of anaesthesia are the same as for inpatient care. It requires high quality induction, maintenance and recovery. The recovery should be free from side effects. Anaesthesia should be performed by an experienced anaesthetist. The use of local anaesthetic techniques should be encouraged.

Discharge criteria

Prior to discharge from the day case unit patients should:

- Have stable vital signs
- Be alert and orientated
- Be comfortable/pain free
- Be able to walk
- Be able to tolerate oral fluids
- Have minimal nausea and vomiting

Adequate follow-up arrangements should be made. Patients should be provided with information sheets and have a contact telephone number in case of problems.

Endoscopic surgery and laparoscopy

Minimal access surgery presents the opportunity of reduced trauma associated with access to body cavities without compromising exposure of the operative field. Minimal access surgery can be performed using the following approaches:

- Laparoscopic
- Thoracoscopic
- Endoluminal
- Intra-articular joint surgery
- Combined approaches

The advantages of minimal access surgery are:

- Less tissue trauma
- Less postoperative pain
- Faster recovery
- Fewer postoperative complications
- Better cosmesis

The disadvantages of minimal access surgery are:

- Lack of tactile feedback
- Increased technical expertise required
- Possible longer duration of surgery
- Increased risk of iatrogenic injuries
- Difficult removal of bulky organs
- More expensive

Pneumoperitoneum

Laparoscopic surgery invariably requires the establishment of a pneumoperitoneum. The ideal gas for insufflation during laparoscopy must have the following characteristics:

- Limited systemic absorption across the peritoneum

- Limited systemic effects when absorbed
- Rapid excretion if absorbed
- Incapable of supporting combustion
- High solubility in blood
- Limited physiological effects with intravascular systemic embolism

Carbon dioxide is the best gas available. A pneumoperitoneum can be performed using either a closed or open technique.

The closed technique involves the use of a Veress needle. It is a blind procedure with the potential for complications. Major complications include visceral or vascular puncture. The needle is usually inserted at the umbilicus and is aimed towards the pelvis. Intraperitoneal placement can be checked by either a saline drop test or low-flow gas insufflation. In an adult, insufflation of about 3.5 litres of CO_2 is required to establish an adequate pneumoperitoneum usually with a maximum pressure of 10–12 mmHg. The primary port is then inserted blindly through the umbilicus and the secondary ports are placed under direct vision.

The open (Hasson) technique for establishing a pneumoperitoneum is associated with a reduced risk of visceral injury. The primary port is inserted using a 'cut-down' technique. A subumbilical incision is made and stay sutures are inserted in to the linea alba to provide counter traction. An incision is made in the linea alba and a finger inserted through peritoneum to ensure that there are no adhesions. The primary port is then inserted under direct vision.

Tourniquets

Tourniquets are commonly used in surgical practice to reduce blood loss in the operative field. When properly applied they provide excellent haemostasis. When incorrectly used, they can be dangerous. Cuff failure can be disastrous with rapid systemic absorption of drugs (e.g. local anaesthetics).

The use of a tourniquet requires correct placement and connection. There should be adequate padding and the limb should be exsanguinate before inflation. Their use should involve minimal pressure (usually 100 mmHg above systolic blood pressure) for minimal duration (no longer than 90 minutes). Multiple inflations or deflations should be avoided. Relative contraindications to the use of tourniquets include:

- Previous DVT or pulmonary embolus
- Arterial disease
- Vasculitic disorders
- Sickle cell anaemia

Complications of tourniquet use include:

- Nerve injury
- Vascular injury
- Postoperative embolic events
- Post-tourniquet syndrome
- Myoglobinuria
- Increased blood viscosity
- Increased postoperative pain
- Tourniquet burns

Rubber tubing and surgical gloves are frequently used as tourniquets on fingers. This practice should be condemned as they can inadvertently be left on the digit at the end of the procedure. Specific brightly coloured digital tourniquets are now available.

Surgical drains

Drains are often used to evacuate establish collections of pus, blood or other fluids (e.g. lymph) or to drain potential collections. Their use is contentious.

Arguments for their use include:

- Drainage of fluid removes potential sources of infection
- Drains guard against further fluid collections
- They may allow the early detection of anastomotic leaks or haemorrhage
- They leave a tract for potential collections to drain following removal

Arguments against their use include:

- The presence of a drain increases the risk of infection
- Tissue damage may be caused by mechanical pressure or suction
- Drains may induce an anastomotic leak
- Most abdominal drains become infected within 24 hours

Types of drain

Most modern drains are made from an inert silastic material. They induce minimal tissue reaction. Older red rubber drains induce an intense tissue reaction allowing a tract to form and have specific uses in modern surgical practice. In some situations this may be useful (e.g. biliary T-tube). Drains can be open or closed and can be active or passive. Open drains include corrugated rubber or plastic sheets. The drain fluid collects into a gauze pad or stoma bag. Open drains can be associated with an increased risk of infection. A closed drain consists of a tube draining into a bag or bottle. Examples include chest and abdominal drains. With closed drains the risk of infection is reduced. Active drains are maintained under suction with either low or high pressure. Passive drains have no suction. They function by the differential pressure between body cavities and the exterior.

Nasogastric tubes

Following abdominal surgery, gastrointestinal motility is reduced for a variable period of time. Gastrointestinal secretions accumulate in the stomach and proximal small bowel. This may result in postoperative distension and vomiting and the risk of an aspiration pneumonia. Nasogastric tubes are often used to remove fluid and secretions. There is little clinical evidence available to support their routine use following elective gastrointestinal surgery and they may actually increase the risk of pulmonary complications. They are of proven value for gastrointestinal decompression in intestinal obstruction and following emergency abdominal surgery. Nasogastric tubes are usually left on free drainage and aspirated on an intermittent basis. They should be removed when the volume of nasogastric aspirate has reduced and gastrointestinal motility has returned.

Urinary catheters

A urinary catheter is a form of drain. It is commonly used to alleviate or prevent urinary retention or to monitor urine output. It can be inserted transurethrally or suprapubically. Catheters vary by:

- The material from which they are made (latex, plastic, silastic, Teflon-coated)
- The length of the catheter (38 cm 'male' or '22 cm 'female')

- The diameter of the catheter (10 Fr to 24 Fr)
- The number of channels (two or three)
- The size of the balloon (5 mL to 30 mL)
- The shape of the tip

When using a catheter it should be of an appropriate size, inserted using an aseptic technique and never with the use of force. The balloon should not be inflated until urine has been seen coming from the catheter. The residual volume should be recorded. A catheter introducer should not be used unless the operator has been trained in its use. If difficulty is encountered inserting a urethral catheter consider a suprapubic route. The catheter should be removed as early as possible. Special catheters exist such as:

- Gibbon catheters
- Nelaton catheters
- Tiemann catheters
- Malecot catheters

Indications for a urinary catheter include:

- The management of acute urinary retention or bladder outlet obstruction
- The measurement of urine output in a critically ill patient
- During surgery to assess fluid status
- During and following specific surgeries of the genitourinary tract
- The management of haematuria associated with clots
- The management of an immobilised patients
- The management of patients with a neurogenic bladder
- Intravesical pharmacologic therapy
- Improved patient comfort for end of life care
- The management of patients with urinary incontinence

The only absolute contraindication to the placement of a urethral catheter is the presence of urethral injury. Relative contraindications include a urtethral stricture or recent urinary tract surgery.

Complications of urethral catheterisation include:

- Paraphimosis
- Blockage
- By-passing
- Infection
- Failure of balloon to deflate
- Urethral strictures

Suprapubic catherisation

Suprapubic catheterisation should be used when urethral catheterisation is contraindicated or where it is technically impossible to relieve urinary retention in both acute and chronic conditions. In addition, it may be chosen to improve patient comfort, dignity or convenience, and to prevent complications such as catheter-induced urethral injury. Insertion requires a palpable bladder. Complications include misplacement, bleeding and bowel perforation.

Chapter 5

Evidence-based surgical practice

Evidence-based medicine

The primary purpose of any healthcare system is to secure through the resources available the greatest possible improvement to physical and mental health of the population. To achieve this, decisions about the delivery and provision of healthcare are increasingly being driven by evidence of clinical and cost-effectiveness as well as systematic assessment of actual health outcomes. Evidence-based medicine is the process of systematically reviewing, appraising and using clinical research findings to aid the delivery of optimum clinical care to patients.

Principles of research and clinical trials

Primary research includes:

- Animal or volunteer experiments
- Clinical trials
- Surveys

Secondary research includes:

- Systematic review and meta-analyses
- Guidelines

- Decision analyses
- Economic analyses

The strength of a study depends on its design. A hierarchy of evidence (**Table 5.1**) exists with decreasing strength as follows:

- Systematic review and meta-analysis
- Randomised controlled trials with definitive results
- Randomised controlled trials with non-definitive results
- Cohort studies
- Case–control studies
- Cross sectional surveys
- Case reports

Clinical trials

Purpose of clinical trials

Clinical trials conduct 'human experiments'. Three fundamental principles apply:

- The trial must address a legitimate question
- The patient must be informed and willing to participate
- The patient may decline entry or withdraw at any stage

Hierarchy of evidence	
Level	**Description**
Ia	Evidence from a meta-analysis of randomised controlled trials
Ib	Evidence from at least one randomised controlled trial
IIa	Evidence from at least one well-designed controlled study without randomisation
IIb	Evidence from at least one well-designed quasi-experimental study
III	Evidence from well-designed non-experimental descriptive studies such as comparative studies, correlation studies or case studies
IV	Evidence from expert committee reports or opinions or clinical experiences of respected authorities

Table 5.1 Hierarchy of evidence

Phase 1 study

Phase 1 studies provide basic pharmacological and toxicology information. They are not a test of therapeutic efficacy. They can be performed on either on healthy volunteers or patients whose disease has progressed on all available treatments.

Phase 2 study

Phase 2 studies are used to identify the dose range of a particular drug. The sample size is small and patients usually have end-stage disease. The study is not usually randomised and drug combinations may be tested.

Phase 3 study

Phase 3 studies are randomised and designed to compare the effects of different treatments. One treatment option should be the best currently available. Outcome measures usually include survival, disease-free survival, response and toxicity. These studies usually involve large numbers of patients.

Phase 4 study

Phase 4 studies are less commonly used. They are aimed at evaluating the long-term outcome of established therapies and are often regarded as a post-marketing study.

Randomised controlled trials

In randomised controlled trials (RCTs), participants are randomly allocated to one intervention or another. Both groups are followed up for a specified period. The two groups are analysed in terms of outcome defined at the outset. If the groups are similar at the outset then any difference should be due to the intervention.

The advantages of RCTs are:

- Allow rigorous evaluation of a single variable in a defined patient group
- Potentially eradicate bias by comparing two (or more) identical groups
- Allow for meta-analysis

The disadvantages of RCTs are:

- Expensive and time consuming
- Often have too few patients or too short a follow-up period
- Surrogate endpoints are often used in preference to clinical outcome measures
- Often imperfect randomisation
- Often not all eligible patients are randomised
- Failure to blind assessors to randomisation status of patients

Cohort studies

Cohort studies compare groups exposed to different factors who are followed up to see whether there is a difference in outcome. They are often used to study disease aetiology and assess disease prognosis.

Case–control studies

Case–control studies match patients with a disease to controls. Data are then collected retrospectively to find a difference between the groups.

Statistics
Types of data

Before data analysis can be performed it is necessary to identify the type of data presented. Data can be quantitative or categorical:

- Quantitative and continuous – e.g. height, weight, blood pressure
- Quantitative and discrete – e.g. number of children
- Categorical and ordinal – e.g. Grade of tumour
- Categorical and nominal – e.g. Male/female, blood group

Description of quantitative data

Data can be described by a 'measure of location'

- Median = mid point: 50% of variables above and 50% of variables below
- Mode = most common variable
- Mean = the average i.e. the sum of variable divided by the number

Data can also be described by a 'measure of variation'

- Range = distribution between maximum and minimum value
- Interquartile range = distribution between first and third quartile
- Standard deviation = distribution around mean in a 'normally' distributed population

Data can be either be either normally distributed (**Figure 5.1**) or can have a skewed distribution, (**Figure 5.2**). With a normal

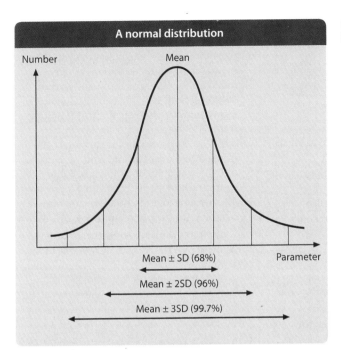

Figure 5.1 A normal distribution.
SD = Standard deviation

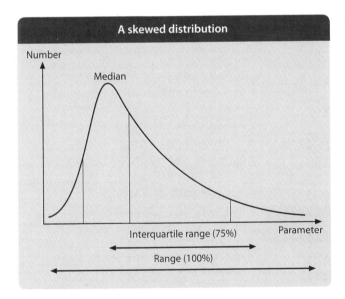

Figure 5.2 A skewed distribution

distribution the median equals the mean and 68%, 95% and 99.7% of variable lies with one, two and three standard deviations of the mean.

Statistical hypothesis

A statistical hypothesis is an assumption about a population parameter. This assumption may or may not be true. The best way to determine whether a statistical hypothesis is true would be to examine the entire population. Since that is often impractical, researchers typically examine a random sample from the population. If sample data are not consistent with the statistical hypothesis, the hypothesis is rejected. There are two types of statistical hypotheses.

- Null hypothesis – is the hypothesis that sample observations result purely from chance
- Alternative hypothesis – is the hypothesis that sample observations are influenced by some non-random cause

Calculation of sample size

The sample size needed to test a hypothesis depends on four factors:

- Expected difference in means between the two groups
- Variability of the data
- Power of the study and the probability that any difference is real (usually 90%)
- Level of significance accepted (usually 5%)

Type I and Type II errors

A Type I error is rejection of null hypothesis when it is in fact true:

- No difference is present between the samples
- The statistical method used identified a difference

A Type II error is rejection of null hypothesis when difference between groups exists:

- A difference is present between the samples
- The statistical method used failed to identify it

Choice of statistical test

Prior to analysing data it is necessary to define the hypothesis being tested. If no hypothesis is proposed then no statistical test can be selected. When selecting an appropriate statistic test it is necessary to decide whether the variables are matched, paired or independent and to define both the input and output variables. Both variable can be categorical or quantitative. Statistical tests for paired or matched variables are shown in **Table 5.2**. Appropriate statistical tests for independent observations and categorical outcome variables are shown in **Table 5.3**. Appropriate statistical tests for independent observations and quantitative outcome variables are shown in **Table 5.4**.

A test of a statistical hypothesis, where the region of rejection is on only one side of the sampling distribution, is called a one-tailed test. A test of a statistical hypothesis, where the region of rejection is on both sides of the sampling distribution, is called a two-tailed test.

Quality of life

Diseases and their treatment have an impact on patient wellbeing. Quality of life (QoL) is a measure of an illness, disease and its treatment on patient welfare. It has dimensions beyond physical measures of patients' progress. No universal definition of QoL exists. It has three fundamental characteristics:

- Multidimensional – physical, social, psychological
- Subjective
- Dynamic

Quality of life assessment

QoL assessment is used to access progress of individual patients. In clinical trials it is used to compare treatment options and determine cost-effectiveness of treatment. The instrument used must be:

- Valid – measure what it is supposed to measure
- Reliable – produce consistent results
- Responsive – be able to detect changes with time

QoL assessments can be either self-administered or by interview and can be repeated on several occasions. Data are usually collected using a structured questionnaire.

Statistical tests for paired or matched variables	
	Test
Nominal	McNemar
Ordinal	Wilcoxon
Quantitative (non-normal)	Wilcoxon
Quantitative (normal)	Paired t-test

Table 5.2 Statistical tests for paired or matched variables

Statistical tests for independent observations and categorical outcome variables			
	Nominal	**Categorical**	**Ordinal**
Nominal	Chi-squared or Fisher	Chi-squared	Chi-squared or Mann–Whitney
Categorical	Chi-squared	Chi-squared	Kruskal–Wallis
Ordinal	Mann–Whitney		Spearman rank
Quantitative – discrete	Logistic regression		
Quantitative – non-normal	Logistic regression		
Quantitative – normal	Logistic regression		

Table 5.3 Statistical tests for independent observations and categorical outcome variables

Statistical tests for independent observations and quantitative outcome variables			
	Quantitative – discrete	**Quantitative – non-normal**	**Quantitative – normal**
Nominal	Mann–Whitney	Mann–Whitney or log-rank	Student's t-test
Categorical	Kruskal–Wallis	Kruskal–Wallis	ANOVA
Ordinal	Spearman rank	Spearman rank	Spearman rank or linear regression
Quantitative – discrete	Spearman rank	Spearman rank	Spearman rank or linear regression
Quantitative – non-normal		Pearson or Spearmen rank	Pearson or Spearman rank
Quantitative – normal		Linear regression	Linear regression

Table 5.4 Statistical tests for independent observations and quantitative outcome variables

Different items on the questionnaire tap various dimensions of QoL. QoL instruments can be either generic or specific.

Generic instruments assess many dimensions and produce a global concept of QoL. Two types of generic questionnaires exist:

- Health profiles (e.g. SF-36)
- Health indices (e.g. Quality adjusted life years)

Specific instruments are used for specified disease or condition. Several types exist including:

- Domain specific (e.g. hospital anxiety and depression scales)
- Disease specific (e.g. EORTC QLQ-C30 for cancer patients)
- Population specific (e.g. children or elderly)
- Symptom specific (e.g. McGill pain questionnaire)

Chapter 6

Surgical pathology and microbiology

Surgical pathology

Necrosis

Cells can be damaged by various processes including:

- Reduced oxygen supply
- Physical agents
- Chemical agents
- Toxins
- Viruses
- Abnormal immunological reactions

Necrosis results from cell death. It results in disintegration of the nucleus, cytoplasmic organelles and the plasma membrane. Intracellular enzymes are released. Necrosis is associated with visible changes – coagulative or colliquative necrosis. In coagulative necrosis the nucleus fades and dissolves (karyolysis), becomes more dense (pyknosis) and fragments (karyorrhexis).

Apoptosis

Apoptosis is programmed cell death. It is a physiological process and affects single cells in a population of healthy cells. It is the mechanism of removing effete and abnormal cells. Normal cells divide to replace lost cells. There is no evidence of inflammation. It provides a balance between cell proliferation and elimination. It is associated with maintenance of organ size in adults, organ development and physiological atrophy or involution.

Atrophy

Atrophy is a decrease in organ size due to a reduction in cell size or number. Causes include:

- Gradual diminution in blood supply
- Reduced functional activity
- Interrupted nerve supply
- Endocrine deficiency
- Pressure

Calcification

Abnormal deposits of calcium salts occur in two circumstances. Dystrophic calcification is deposition of calcium that occurs when necrotic tissue is not absorbed or tissues undergo slow degeneration. Metastatic calcification occurs when serum calcium is elevated for a long period of time. It is associated with increased calcium absorption due to high vitamin D levels, resorption of bone, mobilisation of calcium due to parathyroid hormone excess and chronic renal failure. Calcium is deposited in the arterial walls, kidneys, lungs and stomach wall.

Amyloid

Amyloid is abnormal protein that is deposited in extracellular tissue. It occurs around the basement membrane and capillaries and is resistant to degradation. Two types of amyloidosis are recognised. Primary amyloidosis is due to unknown causes. Secondary amyloidosis is most commonly due to:

- Tuberculosis
- Pyogenic infection
- Rheumatoid arthritis
- Myeloma
- Hodgkin's disease

Amyloidosis affects several organs including the heart, intestinal tract and kidneys. It results in atrophy due to pressure. Transudation of proteins occurs due to increased permeability and is associated with vessel narrowing. Pathologically it can be detected by Lugol's iodine and Congo red dye. With Congo red, tissues show apple green fluorescence in polarised light.

Hypersensitivity reactions

Hypersensitivity reactions are exaggerated immunological response to an antigen by a normal immune system. They require previous exposure to the antigen. Four types are recognised based on the mechanism involved:

- Type I – anaphylactic
- Type II – cytotoxic
- Type III – immune complex
- Type IV – cell mediated or delayed

Various clinical conditions are associated with one or more type of reaction.

Type I hypersensitivity

Immediate or anaphylactic hypersensitivity reaction occurs within 10–15 minutes of exposure to an antigen. The extent of the reaction can range from mild to life-threatening. Clinical features include urticaria, conjunctivitis, rhinitis and bronchospasm. The reaction is mediated via IgE. The main cellular component is the mast cell or basophil. The reaction is amplified by platelets and eosinophils. IgE is produced in response to exposure to an antigen or allergen. IgE binds to cell surface receptors on mast cells. Cross linking or receptors result in mast cell degranulation via a calcium influx. Mediators released include:

- Histamine
- Tryptase
- Kininogenase
- Leukotriene B4
- Prostaglandin D2
- Platelet activating factor

Mast cell degranulation can also be triggered by exercise, stress, chemicals and anaphylatoxins. Reaction to these agents or stimuli is not mediated via IgE. Treatment is by agents that block histamine receptors, inhibit mast cell degranulation and leukotriene receptor blockers. Examples include hay fever and drug allergies.

Type II hypersensitivity

Cytotoxic hypersensitivity affects various organs and tissues. Antigens are normally endogenous and reactions occurs in hours. It is mediated via IgM and IgG antibodies and complement. Phagocytes and K cells play a role. Examples include Goodpasture's syndrome and pemphigus.

Type III hypersensitivity

Immune complex hypersensitivity can be general or affect individual tissues. The reaction occurs several hours after exposure to antigen. It is mediated via soluble immune complexes and complement. Antibodies are of IgG class. Antigen can be exogenous – bacteria, virus or parasites or endogenous. Examples include, systemic lupus erythematosis and rheumatoid arthritis.

Type IV hypersensitivity

Cell mediated or delayed type hypersensitivity reactions peak after about 48 hours. They are mediated via T lymphocytes, monocytes and macrophages with cytotoxic T cells causing direct damage. T helper cells secrete cytokines that recruit and activate macrophages. The major lymphokines involved include monocyte chemotactic factor, interleukin 2 and TNF-α. Examples include many autoimmune and infectious diseases (e.g. tuberculosis, toxoplasmosis).

Surgical microbiology
Abscesses
Superficial and deep abscesses

An abscess is a collection of pus within soft tissues. It occurs when a host's response to infection is inadequate. Predisposing factors include foreign bodies within the wound, haematoma formation and ischaemia.

Pathology

An abscess contains bacteria, acute inflammatory cells, protein exudate and necrotic tissue. It is surrounded by granulation tissue often called the 'pyogenic membrane'. The commonest organisms involved in superficial abscesses are *Staphylococcus aureus* and *Streptococcus pyogenes*. The commonest organisms involved in deep abscesses are Gram-negative species (e.g. *Escherichia coli*) and anaerobes (e.g. *Bacteroides*).

Clinical features

Common superficial abscesses include infected sebaceous cysts, breast and pilonidal abscesses. They show the cardinal features of inflammation – calor, rubor, dolor, tumour

- Heat
- Redness
- Pain
- Swelling

After a few days, superficial abscess become fluctuant and often 'point'. Deep abscesses include diverticular, subphrenic and anastomotic leaks. Patients usually show signs of inflammation including a swinging pyrexia, tachycardia and tachypnoea. Physical signs are otherwise difficult to demonstrate. The site of an abscess may not be clinically apparent. Radiological investigations are often required to make the diagnosis.

Treatment

All abscesses require adequate drainage often under general anaesthesia. Antibiotics have little to offer as tissue penetration is usually poor and prolonged antibiotic treatment can result in a chronic inflammatory mass (an 'antibioma'). Superficial abscesses are usually suitable for open drainage. For deep abscesses closed drainage may be attempted.

Superficial abscesses can usually be drained through a cruciate incision. The position of the incision should allow depended drainage. The loculi within the abscess should be broken down and necrotic tissue excised. Pus should be sent for microbiology. A dressing should be inserted into the wound. Packing is usually not required – it is painful and rarely improves the outcome. Deep abscesses can often be treated by ultrasound or CT guided aspiration, however, success can not always be guaranteed. Percutaneous access may be difficult because of the position of adjacent organs. Multiloculated abscesses may not drain adequately and open drainage may be required.

Psoas abcess

The iliopsoas compartment is an extraperitoneal space. It contains both the psoas and iliacus muscles. The psoas lies close to several abdominal structures and organs (e.g. sigmoid colon, ureter, appendix) and infection in these structures can spread to the muscles. The muscles also have a good blood supply predisposing to haematogenous spread of infection.

Aetiology

A psoas abscess can be classified as primary or secondary. A primary abscess occurs as a result of haematogenous spread of infection and is seen in conditions in which patients are immunocompromised such as in diabetes mellitus, intravenous drug abuse or renal failure.

Secondary abscesses are associated with local pathology. Common causes include:

- Crohn's disease
- Diverticulitis
- Appendicitis
- Urinary tract infection
- Septic arthritis
- Femoral vessel cannulation

In developing countries, most psoas abscesses are primary. In Western countries, about 60% of abscesses are secondary. *Staphylococcus aureus* is the commonest causative organism in primary abscess. Gut-related organisms are the commonest cause of a secondary abscess. Tuberculosis is a rare cause of psoas abscess in developed countries.

Clinical features

The clinical features are non-specific and the diagnosis may be delayed. Typical symptoms and signs include, flank, back or abdominal pain, fever, a limp, malaise and weight loss or a lump in the groin.

Investigation

The white cell count and inflammatory markers may be raised. A plain abdominal x-ray may be normal. Ultrasound has limited use and has a sensitivity of only 60%. CT is the gold standard investigation. MRI may be useful.

Management

Management involves the use of appropriate antibiotics based on the likely cause and drainage of the abscess, possibly by a percutaneous route. Antibiotics can be changed when sensitivities are known. Surgery may be more appropriate in secondary abscesses when the underlying pathology may require surgical correction.

Cellulitis

Cellulitis is a spreading infection in the subcutaneous tissue. It often occurs after a skin abrasion or other similar minor trauma. It is usually due to infection with β haemolytic Streptococcus or Staphylococcus aureus. Both produce enzymes that degrade tissue and allow spread of infection.

Clinical features

Cellulitis usually presents with a well-demarcated area of inflammation. It is often associated with malaise, fever and a raised white cell count. If not rapidly treated, it can progress to lymphangitis and lymphadenitis. Localised areas of skin necrosis may occur. Predisposing factors for infection include lymphoedema, venous stasis, diabetes mellitus and surgical wounds.

Management

Treatment should be by rest and elevation of the affected limb. Antibiotics may initially be given orally but consideration should be given to intravenous administration if there is no early improvement. Benzylpenicillin and flucloxacillin are usually the antibiotics of choice.

Necrotising soft tissue infections

Necrotising soft tissue infections are the result of skin and subcutaneous infections with virulent bacteria. Bacterial toxins can cause widespread skin and fascial necrosis.

Meleney's synergistic gangrene

Meleney's synergistic gangrene results from synergistic infection affecting principally the skin. It usually occurs around surgical wounds, stomas and cutaneous fistulae. It is due to infection with both Staphylococcus aureus and anaerobic streptococci. The initial clinical features are often initially indistinguishable from cellulitis. However

it spreads slowly and often results in skin ulceration. It lacks the severe systemic toxicity seen with necrotising fasciitis. Treatment should be with antibiotics including benzylpenicillin. Surgical debridement of the affected area may be required.

Necrotising fascitis

Necrotising fasciitis is usually seen in immunocompromised patients such as diabetics, alcoholics or intravenous drug abusers. It occurs at several characteristic sites including the limbs after cuts, abrasions or bites, around postoperative abdominal surgical wounds, in the perineum secondary to anorectal sepsis or in the male genitalia (Fournier's gangrene). It occurs as a result of a polymicrobial infection involving facultative aerobes, Streptococcal species or Escherichia coli and anaerobes. The exotoxins produced by the organisms result in severe systemic toxicity.

Clinical features

The early clinical features are often similar to cellulitis but warning features include severe pain – out of proportion to the clinical signs, systemic toxicity, cutaneous gangrene or haemorrhagic fluid leaking from a wound. Untreated, it rapidly progresses to multiple organ failure and overall has a mortality of about 30%. A plain x-ray may show gas in the subcutaneous tissue.

Management

Early and rapid treatment requires a high degree of clinical suspicion. Patients should be managed in a high dependency unit as they will need vigorous fluid resuscitation and organ support. Early surgical debridement is essential. Excision should extend well into apparently normal tissue. Amputation or fasciotomies may be required. A defunctioning colostomy may be required for perineal sepsis. Antibiotic cover should include benzylpenicillin, metronidazole and gentamicin. Hyperbaric oxygen therapy may be of benefit.

Wound infection

About 75% of nosocomial infections occur in surgical patients. Most postoperative infections arise from the patient's own bacterial flora. The commonest sites of infection are the urinary tract (40%), wounds (35%), the respiratory tract (15%) and bacteraemia (5%). Wound contamination can occur from direct inoculation from the patient's residual flora or skin contamination from the surgeon's hands, contaminated instruments, dressings, drains, catheters or intravenous lines. Airborne contamination can occur from the skin and clothing of staff or from air flow in the operating theatre or ward. Haematogenous spread can occur from intravenous lines and sepsis at other anatomical sites.

Definition

Wounds infections can be defined as:

- Surgical site infections
- Superficial incisional infections
- Deep incisional infections
- Organ space infections

To meet the definition, surgical site infections must occur within 30 days of surgery and the infection must involve only the skin and subcutaneous tissue. There must be either purulent discharge from a superficial infection or organisms isolated from aseptically obtained wound culture. There must also be signs of inflammation. Several predisposing factors for wound infection are well-recognised (**Table 6.1**).

Microbiology

Aerobic pathogens found in wound infections include:

- *Staphylococcus aureus* (17%)
- Enterococci (13%)
- Coagulase-negative staphylococci (12%)
- *Escherichia coli* (10%)
- *Pseudomonas aeruginosa* (8%)
- *Enterobacter* species (8%)
- *Proteus mirabilis* (4%)
- *Klebsiella pneumoniae* (3%)
- *Candida* species (2%)

Prevention

Exogenous methods of preventing wound infections include:

- Sterilisation of instruments and sutures
- Positive pressure ventilation of operating theatres
- Laminar air flow in high-risk areas
- Exclusion of staff with infections

Endogenous methods of preventing wound infections include:

- Skin preparation
- Mechanical bowel preparation
- Antibiotic prophylaxis
- Good surgical technique

Wound infection rates

The risk of wound infection varies with the type of surgery. Four categories of surgery have been defined:

- Clean
- Contaminated
- Clean-contaminated
- Dirty

A clean wound involves an incision though non-inflamed tissue and the wound is

Predisposing factors to wound infection		
General factors	**Local factors**	**Microbiological contamination**
Age, obesity, malnutrition	Necrotic tissue	Type and virulence of organism
Endocrine and metabolic disorders	Foreign bodies	Size of bacteriological dose
Hypoxia, anaemia	Tissue ischaemia	Antibiotic resistance
Malignant disease	Haematoma formation	
Immunosuppression	Poor surgical technique	

Table 6.1 Predisposing factors to wound infection

primarily closed. There is no breach in aseptic technique and no viscus is opened. Examples include mastectomy and hernia repair and wound infection rates are typically 1–2%. A clean-contaminated wound is created at emergency surgery or by reoperation via a clean incision within 7 days of the original surgery. A viscus may be opened but no spillage of gut contents has occurred. There can be a minor break in aseptic technique. Examples include right hemicolectomy and cholecystectomy. Infection rates are usually less than 10%. A contaminated wound is one that is left open or created by penetrating trauma less than 4 hours old. A viscus may be opened with inflammation or spillage of contents or there has been a major break in sterile technique. Examples include appendicectomy and stab wounds and infection rates are often about 15–20%. A dirty wound has the presence of pus, intraperitoneal abscess formation or visceral perforation. It can also be caused by penetrating trauma more than 4 hours old. Examples include all perforated abdominal viscera and infection rates are often more than 40%.

Antibiotic prophylaxis

Wound infection rates can be reduced with antibiotic prophylaxis. Prophylaxis is the use of antibiotics to prevent infection. Treatment is their use to eradicate established sepsis. Prophylaxis is important in surgery with a high incidence of postoperative infection (e.g. colonic surgery) or where infection would be disastrous (e.g. prosthetic valves). It is necessary to consider the use of an appropriate antibiotic based on likely bacteria, tissue penetration and the timing and duration of administration. Antibiotics are usually administered intravenously at induction of anaesthesia and often involves only one or a limited number of doses to cover the period of risk.

Tetanus

Less than 100 cases of tetanus are reported each year in the UK. It develops following a deep or penetrating wound in a relatively avascular area. It is more prevalent in developing countries where it is seen in neonates (tetanus neonaturum) following the use of cow dung on the umbilicus.

Microbiology

Tetanus is due to infection with *Clostridium tetani*. This is a Gram-positive spore forming rod which on microscopy has a typical 'drum-stick' appearance with a terminal spore. It is widely found in the environment and soil. It is a strict anaerobe that produces a powerful exotoxin. The exotoxin is resistant to autoclaving. It is not antigenic and repeat infection can occur. Infection produces few signs of local inflammation.

Pathogenesis

Germination of spores results in the release of the exotoxin. The toxin affects the nervous system and reaches the central nervous system via the peripheral nerves. It acts on the presynaptic terminals of inhibitor nerves and reduces the release of inhibitory neurotransmitters (e.g. glycine). The excess activity of motor neurones produces muscle spasm.

Clinical features

Facial muscle spasm produces trismus. The typical facial appearance is often referred to as 'risus sardonicus'. Back muscle spasm produces opisthotonos. Eventually exhaustion and respiratory failure leads to death. The diagnosis is essentially clinical. Differentiating between contamination and infection on wound swabs is difficult.

Treatment

Tetanus can be prevented by active immunisation with tetanus toxoid with a booster every 5–10 years, adequate wound toilet of contaminated wounds and passive immunisation with hyperimmune immunoglobulin in those at risk. In suspected cases, treatment should involve passive immunisation with anti-tetanus immunoglobulin, adequate wound debridement, intravenous benzylpenicillin and intensive care support. Despite the use of intensive care, the mortality associated with tetanus is about 50%.

Gas gangrene

Clostridial spores are widely distributed in the environment. They may enter traumatic or surgical wounds. Contamination may also occur from the patient's own faecal flora.

Microbiology

Gas gangrene results from the following clostridial species:

- *Clostridium welchii*
- *Clostridium oedematiens*
- *Clostridium septicum*

Microscopy of wound exudate shows Gram-positive bacilli. They are rectangular in shape without spore formation. Anaerobic culture on blood agar show haemolytic colonies (*Clostridium welchii*) and a 'stormy' clot reaction with litmus milk. *Clostridium welchii* also shows a positive Nagler reaction (**Figure 6.1**) due to a lecithinase reaction of α exotoxin.

Clinical features

Patients with gas gangrene are generally toxic and unwell. They often have features of shock, jaundice, haemolysis or acute renal failure. Local signs of gas gangrene include myositis or myonecrosis, gas formation with palpable crepitus and mottled discolouration of the overlying skin. A plain x-ray often shows gas in the subcutaneous tissue and fascial plains. Failure of recognition often results in rapid deterioration.

Treatment

Patients usually require vigorous resuscitation and early surgery. Debridement or amputation should be considered to remove the affected tissue or limb. The organisms responsible are usually sensitive to penicillin. Hyperbaric oxygen may be helpful. Benzylpenicillin antibiotic prophylaxis should be considered in those with contaminated wounds or in diabetics undergoing elective peripheral vascular surgery.

Pseudomembranous colitis

Pseudomembranous colitis is due colonic infection with *Clostridium difficile*. It is a Gram-positive anaerobic bacillus. It was not identified until 1953 because it was 'difficult' to culture. Spores are commonly found in the hospital environment.

Pathophysiology

Normal stool contains more than 500 different bacteria at a concentration of 10^{12} per gram. Antibiotic therapy can change the faecal flora. Broad-spectrum antibiotics are the main culprits and particular problems are seen with lincomycin and clindamycin – but these are rarely used. Changes in the faecal flora allow colonisation by *C. difficile* transmitted by the faecal–oral route. Exotoxins produced by bacteria are cytotoxic. They act via cell membrane receptors and produce mucosal inflammation and cell damage. If severe infection occurs, epithelial necrosis follows and a pseudomembrane is formed. This consists of mucin, fibrin, leukocytes and cellular debris. Approximately 50% of neonates are transient healthy carriers of *C. difficile*. Only 1% of adults are asymptomatic carriers. About 10% patients on antibiotics develop diarrhoea but only 1% develop pseudomembranous colitis.

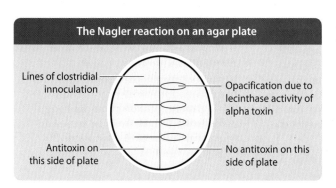

The Nagler reaction on an agar plate

Lines of clostridial innoculation

Opacification due to lecinthase activity of alpha toxin

Antitoxin on this side of plate

No antitoxin on this side of plate

Figure 6.1 The Nagler reaction on an agar plate

Clinical features

The spectrum of symptomatic disease is wide and includes mild diarrhoea, colitis without pseudomembrane formation, pseudomembranous colitis and fulminant colitis. Diagnosis of *C. difficile* infection is confirmed by the detection of the toxin in the stool.

Treatment

Asymptomatic carriers require no active treatment. Those with mild diarrhoea should have their antibiotics stopped. If colitis is present, then active treatment with oral antibiotics is required. Metronidazole is first line therapy. Vancomycin is second line therapy. Symptoms usually improve within 72 hours but it may take 10 days for diarrhoea to stop. About 10% of patients relapse after initial treatment due to either failure of eradication or re-infection. Pseudomembranous colitis requires aggressive resuscitation and treatment. If fulminant colitis occurs with toxic megacolon or perforation, surgery will be required.

Tuberculosis

Tuberculosis is common throughout the world. It causes significant morbidity and mortality, particularly in Africa and Asia. Over 10,000 cases per year occur in UK and it accounts for 1000 deaths mainly in the immigrant Asian population. It is usually due to infection with *Mycobacterium tuberculosis* or *Mycobacterium bovis*.

Primary tuberculosis

Primary tuberculosis is usually a respiratory infection that occurs in childhood. Infection results in a sub-pleural Ghon focus and mediastinal lymphadenopathy. This if often regarded to as the primary complex. Symptoms are often few and resolution of infection usually occurs. Complications of primary tuberculosis include haematogenous spread causing miliary tuberculosis affecting the lungs, bones, joints, meninges or direct pulmonary spread resulting in tuberculosis bronchopneumonia.

Post-primary tuberculosis

Post-primary tuberculosis occurs in adolescence or adult life. It is due to reactivation of infection or repeat exposure and results in more significant symptoms. Reactivation may be associated with immunosuppression (e.g. drugs or HIV infection). Pulmonary infection accounts for 70% of cases of post-primary tuberculosis. It usually affects the apices of either the upper or lower lobes. Cavitation of infection into the bronchial tree results in 'open' tuberculosis. Clinical features include cough, haemoptysis, malaise, weight loss and night sweats. Infection of lymph glands results in discrete, firm and painless lymphadenopathy. Confluence of infected glands can result in a 'cold' abscess. Infection of the urinary tract can cause haematuria and 'sterile pyuria'.

Investigation

Large volume specimens of sputum or urine should be collected, preferably in the early morning. Repeated samples may be required.

Microbiology

If mycobacterial infection is suspected, then samples should be submitted for a Ziehl–Neelsen stain. Mycobacteria appear as red acid-alcohol fast organisms. The organisms also fluoresce with auramine staining. Negative microscopy does not exclude tuberculosis. Mycobacteria can be difficult to culture. To confirm or exclude a diagnosis, one needs to collect adequate and relevant specimens (e.g. early morning urine ×3), concentrate the specimen (e.g. centrifugation), decontaminate the specimen to remove other organisms (e.g. Petroff method). The material should be cultured on Lowenstein–Jensen method at 35–37° for at least 6 weeks to confirm that any mycobacteria cultures are pathological.

Histology

Histological examination shows evidence of a delayed hypersensitivity reaction. The classical appearance is of caseating necrosis. Tuberculous follicles consist of central caseous necrosis, surrounded by lymphocytes, multi-nucleate giant cells and epitheloid macrophages. Organisms may be identified within the macrophages.

Skin tests

A delayed hypersensitivity skin reaction can be used to diagnose tuberculosis. The two commonest tests are the Mantoux and Heaf test. In the Mantoux test, 0.1 mL of purified protein derivative (PPD) is injected intradermally. A positive reaction is a papule of more than 5 mm diameter at 72 hours. In the Heaf test, PPD is placed on the skin. A gun is used to produce multiple punctures. A positive reaction is more than four papules at the puncture sites at 72 hours. Positive skin tests are indicative of active infection or previous BCG vaccination.

Management

First line chemotherapeutic agents are rifampicin, isoniazid and ethambutol. They are given as 'triple therapy' for the first 2 months until sensitivities are available. Rifampicin and isoniazid are then usually continued for a further 7 months. Less than 5% of organisms are resistant to first-line agents. Second line treatment includes pyrazinamide.

Staphylococcal and streptococcal infections

Staphylococcal infections

More than 30 staphylococcal species exist. All are part of the normal skin and mucous membrane flora. They are either coagulase-positive or negative. The most important coagulase-positive species is *Staphylococcus aureus*.

Staphylococcus aureus

About 30% of adults carry *Staphylococcus aureus* in the anterior nares of their nose. Carriers transfer the organism to skin allowing a portal of entry. The organism has several putative determinants of pathogenicity including cell wall constituents, cell surface proteins, toxins (e.g. haemolysins and leukocidins) and enzymes (e.g. coagulase, protease, hyaluronidase). The organism is both aerobic and anaerobic

on blood agar. Microscopically, it is Gram-positive and forms clusters on solid media. There is increasing spread of clones resistant to β-lactam antibiotics (e.g. MRSA).

Staphylococcus aureus produces skin and soft tissue infections including impetigo, folliculitis and cellulitis. Deeper infections may occur after trauma or surgery. Metastatic infection may result in endocarditis, pericarditis, osteomyelitis and lung abscesses. Treatment is with anti-staphylococcal antibiotics (e.g. flucloxacillin). In MRSA, vancomycin is the treatment of choice.

Coagulase-negative staphylococci

Staphylococcus epidermidis and *Staphylococcus saprophyticus* are the commonest human pathogens. *Staphylococcus epidermidis* is a common cause of nosocomial bacteraemia, often associated with indwelling catheters and prosthetic materials. It is a common cause of prosthetic valve endocarditis. It is often multiple antibiotic resistant. Treatment may require removal of the line or prosthesis.

Streptococcal infections

Streptococci are Gram-positive cocci. More than 30 species have been identified. On solid media they grow in pairs or chains. They are catalase negative. β-haemolytic streptococci are classified according to their Lancefield group. The following are human pathogens

- *Strep. pyogenes* (group A streptococcus)
- Group C and G streptococci
- *Strep. pneumoniae* (pneumococcus)
- Group B streptococcus
- viridans group streptococci
- *Enterococcus*

Streptococcus pyogenes

Streptococcus pyogenes is an important human pathogen. It causes various cutaneous and systemic infections including streptococcal pharyngitis, scarlet fever, rheumatic fever and post-streptococcal glomerulonephritis. The bacterium is sensitive to penicillin.

Streptococcus pneumoniae

Streptococcus pneumoniae is a common bacterial pathogen. It is found in the nasopharynx of 20% of adults. On a Gram-stain it appears as a diplococcus. It is α-haemolytic on blood agar. It is a common cause of localised and systemic infections including otitis media, sinusitis, meningitis, pneumonia, endocarditis and osteomyelitis. Infection can be prevented by the pneumococcal vaccine. Resistance to penicillin is increasing worldwide.

Viridans group streptococci

The viridans group of streptococci are a diverse group of organisms. They are respiratory, gastrointestinal and oral cavity commensals. Infection usually occurs in immunocompromised hosts. The principal virulence trait is to adhere to cardiac valves and cause endocarditis. It accounts for 30–40% of cases of endocarditis. Most occur in patients with valvular heart disease. Other risk factors include prosthetic heart valves and intravenous drug abuse. Most viridans streptococcal species are sensitive to penicillin.

Enterococcus species

Enterococci are facultative anaerobes. They are common commensal of the gastrointestinal tract. They are significant cause of nosocomial infection including urinary tract infections, endocarditis and intra-abdominal infection. Risk factors for infection include severe underlying disease, previous surgery, previous antibiotic therapy, renal failure and the presence of vascular or urinary catheters. Mortality from enterococcal infection is high. They are intrinsically resistant to β-lactams and aminoglycosides. They can also acquire resistance to vancomycin. Management of vancomycin-resistant enterococcus is difficult.

Methicillin resistant Staphylococcus aureus

Methicillin resistant Staphylococcus aureus (MRSA) is a major nosocomial pathogen. It causes severe morbidity and mortality worldwide. It is endemic in many European and American hospitals where 40% of nosocomial Staphylococcus aureus infections are methicillin resistant. Many inpatients are colonised or infected and up to 25% hospital personnel may be carriers. It is often found on the inguinal, perineal or axillary skin and anterior nares. It can be spread by hand, usually of healthcare workers. Risk factors for colonisation of patients include:

- Advanced age
- Male gender
- Previous hospitalisation
- Length of hospitalisation
- Stay in intensive care
- Chronic medical illness
- Prior and prolonged antibiotic therapy
- Presence and size of a wound
- Exposure to colonised or infected patient
- Presence of invasive indwelling device

Clinical features

The clinical presentation of MRSA infection is as:

- Pneumonia
- Surgical site infections
- Line sepsis
- Intra-abdominal infections
- Osteomyelitis
- Toxic shock syndrome

Microbiology

Staphylococcus aureus is a Gram-positive coccus which forms clusters on culture medium. Methicillin resistance is mediated by the mecA gene which encodes a single additional penicillin binding protein PBP2a. Expression of mecA can be either constitutive or inducible. The risk of colonisation and infection of patients can be reduced by strict infection control measures including:

- Screening of patients and staff
- Hand washing
- Use of gowns and gloves
- Topical antimicrobials
- Isolation of patients
- Environmental cleaning

Management

Vancomycin is the antibiotic of choice. Teicoplanin may be used if the isolate is resistant to vancomycin. Linezolid is new class of antimicrobial agent active against MRSA and VRE. Quinupristin and dalfopristin are also newer alternatives.

Prevention of infection
Principles of asepsis and antisepsis

Antisepsis is the use of chemical solutions for disinfection. It involves the removal of transient microorganisms from the skin and a reduction in the resident flora. Asepsis is the complete absence of infectious organisms. Aseptic techniques are those aimed at minimising infection. Asepsis usually involves the use of sterile instruments and a gloved no touch technique.

Preoperative skin preparation

The bacterial flora of the patient is the principle source of surgical wound infection. It is important that focal sources of sepsis should be treated prior to elective surgery. In patients with active infection, consideration should be given to delaying surgery. Preoperative showering with an antiseptic solution does not reduce wound infections

Skin shaving

Skin shaving is aesthetic and makes surgery, suturing and dressing removal easier. Wound infection rates are lowest when when skin-shaving is performed immediately prior to surgery. Infection rate increases from 1% to 5% if performed more than 12 hours prior to surgery. Abrasions can cause colonisation which can lead to wound infection. The use of clippers or depilatory creams reduce infection rates to less than 1%.

Skin preparation

70% isopropyl alcohol acts by denaturing proteins. It is bactericidal but short acting. It is effective against both Gram-positive and Gram-negative organisms. It is also fungicidal and virucidal. 0.5% chlorhexidine is a quaternary ammonium compound that acts by disrupting the bacterial cell wall. It is bactericidal but does not kill spore forming organisms. It is persistent and has a long duration of action (up to 6 hours). It is more effective against Gram-positive organisms. 70% povidone–iodine acts by oxidation/substitution of free iodine. It is both bactericidal and active against spore forming organisms. It is effective against both Gram-positive and Gram-negative organisms. It is rapidly inactivated by organic material such as blood. Patient skin sensitivity is occasionally a problem. Chlorhexidine may be more effective than iodine at reducing wound infections.

Surgical preparation

Preoperative washing with bactericidal agent eliminates transient skin flora. A brush should be used on the nails but not on the skin and should only be performed once in a surgical session. The scrub time makes little difference to the incidence of wound infections. Most surgical gloves are made of latex and are disposable and single-use. About 50% of gloves are punctured during surgery. Glove perforation increases the risk of wound infection by a factor of five. Double gloving affords better protection to the surgeon. Face masks protect the surgeon but not the patient. There is no evidence that masks reduce the incidence of wound infections.

Sterilisation and disinfection
Sterilisation

Sterilisation is the removal of viable microorganisms including spores and viruses. It can be achieved by the use of:

- Autoclaves
- Hot air ovens
- Ethylene oxide
- Low-temperature steam and formaldehyde
- Sporicidal chemicals
- Irradiation
- Gas plasma

Autoclaves and hot air ovens

Autoclaves use steam under pressure at high temperature. To be effective against viruses and spore-forming bacteria, it is necessary to have steam in direct contact with the material and for a vacuum to be created. To ensure sterilisation, it is necessary to autoclave for 3 minutes at 134°C or 15 minutes at 121°C. Performance can be checked by colour changes on indicator tape. Autoclaves are highly effective and inexpensive but are not suitable for heat-sensitive objects. Hot ovens are inefficient compared to autoclaves. They require temperatures of 160°C for 2 hours or 180°C for 30 minutes.

Ethylene oxide

Ethylene oxide is highly-penetrative gas that is active against bacteria, spores and viruses. Unfortunately, it is also flammable, toxic and expensive and leaves toxic residue on sterilised items. Instruments therefore need to be stored for prolonged period before use. It is suitable for sterilisation of heat-sensitive items.

Sporicidal chemicals

Sporicidal chemicals are often used as disinfectants but can also sterilise instruments if used for prolonged period. They are inexpensive and suitable for heat-sensitive items. They are toxic and irritant. 2% Glutaraldehyde is the most widely used liquid sporicidal chemical. Most bacteria and viruses are killed within 10 minutes but spores can survive several hours.

Irradiation

Gamma rays and accelerated electrons are excellent at sterilisation and are used as an industrial rather than hospital-based method of sterilisation.

Disinfection

Disinfection is a reduction in the number of viable organisms. It can be achieved by:

- Low-temperature steam
- Boiling water
- Chemical disinfectants

Low-temperature steam

Most bacteria and viruses are killed by exposure to moist heat. This is usually achieved with dry saturated steam at 73°C for greater than 10 minutes. It is effective and reliable and suitable for instrument with a lumen but is not suitable for heat-sensitive items.

Chemical disinfectants

Chemical disinfectants destroy micro-organisms by chemical or physicochemical means. Different organisms vary in their sensitivity to disinfectants. Gram-positive organisms are highly sensitive where as clostridial and mycobacterial species are very resistant. Disinfectants are suitable for heat-sensitive items but are less effective than heat. Chemicals used for disinfection include:

- Clear soluble phenolics
- Hypochlorites
- Alcohols
- Quaternary ammonium compounds

Surgery in hepatitis and HIV carriers

Hepatitis B

The hepatitis B virus is a single-stranded DNA virus. It consists of 42 nm Dane particle (Hb_sAg) and 22 nm core (Hb_cAg). The hepatitis B surface antigen (Hb_sAg) is also know as the Australia antigen. The virus also contains the hepatitis B 'e' antigen (Hb_eAg). The body produces antibodies to the surface antigen (Hb_sAb).

In the UK, the prevalence of Hb_sAg positivity is about 1–2% and is seen particularly in drug addicts, homosexuals, dialysis patients and occasionally medical staff. In Asia, Middle East and South America the prevalence of Hb_sAg positivity is between 20–30%. It is transmitted by vertical transmission, inoculation, oral and sexual contact. The incubation period is between 6 weeks and 6 months. The period of infectivity is from 6 weeks, before the onset of symptoms and possibly indefinitely after. About 10% of infected patients become chronic carriers. The risk of chronic infection varies with age at which infection is acquired and is greatest in young children.

Clinical features

There are three common clinical pictures:

- Acute hepatitis with clinical recovery
- Acute fulminating hepatitis leading to death
- Chronic active hepatitis with risk of cirrhosis and hepatocellular carcinoma

Serological results

Hb_sAg positivity is the first indicator of infection and is seen throughout the course of the disease. Persistence is a marker of failure to clear infection. Hb_sAb positivity is a marker of protection due to either previous infection or immunisation. Hb_eAg positivity is closely associated with infectivity of the patient.

Prevention of infection

It is important to avoid contact with the virus. It requires care with needles and body fluids. After a needle stick injury from a high-risk patient, hyperimmune anti-hepatitis B IgG should be given, ideally within 24–48 hours after exposure and repeated at 1 month. All paramedical staff should be immunised. Hepatitis B vaccine should be given and repeated at 1 and 6 months. A Hb_sAb levels of more than 1000 µ/L indicates an adequate response and confers protection for up to 5 years .

Hepatitis C

The hepatitis C virus (HCV) is a small, enveloped, single-stranded RNA virus. The infection is often asymptomatic, but chronic infection can occur. The HCV is spread by blood-to-blood contact. The virus persists in the liver in about 85% of those infected. During the first 12 weeks after infection with HCV, most people suffer no symptoms. For those who do, the main manifestations of acute infection are generally mild and vague, and rarely point to a specific diagnosis of hepatitis C. The HCV is usually detectable in the blood by PCR within 1 to 3 weeks after infection, and antibodies to the virus are generally detectable soon after that. Chronic hepatitis C is defined as infection with the hepatitis C virus persisting for more than 6 months. Clinically, it is often asymptomatic, and it is mostly discovered accidentally, following the investigation of elevated liver enzyme levels. One-third of untreated patients will progress to cirrhosis within 20 years. Treatment is generally recommended for patients with proven hepatitis C virus infection and persistently abnormal liver function tests. Current treatment is a combination of interferon-α-2a and the antiviral drug ribavirin.

HIV infection

Acquired immunodeficiency syndrome (AIDS) was first recognised in the USA in the 1970s and the human immunodeficiency virus (HIV) was isolated in 1983. In 1984, a serological test for antibodies to the virus became available. About 30–50% of HIV positive patients are unaware of their infection. HIV is a treatable disease. Where therapy is available, infected individuals have the same rate of death as aged-matched uninfected controls.

Immunology

HIV is a double-stranded RNA retrovirus that attaches to human immune cells through the CD4 molecule. It produces DNA by the use of the enzyme reverse transcriptase. DNA is then incorporated into host cells. The incorporated viral DNA produces new viral components which are spliced and assembled using a viral protease. HIV infection results in widespread immunological dysfunction. It results in a fall in CD4 lymphocytes, monocytes and antigen-presenting cells. Immunological dysfunction results in opportunistic infections and increases the risk of malignancy. The virus is transmitted in bodily fluids by:

- Heterosexual intercourse
- Homosexual intercourse
- Blood transfusions
- Intravenous drug abuse
- Perinatal transmission

Natural history

Up to 3 months after infection, there is often an asymptomatic viraemia and patients are infective during this period. The ELISA test for HIV antibodies is negative. At seroconversion an acute seroconversion illness (ASI) can occur and may be followed by persistent generalised lymphadenopathy (PGI). Progression to symptomatic disease occurs within several years. AIDS develops within 5 to 10 years. AIDS is diagnosed by the presence of an AIDS indicator disease with a positive HIV test. The median survival with AIDS is 5 years. The virological, serological and clinical response to HIV infection is shown in **Figure 6.2**. AIDS indicator diseases include:

- Multiple recurrent bacterial infections
- Tracheal or bronchial candidiasis
- Invasive cervical carcinoma
- Extrapulmonary or disseminated coccidioidomycosis
- Cryptosporidiosis
- Cytomegalovirus retinitis

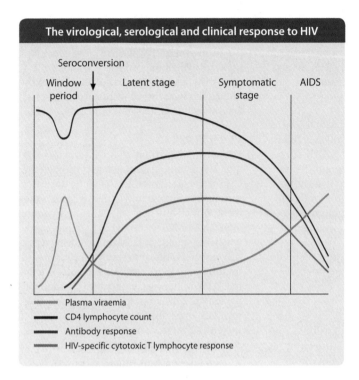

Figure 6.2 The virological, serological and clinical response to human immunodeficiency virus infection. AIDS = Acquired immunodeficiency syndrome

- HIV encephalopathy
- Disseminated or extrapulmonary histoplasmosis
- Kaposi's sarcoma
- Lymphoma
- Disseminated mycobacteriosis
- *Pneumocystis carinii* pneumonia
- Progressive multifocal leukoencephalopathy
- Cerebral toxoplasmosis

Sites of pyogenic infections in AIDS include:

- Thoracic empyema
- Anorectal abscesses
- Skin boils, carbuncles and cellulitis
- Necrotising fasciitis
- Pyomyositis
- Osteomyelitis
- Septic arthritis
- Epididymo-orchitis
- Pelvic inflammatory disease
- Appendicitis

Management

HIV therapies are available that prevent virus entry into cells, inhibit the viral reverse transcriptase and viral protease. Combination therapy with anti-HIV drugs inhibits viral replication, reduces viraemia to undetectable levels, leads to reconstitution of immune dysfunction and prevents opportunistic disease. Stopping therapy often leads to re-emergence of the viraemia.

Chapter 7

Emergency medicine and the management of trauma

Pathophysiology of trauma
Metabolic response to injury

A similar metabolic response is seen following trauma, burns, sepsis and surgery. It involves both local and systemic reactions with the extent of the response being proportional to the severity of insult. An appropriate response maintains homeostasis and allows wound healing to occur. An excessive response can produce a systemic response. This can cause the systemic inflammatory response syndrome (SIRS) and multiple organ dysfunction syndrome (MODS).

Initiation of response

Several factors can initiate the physiological response to trauma and multiple simultaneous factors can have a synergistic effect. Important factors are:

- Tissue injury
- Infection
- Hypovolaemia
- Hypoxia or hypercarbia

Control of response

Four systems control the response to trauma:

- Sympathetic nervous system
- Acute phase response
- Endocrine response
- Vascular endothelium

Sympathetic nervous system

The sympathetic nervous system has direct actions via the release of noradrenaline from sympathetic nerves and has indirect action via the release of adrenaline from the adrenal medulla. It produces cardiovascular, visceral and metabolic actions. Blood is diverted from the skin and visceral organs. The heart rate and myocardial contractility are increased. Bronchodilation occurs and gastrointestinal motility is reduced. Insulin production is reduced and glucagon production is increased. Increased glycogenolysis increases blood sugar levels.

Acute phase response

Tissue injury results in cytokine release. Important cytokines include tumour necrosis factor-alpha (TNF-α), interleukins (IL-1, IL-2, IL-6), interferon and prostaglandins. Cytokines have mainly paracrine actions and are important in regulating the inflammatory response. Overflow of cytokines into systemic circulation is important factor in SIRS. Cytokines stimulate the production of acute phase proteins such as C-reactive protein, fibrinogen, complement C3 and haptoglobin.

Endocrine response

The hypothalamus, pituitary, adrenal axis is important in the endocrine response to trauma. Trauma increases ACTH and cortisol production. Steroids have a permissive action in many metabolic responses. Catabolic action increases protein breakdown. Insulin antagonism increases blood sugar levels. Anti-inflammatory actions reduce vascular permeability. Aldosterone increases sodium reabsorption. Vasopressin increases water reabsorption and produces vasoconstriction. Histamine increases vascular permeability. Total T4, total and free T3 levels are reduced.

Vascular endothelium

Nitric oxide production by the vascular endothelium produces vasodilatation. Platelet activating factor (PAF) augments the cytokine response. Prostaglandins produce vasodilatation and induce platelet aggregation.

Outcome of response

The inflammatory response produces clinically apparent local and systemic effects.

The local response is usually the cardinal signs of inflammation. The systemic response includes:

- Increased ECF volume and hypovolaemia
- Increased vascular permeability and oedema
- Early reduced urine output and increased urine osmolality
- Reduced 'free' water clearance
- Late diuresis and increased sodium loss
- Pyrexia in the absence of infection
- Early reduction in metabolic rate
- Late increased metabolism, negative nitrogen balance and weight loss
- Lipolysis and ketosis
- Gluconeogenesis via amino acid breakdown
- Reduced serum albumin
- Hyponatraemia due to impaired sodium pump action
- Acid–base disturbance – usually a metabolic alkalosis or acidosis
- Immunosuppression
- Hypoxia and coagulopathy

The inflammatory response can be limited by:

- Reducing the degree of trauma with appropriate and careful surgery
- Reducing infection with wound care and antibiotics
- Maintaining enteral nutrition
- Controlling pain
- Correcting hypovolaemia
- Correcting acid–base disturbance
- Correcting hypoxia

Initial assessment of the trauma patient

Prehospital trauma care

Epidemiology of trauma

Trauma is the commonest cause of death in young adults. Road traffic accidents each year in UK result in 320,000 minor injuries, 40,000 serious injuries and 3400 deaths. Up to 30% of prehospital deaths may be preventable. Prehospital care is important. The philosophy of prehospital care varies between countries. In the USA, only basic resuscitation is performed at the scene. This has been described as 'scoop and run'. In France,

mobile intensive care units often attend the scene of an accident. This has been described as 'stay and play'.

Initial action

Potential problems at the scene of an accident depend on the hostility of the environment, the lack of familiarity with surroundings and the presence of intrusive onlookers. It is important to assess the ongoing safety of the emergency services and any casualties and if necessary, it is vital to make the accident site as safe as possible before treating any casualties. It is important to determine the nature of the accident and likely mechanism of injuries. At road traffic accidents, the number, direction and types of vehicles involved and the degree of intrusion of damages vehicles should be assessed along with whether occupants were wearing seatbelts.

Important indicators of potential significant trauma are:

- Penetrating injury to chest and abdomen
- Two or more proximal long bone fractures
- Burns involving more than 15% of body surface area
- Burns to face and airway
- Abnormal physiological variables

Evidence of high-energy impact include:

- Fall more than 6 m
- Crash speed greater than 20 mph
- Inward deformity of car of more than 0.6 m
- Rearward displacement of front axle
- Ejection of passenger from vehicle
- Rollover of vehicle
- Death of another car occupant
- Pedestrian hit at great than 20 mph

Prehospital resuscitation

Prehospital resuscitation should follow the same principles as that in hospital but will need to be adapted to circumstances. Airway management can be difficult but an airway can usually be maintained with basic measures. Intubation without anaesthesia and rapid sequence induction is ill advised as it can induce vomiting and raise intracranial pressure. The cervical spine should be immobilised with a hard collar. Oxygen should be given. Haemorrhage should be controlled with direct pressure.

If a casualty is entrapped it is important to ensure good venous access before releasing him or her from the vehicle. Fluid resuscitation should be give to maintain a systolic blood pressure of 90 mmHg. If venous access is difficult, consideration should be given to 'scoop and run' rather than delay transfer. Analgesia can be achieved with Entonox or ketamine. Entonox is contraindicated if there is a possibility of a pneumothorax or basal skull fracture. Extrication requires close co-ordination between medical and fire services. The casualty should be 'packaged for transport'. This will require hard collar, head blocks, limb splints, scoop stretcher or a vacuum mattress.

Major incident triage

If faced with a large number of casualties, it is important to prioritise management. The overall aim is to 'do the most for the most'. Triage is the sorting of casualties by priority of treatment. Triage can be performed rapidly by assessing ability to walk, airway, respiratory rate, pulse rate or capillary return. In a mass casualty situation it should be performed by a 'Triage officer' who assesses casualties without giving treatment. He or she should divide patients into categories according to the severity of the injuries (**Table 7.1**). Casualties may be given a coloured triage label to help with their subsequent management.

Clinical assessment and resuscitation

Trauma deaths have a trimodal distribution. The first peak occurs within minutes of injury and is due to major neurological or vascular injury. Medical treatment can rarely improve the outcome for these patients. The second peak occurs during the 'golden hour' and is due to intracranial haematoma, major thoracic or abdominal injury. This time period is the primary focus of intervention for the Advanced Trauma Life Support (ATLS) methodology. The third peak occurs after days or weeks and is due to sepsis and multiple organ failure. The assessment of patients with major trauma should involve a primary survey and resuscitation, secondary surgery and definitive treatment. The primary survey involves:

- A = Airway and cervical spine
- B = Breathing
- C = Circulation and haemorrhage control
- D = Dysfunction of the central nervous system
- E = Exposure

Primary survey and resuscitation

Airway and cervical spine

In patients with major trauma, it is prudent to assume that they have a cervical spine injury until proved otherwise. They should be placed in a hard collar which should be kept on until the cervical spine has been 'cleared'. If the patient can talk, then he or she is able to maintain their own airway. If the airway appears compromised, an initial attempt should be made to improve it with a chin lift and by clearing the airway of any foreign bodies. If a gag reflex is present, then consideration should be given to insertion of a nasopharyngeal airway. If no gag reflex is present, then the patient will

Triage categories			
Category	Definition	Colour	Treatment
P1	Life-threatening	Red	Immediate
P2	Urgent	Yellow	Urgent
P3	Minor	Green	Delayed
P4	Dead	White	

Table 7.1 Triage categories

need endotracheal intubation. If it proves impossible to intubate the patient, then perform a cricothyroidotomy. Once a secure airway has been achieved, 100% oxygen should be given through a Hudson mask.

Breathing

It is important to assess the position of the trachea, respiratory rate and air entry. If there is clinical evidence of a tension pneumothorax, then place a venous cannula through the second intercostal space in the mid-clavicular line on the affected side. If there is an open chest wound, seal it with an occlusive dressing.

Circulation and haemorrhage control

It is important to check the pulse, capillary return and state of neck veins. Identify any exsanguinating haemorrhage and apply direct pressure. Place two large calibre intravenous cannulas in the antecubital fossae and take venous blood for measurement of a full blood count, electrolytes and a cross match. Take a sample for arterial blood gas analysis. Boluses of intravenous fluids should be given and the patient should be attached to an ECG monitor. A urinary catheter should be inserted.

Dysfunction and exposure

Once problems related to the airway, breathing, and circulation have been addressed, it is necessary to perform a focused neurologic examination. The level of consciousness should be rapidly assessed using AVPU method:

- A = alert
- V = responding to voice
- P = responding to pain
- U = unresponsive

This should be followed by recording of the patient's level of consciousness using the Glasgow Coma Scale (GCS) score, and assessments of pupillary size and reactivity, gross motor function and sensation. The patient should be fully undressed and other signs of injury should be sought. Steps should be taken to avoid hypothermia. If hypothermia is identified then it should be corrected.

Radiological investigations

Plain radiographs play an important role in the primary evaluation of the unstable trauma patient. For haemodynamically unstable patients proceeding directly to surgery after the primary survey, plain x-rays of the lateral cervical spine, chest, and pelvis can detect life-threatening injuries that might otherwise be missed. A chest x-ray should be obtained in patients with penetrating injuries of the chest, back, or abdomen. It the patient is haemodynamically stable and a CT scan is indicated, then plain x-rays can often be omitted.

Airway and ventilation

Airway assessment and management

The patient should be asked a simple question. If he responds appropriately, the airway is patent, ventilation is intact and the brain is being adequately perfused. Agitation is often a sign of hypoxia. The aims of airway management are:

- To secure an intact airway
- To protect a jeopardised airway
- To provide an airway when none is available

These can be achieved with basic, advanced and surgical techniques.

Basic life support

Foreign bodies should be removed from the mouth and oropharynx. Secretions and blood should be removed with suction. The airway can usually be secured with a chin lift or jaw thrust. An oropharyngeal or nasopharyngeal airway may be required. Oxygen should be delivered at a rate of 10–12 L/min. It should be administered via a tight fitting mask with reservoir (e.g. Hudson mask). An F_iO_2 of 85% should be achievable.

Advanced measures

If a gag reflex is absent, endotracheal intubation is required. If no cervical spine fracture is suspected then orotracheal intubation is preferred. If cervical spine injury can not be excluded, then consider nasotracheal intubation. The position of the tube should be checked. Complications of tracheal intubation include:

- Oesophageal intubation
- Intubation of right main bronchus
- Failure of intubation
- Aspiration

Surgical airways

If the patient is unable to be intubated, then a surgical airway is required. There are few indications for an emergency tracheostomy. A surgical airway can be achieved with a needle or surgical cricothyroidotomy.

Needle cricothyroidotomy

In a needle cricothyroidotomy, the cricothyroid membrane is punctured with a 12 or 14 Fr cannula. It is connected to an oxygen supply via a Y connector. Oxygen is supplied at a rate of 15 L/min. Jet insufflation is achieved by occlusion of the Y connection. Insufflation is provided 1 second on and 4 seconds off. Jet insufflation can result in significant hypercarbia and should only be used for 30–40 minutes until a more secure airway can be achieved.

Surgical cricothyroidotomy

To create a surgical cricothyroidotomy, a small incision is made over the cricothyroid membrane. A 5 mm incision made in the cricothyroid membrane and a small tracheostomy tube is inserted. Complications of surgical airways include:

- Aspiration
- Haemorrhage/haematoma
- Cellulitis
- False passage

- Subglottic stenosis
- Mediastinal emphysema

Ventilation

In a non-intubated patient, ventilation can be achieved either mouth to mouth using a face-mask. This is more efficient if performed with a two person technique. One person maintains the face seal and the other ventilates the patient. If endotracheal intubation is required, it should be performed with cricoid pressure. If rib fractures are present, it is necessary to insert a chest drain on side of the injury to prevent a tension pneumothorax.

Hypovolaemic shock

Clinical features

The clinical features of hypovolaemic shock depend on the extent of the blood loss and the age of the patients. Signs of hypovolaemia include tachycardia, a reduction in pulse pressure and hypotension. In young fit patients, there can be significant hypovolaemia with few physical signs. Young patients can maintain an adequate blood pressure until their physiological reserve is exhausted. At this point they can become profoundly hypotensive. The grading of hypovolaemic shock is shown in **Table 7.2**.

Fluid resuscitation

Early intravascular volume replacement is essential in trauma patients. The ideal resuscitation fluid remains uncertain.

The grading of hypovolaemic shock		
Grade	Blood loss	Clinical features
Grade 1	Up to 15%	Mild resting tachycardia
Grade 2	15–30%	Moderate tachycardia, fall in pulse pressure, delayed capillary return
Grade 3	30–40%	Hypotension, tachycardia, low urine output
Grade 4	40–50%	Profound hypotension

Table 7.2 The grading of hypovolaemic shock

Crystalloid versus colloid resuscitation

More than 40 randomised controlled trials of crystalloid versus colloid resuscitation have been published. None has shown the use of either type of fluid to be associated with a reduction in mortality. No single type of colloid has been shown to be superior another. Albumin solution may be associated with a slight increase in mortality. Colloids can more rapidly correct hypovolaemia. They also maintain intravascular oncotic pressure. Crystalloids require large volume but are equally effective. They are cheaper and have fewer adverse side effects.

Hypertonic solutions

Hypertonic solutions have been subjected to recent intensive investigation. They can be used to resuscitate patient rapidly with a reduced volume of fluid and they may reduce cerebral oedema in patients with severe head injuries.

Packed red blood cells

Packed red blood cells provide the best volume expansion and oxygen carrying capacity. They do however need cross-matching and are not immediately available. Dilutional coagulopathy occurs with massive transfusion.

Oxygen therapeutic agents

The use of oxygen therapeutic agents is currently being investigated. The potential advantages over blood include that they are free from potential viral contamination, have a longer shelf life and have universal ABO compatibility. They have similar oxygen carrying capacity to blood. Agents being studied include:

- Perflurocarbons
- Human haemoglobin solutions
- Polymerised bovine haemoglobin

Intraosseous infusion

Venous access can be difficult in the hypovolaemic child. If difficulty is experienced, then the intraosseous route can be used as an alternative. The medullary canal in a child has a good blood supply. Drugs and fluids are absorbed into the venous sinusoids of the red marrow. Red marrow is replaced by yellow marrow after 5 years of age and therefore intraosseous infusion is less effective in older children. The technique is generally safe with few complications. Indications for intraosseous infusion include:

- Major trauma
- Extensive burns
- Cardiopulmonary arrest
- Septic shock

Contraindications include ipsilateral lower limb fracture or vascular injury.

Technique

Intraosseous access is achieved with specially designed needles. A short shaft allows accurate placement within the medullary canal. The technique of intraosseous needle insertion is shown in **Figure 7.1**. A handle allows controlled pressure during introduction. The needle is usually inserted into the antero-medial border of tibia, 3 cm below tibial tubercle. Correct placement can be checked by aspiration of bone marrow. Both fluids and drugs can be administered. Fluid often needs to be administered under pressure. Once venous access is achieved the intraosseous needle should be removed.

Complications

Complications of intraosseous needle insertion are rare but needles are incorrectly placed or displaced in about 10% patients. Potential complications include:

- Tibial fracture
- Compartment syndrome
- Fat embolism
- Skin necrosis
- Osteomyelitis

Traumatic wounds
Gunshot and blast wounds

Gunshot and blast wounds are well known to military surgeons but are now increasingly seen in civilian practice. However, military and civilian wounds differ in several key respects. Military wounds are often heavily contaminated with delays in treatment. Despite this, the same principles apply to their treatment.

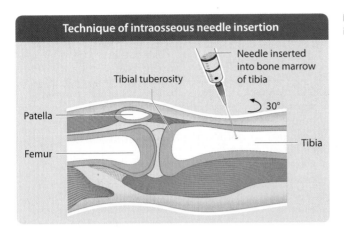

Technique of intraosseous needle insertion

Needle inserted into bone marrow of tibia

Tibial tuberosity

30°

Patella

Femur

Tibia

Figure 7.1 Technique of intraosseous needle insertion

Physical properties

Penetrating missiles include both munition fragments and bullets. Often divided into 'high' and 'low' velocity. However, velocity per se is not important. The amount of kinetic energy transferred to the tissues is the key factor. Kinetic energy transfer depends on velocity, the presenting area of the fragment and the mechanical properties of tissue.

Munition fragments are usually small and numerous. They are of low velocity (100–500 m/s) and low energy (10–100 J). They have poor tissue penetration. Injuries are often numerous but are usually limited to the fragment track. Hand gun bullets are of low velocity (< 250 m/s) and low energy (200–300 J). Rifle bullets are high velocity (750–1000 m/s) and high energy (2–3 kJ). The physiological effects depend on the degree of energy transfer. If little energy is dissipated, high velocity bullets can result in low energy transfer wounds.

Pathophysiology

The effects of bullets can result from both direct and indirect effects. In low energy transfer wounds, injury results from direct effects along the bullet track. In high energy transfer wounds, indirect effects are more important. Radial forces perpendicular to tract result in cavitation. This generates contusions and lacerations away from tract. Negative pressure within the cavity can suck in environmental contaminants. Rifle bullets

also tumble (yaw) within the wound. This increases the presenting area of the bullet and increases energy transfer. It can result in small entry and exit wounds but large wound cavity. Radial energy transfer can also cause indirect fractures. Bullet and bone fragmentation can cause secondary tracts and further unpredictable damage.

Treatment

In the military environment, the standard treatment of gunshot wounds has involved, wound debridement, wound excision, antibiotic prophylaxis with dressing change and delayed primary suture at 5 days. Similar wound management protocols have been advocated by the Red Cross. This approach may be modified in civilian environment.

Abdominal stab wounds

Abdominal stab wounds cause less trauma than gunshot wounds and therefore the associated morbidity and mortality is reduced. The upper abdomen is most commonly involved, particularly the left upper quadrant. Peritoneal violation occurs in up 70% of abdominal stab wounds, but only half of those with peritoneal violation sustain an intra-abdominal injury requiring perative intervention. The liver and small bowel are the commonest organs injured. Multiple stab wounds are present in up to 20% of patients and 10% of abdominal stab wounds enter the chest. Potential intrathoracic injuries include pneumothorax and pericardial tamponade.

Clinical features

Assessment should gain knowledge of the implement used, its site of entry and likely track. Examination should look for signs of evisceration, haemorrhage and peritonitis. Digital exploration or probing of the wound will determine whether the peritoneum has been breached. A plain abdominal x-ray may show signs of free gas but this investigation has limited sensitivity. Abdominal CT is better at assessing peritoneal penetration and the extent of intra-abdominal injury.

Management

In the past surgical dictum mandated exploratory laparotomy for all patients with abdominal stab wounds. However, new diagnostic techniques have rendered such a dogmatic approach obsolete and reduced the number of non-therapeutic laparotomies. Evisceration, hypovolaemia and peritonitis are indications for a laparotomy without the need for extensive investigation. If the penetrating object is still *in-situ*, it should remain so until after induction of anaesthesia. If there are no clinical or radiological signs of bleeding or visceral perforation, then most abdominal stab wounds can be managed conservatively. Patients should be actively observed for 24–48 hours.

Compartment syndromes
Limb compartment syndromes

The deep fascia envelops the limbs and other fascial planes divide the limbs into compartments. The forearm has two fascial compartments. The thigh has three fascial compartments. The lower limb has four fascial compartments (**Figure 7.2**).

Compartment syndrome

A compartment syndrome is a condition in which the circulation and function of the tissues within a closed space is compromised by an increase in pressure within the space. The normal lower limb venous pressure is up to 10 mmHg. Compartmental pressure does not normally interfere with blood flow. Swelling within a fascial compartment results in increased intracompartmental pressure. Initial venous compromise may progress to reduced capillary flow. This exacerbates the ischaemic insult and further increases the compartment pressure. A vicious cycle of increasing pressures can be initiated. Arterial inflow is rarely reduced unless the pressure exceed systolic blood pressure. If this occurs, irreversible muscle ischaemia will occur within 6 to 12 hours. Surgical treatment within 6 hours of onset usually results in a positive outcome.

Aetiology

Causes of compartment syndromes include:

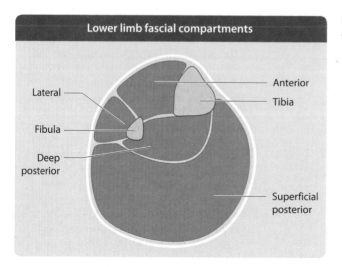

Lower limb fascial compartments

Lateral

Fibula

Deep posterior

Anterior

Tibia

Superficial posterior

Figure 7.2 Lower limb fascial compartments

- Fractures (especially comminuted fractures)
- Ischaemia–reperfusion injury
- Haemorrhage
- Phlegmasia caerulea dolens
- Intravenous or intra-arterial drug injection
- Soft-tissue injury
- Burns

Clinical features

Compartment syndromes are normally seen within 48 hours of injury. Clinical features include increasing pain despite immobilisation of fracture, altered sensation in the distribution of nerves passing through the compartment, muscle swelling and tenderness and excessive pain on passive movement. It is important to note that peripheral pulses may still be present.

Pressure monitoring

Intracompartmental pressure (ICP) can be measured by several means including:

- Wick catheter
- Simple needle manometry
- Infusion techniques
- Pressure transducers
- Side-ported needles

The critical pressure for diagnosing a compartment syndrome is unclear. Different authors recommend surgical intervention if the:

- Absolute ICP is greater than 30 mmHg
- Difference between diastolic pressure and ICP is less than 30 mmHg
- Difference between mean arterial pressure and ICP is less than 40 mmHg

Management

Constricting casts and splints should be removed if there is any clinical suspicion of a compartment syndrome. If there is no improvement, prompt fasciotomies are required. It is necessary to divide both the skin and deep fascia for the whole length of the compartment. Wounds should be left open and may require delayed closure or skin grafting at a later date.

Fasciotomies

Several surgical approaches for fasciotomies have been described. The goal is prevention

of disability. Decompression should not be compromised by a desire for good cosmesis. All compartments should be decompressed. All four compartments of the lower leg can be decompressed through two incision. Skin incisions of about 15–20 cm in length are required. Timely surgery produces a good functional outcome. Delayed surgery results in muscle ischaemia and necrosis. Muscle fibrosis produces the typical Volkmann's ischaemic contracture.

Fat embolism

Fat embolism is due to fat entering torn venous channels at the site of a fracture. Chylomicrons may also aggregate due to lipase release. Fat embolism presents with pyrexia, tachycardia, tachypnoea and reduced consciousness. Patients may develop a petechial rash. Clotting may be deranged with features of disseminated intravascular coagulation. Arterial gases often show hypoxia and hypercapnia. Patients may require ventilation. Mortality can be as high as 15%.

Abdominal compartment syndrome

An abdominal compartment syndrome occurs when the abdomen is subject to increased intracompartmental pressure, usually defined as a pressure above 20 mmHg. It is often the result of retroperitoneal haemorrhage, trauma or sepsis. Intraperitoneal or retroperitoneal fluid accumulation reduces the compliance of the abdominal wall. Once the abdominal wall can no longer expand, any further fluid leaking into the tissue or peritoneum results in a rapid rise in the pressure. Increased intra-abdominal pressure reduces blood flow to the abdominal organs and impairs pulmonary, cardiovascular, renal, and gastrointestinal function.

Clinical features

In the unconscious ventilated patient it can be difficult to recognise. Clinically, it is characterised by a reduce cardiac output, increased central venous pressure, a fall in urine output and the need to increase ventilation pressures. Untreated it can lead to multiple organ dysfunction and death. The diagnosis can be confirmed by the measurement of intra-abdominal pressure. This may be done using simple manometry through a Foley catheter in the bladder.

Management

The development of an abdominal compartment syndrome can often be anticipated. In these situations it often best to leave the abdomen open. The abdomen should not be closed under extreme tension. Exposed bowel can be covered with a 'Bogota bag' or vacuum-assisted temporary abdominal closure can be performed. In those suspected of developing an abdominal compartment syndrome, the abdomen should be decompressed. However, sudden release of an abdominal compartment syndrome may lead to an ischaemia–reperfusion injury causing acidosis, vasodilatation, cardiac dysfunction and cardiac arrest.

The eye – trauma and common infections

The eye is well-protected by the bony orbit and reflex closure of the eye lid. Corneal trauma is common but more major injuries to eye and orbit are rare.

Corneal foreign body

Corneal foreign bodies occur due to fragments hitting the cornea at high speed. They often occur as a result of hammering or drilling. Corneal foreign bodies usually causes pain, photophobia and profuse lacrimation. Local anaesthesia may be required in order to examine the eye. The foreign body is often readily seen. If a metallic foreign body is present for more than a few hours is often results in a 'rust ring'. The object can often be removed with sterile needle under local anaesthesia. Antibiotic ointment and cycloplegic drops should be instilled into the eye. A pad should be applied.

Subtarsal foreign body

Foreign bodies occasionally become embedded in the subtarsal conjunctiva of the upper lid. They cause pain and lacrimation. Examination may show fine, vertical linear corneal abrasions. Eversion of the upper eyelid with a cotton bud will often show the foreign body. They can be removed with a needle. Foreign body sensation may persist for a while after removal.

Corneal abrasion

Corneal abrasions are often causes by twigs, fingernails and the edges of pieces of paper. They causes intense pain and lacrimation. The abrasion can be confirmed with the aid of fluorescein. Antibiotic ointment and cycloplegic drops should be instilled into the eye. A pad should be applied. Most abrasions heal within 48 hours.

Blunt trauma

Blunt ophthalmic trauma can result in:

- Black eye
- Subconjunctival haemorrhage
- Corneal abrasion
- Traumatic mydriasis
- Hyphaema
- Iridoialysis
- Concussion cataract
- Lens subluxation
- Retinal tear
- Vitreous haemorrhage
- Commotio retinae
- Choroidal rupture
- Blow-out orbital fracture

Hyphaema

Hyphaema is blood in the anterior chamber of the eye. It is due to rupture of the iris blood vessels and presents with a reduction in visual acuity. The red reflex is lost. Within a short period of time the blood settles and produces a fluid level. Most hyphaema settle with conservative treatment. Surgical treatment may be required if the anterior chamber is full of blood. Inadequate treatment can result in glaucoma or blood-staining of the cornea.

Blow-out fracture

Posterior displacement of the globe raises the orbital pressure. The orbit may then fractures at its weakest point. This usually occurs at the orbital floor and soft tissues herniates into the maxillary sinus. Clinical features of a blow-out fracture include, enophthalmos, restriction of eye movement, especially on upward gaze and loss of sensation over the region supplied by infra-orbital nerve. Sinus x-ray will shows clouding of the affected sinus and may be able to identify herniated tissue. CT scanning is able to more clearly define the extent and the site of injury. Surgical correction is often required.

Penetrating injuries

Penetrating injuries can result in:

- Corneoscleral lacerations
- Intraocular foreign bodies
- Sympathetic ophthalmitis

Intraocular foreign bodies

Intraocular foreign bodies are usually caused by metal fragment hitting the eye at high speed. The patient is usually aware of something having stuck the eye. In the early stages after the injury there is no significant visual loss and the clinical signs may be easily missed. An x-ray of the orbit is essential. Foreign body may also be identified on CT or ultrasound. Retained iron and copper foreign bodies can give rise to serious chemical reactions. Siderosis from iron causes staining of the iris, cataract formation and retinal atrophy. Chalcosis from copper deposition causes endophthalmitis and rapid visual loss. Ferrous foreign bodies can be removed with a powerful electromagnet. Non-magnetic foreign bodies should be mechanically removed.

Acute red eye

Common causes of an acute red eye include:

- Conjunctivitis
- Keratitis
- Iritis
- Acute glaucoma
- Episcleritis
- Scleritis

Chalazion

A chalazion is due to inflammation of the meibomian gland. It presents as a painless, hard lump close to margin of eye lid. It is more common in the upper lid and can increases in size over days or weeks. Small lesions require no treatment. Large symptomatic lesions can be incised and curetted. This can be performed under local anaesthesia via a conjunctival incision.

Chapter 8

Principles of surgical oncology

Cell proliferation

In health, growth factors are made by one cell type to stimulate another. In contrast, malignant cells generate their own stimulatory growth factors, losing negative feedback mechanisms. Positive feedback cycles can occur by alteration of growth factors, receptors or intracellular signaling pathways. Cell proliferation can be regarded as neoplastic or non-neoplastic.

Non-neoplastic proliferation

There are several types of non-neoplastic proliferation.

Hyperplasia

Hyperplasia is an increase in tissue or organ size due to cell proliferation (e.g. benign prostatic hyperplasia). Causes include chronic infection and increased hormonal activity.

Hypertrophy

Hypertrophy is an increase in tissue or organ size due to enlargement of cell size (e.g. left ventricular hypertrophy in hypertension). There is no increase in cell number and it is due to increased functional requirements.

Metaplasia

Metaplasia is a change of one type of differentiated tissue to another (e.g. squamous metaplasia in the bronchial epithelium). It is usually of the same class of tissue but the new tissue type may be less specialised. It occurs in both epithelial and connective tissue and is often associated with hyperplasia.

Dysplasia

Dysplasia is disordered cell development that may accompany hyperplasia or dysplasia. It is due to increased mitosis. Cells become increasingly abnormal. It is a pre-malignant condition.

Neoplastic proliferation

Neoplasia is an abnormal, uncoordinated and excessive growth that persists after the initiating stimulus has been withdrawn. Neoplastic proliferation is characterised by being:

- Progressive
- Purposeless
- Regardless of surrounding tissues
- Not related to body needs
- Parasitic

Carcinogenesis

All cells have mechanisms for regulating their growth, differentiation and death. Cancer develops when cells escape from the normal control mechanism and proliferation is uncontrolled. Cells develop the ability to invade and metastasise. Carcinogenesis is a multi-step process. Cells accumulate a succession of gene mutations. Each mutation overcomes natural anti-cancer defence mechanisms. Growth regulation is lost. Most cancers result from a series of genetic errors.

Cancer genes

Genes related to cancer development may be divided into oncogenes and tumour suppressor genes. In health, the activity of these genes is closely regulated. They allow differentiated growth of normal tissues. In cancer, the balanced control of growth is lost.

Oncogenes

Oncogenes are regulatory genes whose activity is abnormally increased after a genetic alteration. Oncogene activation may occur after chromosomal translocation, gene amplification or mutation within a coding sequence of an oncogene. Oncogenes act in a dominant fashion. Examples of oncogenes include:

- ras on chromosome 11 – mediates signal transduction
- erbB2 on chromosome 7 – growth factor receptor
- src on chromosome 20 – tyrosine kinase
- myc on chromosome 8 – transcription factor

Tumour suppressor genes

Tumour suppressor genes code for inhibitory proteins. There normal function is to prevent cell growth. In cancer, the suppressor function is lost. Most tumour suppressor genes are recessive. Inactivation of tumour suppressor genes can occur by gene mutation causing loss of the gene product, prevention of binding of a gene product to its target site or inactivation by other proteins. Examples of tumour suppressor genes include:

- Rb on chromosome 13 – control of cell cycle
- p53 on chromosome 17 – DNA repair and apoptosis
- Bcl2 on chromosome 18 – apoptosis
- APC on chromosome 5 – regulation of co-transcriptional activators

Mutation of tumour suppressor genes is seen in many familial cancers.

- Rb – childhood retinoblastoma
- p53 – Li–Fraumeni syndrome
- APC – familial colon cancer
- BRCA1/2 – familial breast cancer

Cancer genetics

Several germline mutations have been shown to increase cancer risk. More than 50 genetic abnormalities have been identified. Most are inherited in an autosomal dominant fashion. Most genetic abnormalities involve tumour suppressor genes. Hereditary cancer syndromes result from a germline mutation in one copy of the suppressor gene. Somatic mutation in the second copy of the gene results in the development of cancer.

Breast cancer genetics

About 5% breast and ovarian cancers are due to a germ-line mutation. The remaining 95% are sporadic. The BRCA1 and BRCA 2 are tumour suppressor genes. The commonest abnormality is in the BRCA 1 gene found on long arm of chromosome 17. A mutation is seen in 50% of families with four or more affected members less than 60 years. More than 100 BRCA mutations have been described. The highest carrier rate is in Ashkenazi Jews. If a patient is BRCA 1 positive she has:

- 50% risk of developing breast cancer by 50 years
- 85% risk of developing breast cancer by 70 years
- 70% risk of developing contralateral breast cancer
- 50% life time risk of developing ovarian cancer

Tumour markers

Tumour markers are molecules occurring in blood that are associated with cancer and whose measurement or identification may be useful in patient diagnosis or clinical management. They are usually glycoproteins detected by monoclonal antibodies. The ideal tumour marker would be present in the blood, undetectable in health, produced only by malignant tissue, be organ specific and would have circulating levels proportional to tumour mass. The ideal tumour marker does not exist. Tumour markers can be used for:

- Screening for primary disease
- Diagnosis of primary disease
- Monitoring response to treatment
- Establishing prognosis
- Detection of recurrence

Commonly measured tumour markers include:

- CA-125 – ovary
- CEA – colon, pancreas, stomach
- PSA – prostate
- α-fetoprotein – teratoma, hepatoma
- β-hCG – seminoma, choriocarcinoma
- CA19.9 – pancreas
- CA15.3 – breast

Epidemiology of common cancer

There are more than 200 types of cancer, each with different causes, symptoms and treatments. There are approximately 300,000 new cases of cancer diagnosed in the UK each year. Every 2 minutes someone is diagnosed with cancer and more than 1 in 3 people will develop some form of cancer during their lifetime. Breast, lung, bowel and prostate cancers together account for over half of all new cancers each year. Cancer can develop at any age, but is most common in older people. More than 60% of cancers are diagnosed in people aged 65 and over. Approximately 1% of cancers occur in children, teenagers and young adults.

Overall, cancer incidence rates have increased by more than a quarter since the late 1970s, but the rates have been fairly stable since the late 1990s. Cancer incidence rates have risen by 16% in males and by 34% in females. There have been increases in the incidence of renal cell, malignant melanoma, oral and endometrial cancers. Over the last decade the incidence rate of stomach cancer has decreased by more than a quarter in both sexes. Cervical and ovarian cancer have each decreased by more than 10% and the lung cancer incidence rate in males decreased by almost a fifth.

Prostate cancer has overtaken lung cancer as the commonest cancer diagnosed in men. The apparent incidence of prostate cancer is rising due to the widespread use of PSA testing. Lung cancer is the second most common cancer in men. The incidence of lung cancer in men is falling. Breast cancer is the commonest cancer in women and accounts for 30% of all female cancer. The second commonest cancer in women is colorectal cancer.

NHS cancer screening programmes

Criteria for an effective screening programme

To justify establishing a screening programme, the World Health Organization has recommended that the following criteria be met:

- The disease screened for must be an important problem

- The natural history of the disease should be well understood with a recognisable early stage
- A specific and sensitive test for the early detection of the disease must be available
- There should be good evidence that the screening test can result in reduced mortality and morbidity in the targeted population
- The test must be acceptable, producing a high participation rate
- There should be suitable facilities for diagnosis and treatment of detected abnormalities
- There should be appropriate treatment options
- The benefits of screening should outweigh any adverse effects
- The benefit must be of an acceptable financial cost
- The results of the implementation require audit to ensure they meet the above criteria

Bias within screening programmes

Various biases exist which can skew the apparent success of a screening programme:

- Selection bias – patients select themselves into one group by attending
- Lead time bias – early detection appears to improve survival by increasing the time from diagnosis to death, yet mortality is unchanged. The patient is simply aware that they have the disease for longer
- Length bias – Slower growing better prognosis tumours are more likely to be detected by screening

Sensitivity and specificity

A screening test can give a positive or negative result. It does not imply that the patient has or does not have the disease. The test results can be:

- True positive (TP) = A positive test result in the presence of the disease
- True negative (TN) = A negative test result in the absence of the disease
- False positive (FP) = A positive test result in the absence of the disease
- False negative (FN) = A negative test result in the presence of the disease

The sensitivity of a test is the ability of the test to identify the disease in the presence of the disease (=TP/(TP + FN)). The specificity of a test is the ability of the test to exclude the disease in the absence of the disease (=TN/(TN + FP)). The positive predictive value (PPV) is the probability of a positive test reflecting the true presence of the disease. The negative predictive value (NPV) is the probability of a negative test reflecting the true absence of the disease.

National heath service breast screening programme

The National Health Service Breast Screening Programme was introduced in 1988 following the Forest Report in 1986. All women between 50 and 70 years are invited for 3-yearly two-view mammography. The age limit is being extended from 47-73 years. If an abnormality is seen on a mammogram women are recalled to a screening assessment clinic for a clinical examination, further imaging and fine needle aspiration cytology or core biopsy as required. About 70% of screen detected abnormalities are shown to be of no clinical significance following assessment.

National health service cervical screening programme

The National Health Service Cervical Screening Programme was established in 1988. Women are screened between 25 and 64 years, 25–49 every 3 years and 50–64 every 5 years. Cervical cells are obtained by either a smear or brush. Brush samples are analysed by liquid based cytology. About 1:10 smear tests are abnormal. Non-neoplastic causes of an abnormal smear include:

- Infection
- Presence of blood or mucus
- Inadequate specimen
- Poorly preserved specimen

Abnormal smears are reported as:

- CIN 1 = Mild dyskariosis
- CIN 2 = Moderate dyskariosis
- CIN 3 = Severe dyskariosis

National health service bowel cancer screening programme

The NHS Bowel Cancer Screening Programme started being rolled out in July 2006 and achieved nation wide coverage by 2010. If offers screening by faecal occult blood (FOB) testing every 2 years to all men and women aged 60 to 69. Patient with a positive result are invited for a colonoscopy. About 1 in 50 FOB tests are abnormal.

Clinicopathological staging of cancer

Staging is the clinical or pathological assessment of the extent of tumour spread. Clinical staging is a preoperative assessment. It is based on clinical, radiological and operative information and is used to determine treatment offered to the patient. Pathological staging is a postoperative assessment. It provides useful prognostic information. It allows decisions to be made regarding adjuvant therapy and comparison of treatment outcomes.

Staging systems

The ideal staging system should be:

- Easy to use and remember
- Reproducible – not subject to inter or intra-observer variation
- Based on prognostically important pathological factors

TNM system

The TNM system is based on the anatomical extent of spread:

- T refers to the extent of primary tumour
- N refers to the extent of nodal metastases
- M refers to the presence or absence of distant metastases

Two classifications are described for each site:

- Clinical classification (TNM)
- Pathological classification (pTNM)

The TNM system is generally accepted but does not recorded all factors (e.g. grade, contiguous organ involvement) that are prognostically important.

T - primary tumour

- T_x = Primary tumour can not be assessed
- T_o = No evidence of primary tumour
- T_{is} = Carcinoma in situ
- T_{1-4} = Increasing size and local extent of primary tumour

N – regional lymph nodes

- N_x = Regional lymph nodes can not be assessed
- N_0 = No regional lymph node metastases
- N_{1-3} = Increasing involvement of regional lymph nodes

M – distant metastases

- M_x = Distant metastases can not be assessed
- M_0 = No distant metastases
- M_1 = Distant metastases present

Principles of cancer treatment

Radiotherapy

Radiotherapy is the use of ionising radiation to treat malignancy. It attempts to deliver a measured radiation does to a defined tumour volume, whilst limiting the dose to the surrounding normal tissue. Radiotherapy may be radical (with curative intent), palliative or adjuvant. Brachytherapy is the use of intracavity irradiation.

Physics

Radiation may be electromagnetic or particulate. Linear accelerators are used to generate high energy x-rays (electromagnetic) created by electrons hitting a fixed target. The depth of tissue penetration depend on the x-ray voltage. 10–125 KeV x-rays are absorbed by superficial tissues. 4–24 MV x-rays are absorbed in deeper tissues. The use of MV x-rays reduces the risk of significant skin toxicity. High energy electrons may be used instead of x-rays but electrons have limited tissue penetration. CT planning of radiotherapy fields reduces the radiation dose delivered to normal tissue.

Biology

Radiation damages DNA. It either causes direct damage to DNA or acts via the production of free radicals. Double-stranded DNA breaks and prevents cell replication, inducing cell death. The tissue response depends on the degree of cellular differentiation. Terminally differentiated cells (e.g. muscle and nerves) are resistant to damage. The most significant effects are seen in rapidly dividing cells (e.g. gut, bone marrow) and tumours. Acute toxicity occurs within days and depends on the overall treatment time. Acute toxicity includes mucositis, bone marrow suppression and skin reactions. Late toxicity occurs after weeks or months and depends on total dose and fractionation. Late toxicity includes tissue necrosis or fibrosis.

Fractionation

A higher total dose of radiation can be given if smaller repeated doses are administered. This allows a degree of repair of normal tissues. A high total dose increases the probability of tumour control. Hypofractionation is a small number of large doses. Accelerated fractionation is a standard dose given over a short interval. Hyperfractionation is a large number of small doses.

Uses of radiotherapy

Radiotherapy is used with curative intent and as the sole treatment in:

- Head and neck cancers
- Carcinoma of the cervix
- Seminomas
- Hodgkin's and non-Hodgkin's lymphomas
- Bladder cancer
- Early prostate cancer
- Early lung cancer
- Anal and skin cancer
- Medulloblastoma and other brain tumours
- Thyroid cancer

It is used as a component of multimodality therapy in:

- Breast cancer
- Rectal cancer
- Soft tissue sarcomas
- Advanced head and neck cancers
- Whole body irradiation before bone marrow transplantation

It is used with palliative intent in:

- Pain – especially bone metastases
- Spinal cord compression
- Cerebral metastases
- Venous or lymphatic obstruction

Chemotherapy

The aims of chemotherapy are to selectively destroy tumour cells whilst attempting to minimise the toxicity on normal cells. This is achieved by the specific growth characteristics of most tumours.

Mechanism of action

A cell synthesising DNA goes through a regular cycle with different phases know as the cell cycle (**Figure 8.1**) as follows:

- G_0 is a resting phase outside the cell cycle
- G_1 is a phase of protein and RNA synthesis
- S is a phase of DNA synthesis
- G_2 is a phase of RNA synthesis
- M is mitosis

Cells in G_0 are resistant to the effects of cytotoxic drugs. The faster cells are growing the more likely are that cytotoxic drugs are to 'catch' them. This also accounts for the toxicity that occurs on rapidly growing normal tissues such as the gastrointestinal mucosa and bone marrow. Most drugs kill a fixed proportion of cells rather than fixed number. Large tumours are relatively unresponsive to chemotherapy as more cells are in G_0 and drug penetration is less reliable.

Different drugs act at different phases of the cell cycle. As a result, combinations of drugs are more likely to be effective. The modes of action of chemotherapeutic agents include inhibiting:

- DNA polymerase causing breakage of single stranded DNA
- RNA synthesis by intercalating between DNA base pairs
- DNA synthesis by cross-linking DNA strands
- Dihydrofolate reductase
- The metaphase of mitosis by binding to tubulin

Non-phase dependent drugs kill cells exponentially with increasing dose. They are equally toxic for cell within the cell cycle or G_0 phase. Examples include:

- Alkylating agents – cyclophosphamide, cisplatin
- 5 Fluorouracil
- Anthracyclines – doxorubicin

Phase dependent drugs kill cells at a lower dose. They act within a specific phase of the cell cycle. Examples include:

- Methotrexate
- Vinca alkaloids – vincristine, vinblastine

Toxicity

Some general side effects occur with many cytotoxic agents and these include:

- Nausea and vomiting
- Bone marrow toxicity
- Gastrointestinal toxicity
- Alopecia
- Gonadal effects
- Hyperuricaemia

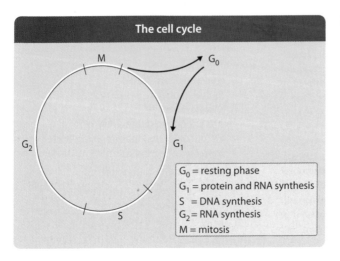

Figure 8.1 The cell cycle

Specific side effects that are seen with certain agents include:

- Pulmonary fibrosis – bleomycin
- Haemorrhagic cystitis – cyclophosphamide
- Cardiomyopathy – doxorubicin
- Hepatic damage – methotrexate
- Skin pigmentation – 5-flurouracil

Uses of chemotherapy

Chemotherapy is used with curative intent in:

- Acute lymphoblastic leukaemia
- Germ cell tumours
- Choriocarcinoma
- Hodgkin's disease
- Wilms' tumour

A significant response to chemotherapy is seen in:

- Breast carcinoma
- Ovarian carcinoma
- Lymphoma
- Osteosarcoma

Tumours that are poorly responsive to chemotherapy include:

- Pancreatic carcinoma
- Melanoma
- Soft tissue sarcomas
- Colorectal carcinoma
- Gastric carcinoma

Hormonal treatment

Hormonal treatment is used in that management of several cancers. It usually works by reducing steroid hormone production.

Breast cancer

The aim of hormonal treatment in breast cancer is to reduce oestrogenic growth stimulation of cancer cells. Hormonal treatment is effective in women with oestrogen and/or progesterone receptor-positive tumours. About 60% of breast cancers are ER positive and 80% of receptor-positive tumours will respond to hormonal manipulation. The response in hormone receptor-negative tumours is minimal. The types of hormonal treatment include:

- Ovarian ablation – surgical, LH–RH analogues

- Selective oestrogen receptor modulators – tamoxifen, raloxifene
- Aromatase inhibitors – anastrozole, letrozole and exemestane
- Progestogens – megestrol acetate

Uses of hormonal treatment

Hormonal treatment in breast cancer can be used as adjuvant treatment or in metastatic disease. In the adjuvant setting, tamoxifen or an aromatase inhibitor are given for 5 years. They have been shown to reduce the risk of recurrence, reduce the risk of contralateral breast cancer and improve survival. In patients with metastatic disease, the use of hormonal therapy depends on the ER status of the tumour, the duration of disease-free interval, the location of metastases, previous therapy and the patient's performance status.

Prostate cancer

The aim of hormonal treatment in prostate cancer is to ablate androgen production. About 80% of prostate cancers respond to medical or surgical androgen ablation. Surgical ablation is by orchidectomy and produces a rapid reduction in testosterone levels. Medical ablation is reversible and the effect may take several weeks to occur. The side effects of androgen ablation include impotence, loss of libido, osteoporosis, gynaecomastia and hot flushes. The site of action of hormonal treatment are:

- Pituitary gland – LH-RH analogues, stilbeostrol, cyproterone acetate
- Adrenal gland – ketoconazole, aminoglutethamide
- Prostate – flutamide, cyproterone acetate
- Testis – orchidectomy

Uses of hormonal treatment

Androgen ablation is used in both the neoadjuvant setting and in metastatic disease. In neoadjuvant setting is used in combination with external beam radiotherapy. LH-RH analogues are commonly used in metastatic disease. The median duration of response is about 18 months and about 20% patients achieve a response that may last several years. The response can be measured by assessing the PSA level. LH-RH analogues are give by monthly injection. The first injection my induce LH-RH release, a rise in PSA and worsening of symptoms. Cyproterone acetate should be give for first 2 weeks of treatment to reduce this effect.

Palliative care

Principles of palliative care

Palliative care is the active, total management of patients at a time when their disease is no longer responsive to curative treatment and when control of pain (or other symptoms) is of paramount importance. Dealing with psychological, social and spiritual problems is important. It affirms life and regards dying as normal. It neither hastens nor postpones death. It perceives the patient and family as a unit and creates a caring, comforting environment. It coordinates care and provides relief from distressing symptoms. It aims to maintain the independence of the patient for as long as possible, provide information and endeavours to reduce fear and anxiety. It promotes an atmosphere where an open and honest exchange of views can take place and helps the patient to come to terms with impending death. It offers a support system to the family to help them cope with illness and bereavement.

Liverpool Care Pathway

The Liverpool Care Pathway for the dying patient was developed to transfer good practice from the hospice model to other care settings such as hospitals. The key aims are to:

- Discontinue or alter delivery of medications
- Discontinue interventions
- Document cardiopulmonary resuscitation status
- Deactivate implanted cardiac defibrillators
- Discontinue inappropriate nursing interventions
- Communicate with the patient and assess their insight
- Assess and meet religious and spiritual needs
- Keep the family informed
- Provided bereavement advice for relatives

Pain

Pain is the commonest and most feared symptom associated with cancer. Chronic pain can be controlled in more than 80% of patients. The WHO analgesia ladder (**Figure 8.2**) forms the most common template for pain control and consists of a 'three-stepped ladder'. With increasing pain, increasing strength of analgesia is required. On each step of the ladder the maximum dose and frequency should be used.

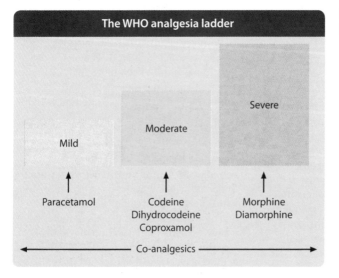

Figure 8.2 The WHO analgesia ladder

The WHO analgesia ladder

Severe

Moderate

Mild

↑ Paracetamol

↑ Codeine Dihydrocodeine Coproxamol

↑ Morphine Diamorphine

◄——— Co-analgesics ———►

Drugs should be prescribed on a regular basis not 'as required'. Co-analgesic agents often have a synergistic effect and may increase the efficacy of a particular analgesic agent.

Control of pain

Morphine

Morphine is the most commonly used strong analgesic in palliative care. It should initially be prescribed as an immediate release preparation (e.g. Oramorph) and can be given as required every 4 hours. The dose can be increased every 24 hours until pain is adequately controlled. Once pain has been controlled the total daily dose can be calculated. Immediate release can then be substituted for delayed release preparations. Immediate release preparations can still be given for breakthrough pain. No ceiling exists for the maximum permissible dose of morphine. Laxative should be prescribed to prevent constipation. Patients may also require an antiemetic. Complications of opiate analgesia include itch, hallucinations and dry mouth, but respiratory depression is rarely a problem. Physical dependence may occur. Psychological dependence and addiction are not a problem in the palliative care setting. If the oral route is unavailable subcutaneous or percutaneous administration may be appropriate.

Co-analgesia

Co-analgesics have little intrinsic analgesic activity but have additive effects to analgesic agents.

Non-steroid anti-inflammatory drugs may be useful in bone pain. Anticonvulsants and antidepressants are useful in neuropathic pain. Steroids increase wellbeing and benzodiazepines reduce muscle spasm.

Other symptoms

Bone pain

Bone pain is often well controlled with a single fraction of radiotherapy and non-steroid anti-inflammatory drugs may have useful co-analgesic effect. Bisphosphonates reduce osteoclastic activity and reduce bone pain.

Neuropathic pain

Neuropathic pain is often resistant to treatment. Anticonvulsants and antidepressants may have useful effect. Neurolytic blocks may be considered if the pain fails to respond to pharmacological agents.

Liver capsule pain

Liver capsule pain is often distressing and non-steroidal anti-inflammatory drugs often have excellent additive effects in this situation. Steroids can reduce swelling, inflammation and pain. Dexamethasone is usually the drug of choice.

Dyspnoea

Dyspnoea is not always due to underlying malignancy and consideration should be given to treatment of any underlying infection or cardiac failure. Causes of breathlessness related to malignancy include pleural effusion, lymphangitis carcinomatosis, intrapulmonary metastases and constricting chest wall disease. Aspiration of a pleural effusion often produces symptomatic improvement. Pleurodesis with talc or bleomycin is only effective if the pleural effusion can be drained to dryness. A pleuro-peritoneal shunt may produce symptomatic improvement. Steroids produce symptomatic improvement in those with lymphangitis and intrapulmonary metastases. The respiratory depressant effect of morphine will also reduce dyspnoea.

Nausea and vomiting

Nausea and vomiting is usually multifactorial in origin and causes include, hypercalcaemia, liver metastases, constipation, drug side effects and intestinal obstruction. Metoclopramide, domperidone and cyclizine are useful if there is gastric stasis or intestinal obstruction. $5-HT_3$ blockers (e.g. ondansetron) are useful for chemotherapy-induced nausea. Haloperidol is useful in morphine-induced nausea.

Constipation

Treatment of constipation should be continuous and anticipatory. It is often a predictable side effect of opiate analgesia. It can be worsened by inactivity, dehydration and hypercalcaemia. Opiate-induced constipation is best treated with compound preparations containing both a stool softener and stimulant (e.g. co-danthrusate).

Applied basic sciences
Anatomy of the heart

The heart is situated in the middle mediastinum. It lies freely within the pericardium. It is pyramidal in shape with its base lying posteriorly. The apex is anterio-inferior and points to the left. The heart has three surfaces. The strenocostal surface is formed by the right atrium and ventricle and by parts of the left ventricle and atrium. The diaphragmatic surface is formed by the right and left ventricles. The base is formed by the left atrium. It is connected to the great vessels at the base. The atrioventricular groove separates the right and left atrium from the ventricles. The anterior and posterior interventricular grooves join each other. Important lateral relations of the heart include the phrenic nerves which run adjacent to the pericardium. Posterior relations include the oesophagus, the descending thoracic aorta, the azygos vein and the thoracic duct.

Blood supply
Left coronary artery

The left coronary artery arises from the left posterior aortic sinus (**Figure 9.1**). It passes behind the pulmonary trunk and then lies under the left auricle. It divides into anterior interventricular and circumflex branches. The anterior interventricular artery is also known as the left anterior descending artery and continues in the anterior interventricular groove. It anastomoses with the posterior interventricular branch of the right coronary artery and also gives the diagonal branch. The circumflex artery winds (circumflexes) around the left heart border. It passes in the atrioventricular groove and anastomoses with the right coronary artery.

Right coronary artery

The right coronary artery arises from the anterior aortic sinus. It passes between the pulmonary trunk and the right atrium and traverses the atrioventricular groove. It ends by anastomosing with the branches of circumflex artery. Branches of the right coronary artery supply the sino-atrial node and the left atrium. It also supplies the right marginal artery and the posterior interventricular artery, also known as posterior descending artery.

'Dominance' of the coronary circulation

Dominance of the coronary circulation arises from variation in the blood supply. Right dominance occurs when the posterior interventricular artery arises from the right coronary artery (80%). Left dominance occurs when the posterior interventricular artery arises from left coronary artery (10%). Codominance occurs when the posterior interventricular artery is formed by both the right and left coronary arteries (10%).

Blood supply to the conducting system of the heart

The sino-atrial node is supplied by a branch of the right coronary artery in 60% of the population. The atrio-ventricular node is supplied from the posterior interventricular artery.

Venous drainage

The coronary sinus receives most of the blood from the heart. It lies in the posterior part of the atrioventricular groove and opens into the right atrium. It is a continuation of the great cardiac vein. Tributaries included the middle and small cardiac veins. The anterior cardiac vein opens directly into the right atrium. The venae cordae minimae drain directly into the chambers of the heart.

Nerve supply

The sympathetic nerves supply of the heart arises from the cervical and upper thoracic portions of the sympathetic chain through the stellate ganglion. Afferent fibres run with the sympathetic fibres that conduct pain. The parasympathetic supply is via the vagus

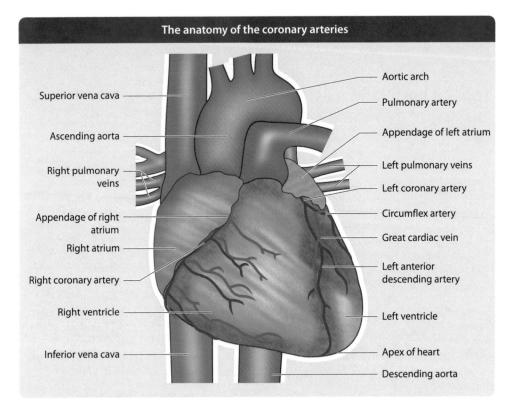

The anatomy of the coronary arteries

- Superior vena cava
- Ascending aorta
- Right pulmonary veins
- Appendage of right atrium
- Right atrium
- Right coronary artery
- Right ventricle
- Inferior vena cava
- Aortic arch
- Pulmonary artery
- Appendage of left atrium
- Left pulmonary veins
- Left coronary artery
- Circumflex artery
- Great cardiac vein
- Left anterior descending artery
- Left ventricle
- Apex of heart
- Descending aorta

Figure 9.1 The anatomy of the coronary arteries. (Reproduced from James S and Nelson K. Pocket Tutor ECG Interpretation. London: JP Medical Ltd, 2011.)

nerves. The sympathetic and parasympathetic nerves form cardiac plexuses. The superficial cardiac plexus lies in front of the right pulmonary artery. The deep cardiac plexus lies in front of the tracheal bifurcation.

Conduction system

The conduction system of the heart is by specialised muscle fibres. The sinoatrial (SA) node is located in the wall of the right atrium just to the right of the opening to the superior vena cava. This node gives a spontaneous impulse that spreads in all directions through the myocardium of the atria and causes the atrial muscle to contract. The atrioventricular node is located on the lower part of the atrial septum, just above the tricuspid valve. It is activated by the excitation wave that passes through the atria from the sinoatrial node. From this node the impulse moves to the atrioventricular bundle, from where it travels on down through the ventricles.

The atrioventricular bundle is also known as the Bundle of His. It is the only normal pathway that connects the myocardium of the atria and the ventricles. It descends through the fibrous skeleton of the heart. At the lower part of the membranous portion of the ventricular septum it divides into two branches, one for each ventricle. The right bundle branch travels down the right ventricle wall. The left bundle branch travels down the left ventricular wall and splits into anterior and posterior branches. Purkinje fibres cover the ventricle wall and ensure that the whole of each ventricle contracts at once.

Pericardium

The pericardium is a made up of two fibroserous layers that enclose the heart and roots of the great vessels. The serous layer has an inner visceral layer and outer parietal layer. Both layers are continuous around the great vessels and the pulmonary veins. This leads to the formation of the two pericardial sinuses – an oblique sinus and transverse sinus. These lie on the posterior surface of the heart.

Cardiac physiology

Myocyte action potential

Normally, the SA node cells have the highest rate of depolarisation. As a result, the SA node acts as the cardiac impulse generator. Cells of the SA node automatically depolarise slowly after each repolarisation. This is due to the gradual influx of calcium through T channels. Once the threshold potential is reached, sudden depolarisation results. This is due to the rapid influx of sodium. Repolarisation is brought about by the efflux of potassium. The phases of the myocyte action potential are shown in **Figure 9.2**.

The action potential spreads from SA node to other cells of the conducting system and the myocytes. Its rapid spread between the myocytes is aided by the presence of gap junctions. As a result, the heart muscle contracts as a syncytium. During the absolute refractory period, the myocyte cannot be stimulated. This lasts from phase 1 through to the middle of phase 3. During the relative refractory period, myocytes can be stimulated only by a supranormal stimulus. This lasts from when the absolute refractory period ends until phase 4.

Cardiac cycle

The cardiac cycle describes the events related to the flow of blood through the heart during one complete heartbeat. It has certain well-described phases (**Figure 9.3**).

- Phase 1 – Atrial contraction
- Phase 2 – Isovolumetric ventricular contraction
- Phase 3 – Rapid ventricular ejection
- Phase 4 – Reduced ventricular ejection
- Phase 5 – Isovolumetric ventricular relaxation
- Phase 6 – Rapid ventricular filling
- Phase 7 – Reduced ventricular filling

During atrial contraction, 25% of the ventricular filling occurs. The AV valves are open and the aortic and pulmonary valves closed. At the end of atrial contraction the AV valves close. During isovolumetric ventricular contraction, the ventricles contract as a closed chamber. The ventricular pressure rapidly rises. At the end of isovolumetric ventricular contraction, the aortic and pulmonary valves open. During rapid ventricular ejection, ventricular contraction continues and blood rapidly passes into the great vessels. About two-thirds of the stroke volume is ejected in the first one-third of systole. During reduced ventricular ejection, ventricular contraction continues but the outflow of blood reduces as the ventricular pressure declines. At the

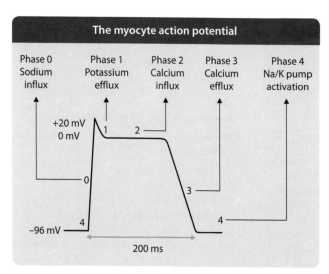

Figure 9.2 The myocyte action potential. (Reproduced from James S and Nelson K. Pocket Tutor ECG Interpretation. London: JP Medical Ltd, 2011.)

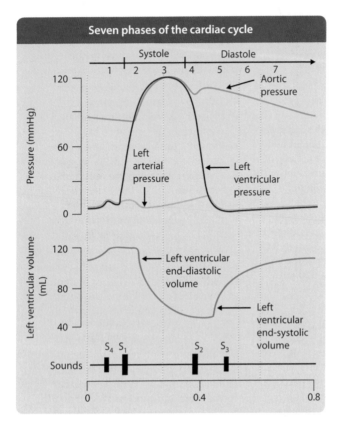

Figure 9.3 Seven phases of the cardiac cycle. AP = Aortic pressure. LVP = Left ventricular pressure. LAP = left atrial pressure. LVEDV = Left ventricular end diastolic volume. LVESV = Left ventricular end systolic volume

end of reduced ventricular ejection, the aortic and pulmonary valves close. During isovolumetric ventricular relaxation, the ventricles relax as closed chambers. When the ventricular pressures reduces to below those in the great veins the AV valves open. During rapid ventricular filling, blood flows into the ventricles from the atria. During reduced ventricular filling the pressure difference between the atria and ventricle reduces and blood slowly keeps flowing into the ventricles.

Heart sounds

There are four heart sounds:

- S1 – due to closure of the atrioventricular valves
- S2 – due to closure of the aortic and pulmonary valves
- S3 – due to rapid ventricular filling
- S4 – due to atrial contraction and blood flow into the ventricle

Cardiac function

Measures of cardiac function that can directly assessed include:

- End diastolic volume
- Stroke volume
- Ejection fraction
- Cardiac output
- Peripheral resistance
- Blood pressure
- Central venous pressure
- Pulmonary capillary wedge pressure

Determinants of stroke volume

The stroke volume depends on several factors including:

- Preload
- Contractility
- Afterload

Preload is a measure of how much the myocyte is stretched before contraction. It is represented by the end diastolic volume or the end diastolic pressure. In the normal heart, cardiac output is directly proportional to preload. Contractility is a measure of the inherent ability of the myocyte to contract. It can be increased by drugs such as digoxin and catecholamines. Cardiac output is directly proportional to the contractility. Afterload is the force against which the ventricle has to contract. Peripheral resistance is a measure of afterload and cardiac output is inversely proportional to afterload. The Frank–Starling curve (**Figure 9.4**) demonstrates that the force of contraction of a myocyte is directly proportional to its initial length up to a level, after which it reduces with any further increase in the initial length.

Regulation of blood pressure
Baroreceptors
Baroreceptors play an important role in the day-to-day regulation of blood pressure, such as in response to postural changes. They are located in the walls of carotid sinus and the arch of the aorta. They are innervated by glossopharyngeal nerve (ninth cranial nerve) and stimulated by increased stretch that occurs following a rise in blood pressure. This leads to inhibition of the vasomotor centre and hence a reduction in blood pressure.

Hormones and catecholamines
Renin–angiotensin, aldosterone, antidiuretic hormone and catecholamines normally play a permissive role in the maintenance of blood pressure but have a more important role in blood pressure regulation in states of shock.

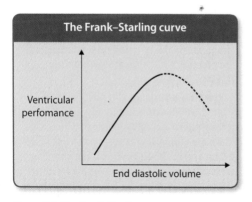

The Frank–Starling curve

Ventricular performance

End diastolic volume

Figure 9.4 The Frank–Starling curve

Anatomy of the lungs
Pleurae
Each pleura has two parts. The parietal layer lines the thorax wall and the diaphragm. The visceral layer covers the outer surface of each lung. They are continuous with each other at root of the lung. They are separated by the pleural cavity containing a small amount of pleural fluid. The pulmonary ligaments at each lung root allow for movement during respiration. The costal pleura is supplied by the intercostal nerves. The mediastinal pleura is supplied by the phrenic nerves. The diaphragmatic pleura is supplied by both the intercostal and phrenic nerves.

Trachea and bronchi
The trachea has a fibroelastic wall with U-shaped hyaline cartilages. It begins below the cricoid cartilage at the level of the C6 vertebra. It ends at the level of the sternal angle at the level of the T4 vertebra. It lies in the superior mediastinum. There are two bronchi. The right main bronchus is wider, shorter and more vertical than the left. It divides at the hilum of the right lung into three branches. The left main bronchus is longer and more horizontal and passes in front of the oesophagus. It divides at the hilum of the left lung into two branches.

Lungs
Each lung is conical in shape and is covered by visceral pleura. They are attached to the mediastinum by the root. The apex extends into the root of the neck. The base of the lung overlies the dome of the diaphragm. The right lung has three lobes – upper, middle and lower. The left lung has two lobes – upper and lower. Each lobe of the lung is divided into bronchopulmonary segments. Each receives a segmental bronchus, artery and vein. The blood supply of the bronchi and their branches are from the bronchial arteries. The bronchial arteries are direct branches of the aorta. The bronchial veins drain into the azygos and hemiazygos veins. Deoxygenated blood enters each lung via the pulmonary artery. Oxygenated blood leaves each lung via the pulmonary vein. At each lung root is

the pulmonary venous plexus. Sympathetic efferent fibres produce bronchodilatation. Parasympathetic efferent fibres produce bronchoconstriction.

Respiratory physiology

The thoracic cage is formed by the 12 thoracic vertebrae, 12 ribs, the sternum and diaphragm. The top 10 ribs are attached directly or indirectly to the sternum. Within the thoracic cage are three compartments. These are the two pleural cavities, each with a lung and the mediastinum, containing the heart. Gases enter and leave the lungs through the mouth and nose, the pharynx and larynx, the trachea, bronchi and bronchioles. These tubes expand at their ends into alveoli, where gas exchange takes place. There are about 23 branchings which lead to a total of about 300 million alveoli.

Respiratory mechanics

Contracting the diaphragm or raising the ribs expands the thoracic cavity. At rest, contraction of the diaphragm accounts for most of inspiration. The diaphragm is supplied by phrenic nerve which originates from cervical spinal cord (C3–C5). The external intercostal muscles also aid inspiration. At rest, expiration is mostly passive and the lungs contract due to their elasticity. During exercise, the internal intercostal muscles and other accessory muscles aid expiration. They pull the ribs downward and inward, reducing the volume of the thoracic cavity.

Pulmonary ventilation

The total amount of air moved in and out of the lungs each minute depends upon the tidal volume (TV) and respiratory rate (RR). Pulmonary ventilation is the product of RR and TV. During exercise both RR and TV can be increased. The extra inspiration available is called the inspiratory reserve volume (IRV). The extra expiration, available is called the expiratory reserve volume (ERV). After maximum expiration some air is still present in the lungs and is know as the residual volume (RV). The maximum volume available for breathing is the vital capacity (VC). Vital capacity is the sum of IRV, TV and ERV.

Oxygen and carbon dioxide transport

Haemoglobin

Haemoglobin consists of four polypeptide chains joined to a porphyrin ring. Haemoglobin A1 consists of two α and two β chains. The porphyrin ring contains iron. Only when the iron is in the ferrous (reduced) state does it binds with oxygen. Haemoglobin with ferric (oxidised) iron is known as methaemoglobin. It cannot take part in oxygen transport. Each haemoglobin molecule can bind up to four molecules of oxygen.

Oxygen is primarily transported bound to haemoglobin. A small amount is transported dissolved free in the plasma. Haemoglobin bound to oxygen is known as oxyhaemoglobin. One gram of haemoglobin can bind with 1.34 mL of oxygen. Therefore, 100 mL of plasma will have about 20 mL of oxygen bound to haemoglobin. The amount of oxygen bound to haemoglobin is expressed as oxygen saturation (SaO_2). This is dependent upon the partial pressure of oxygen (pO_2).

Oxygen dissociation curve

The relationship between pO_2 and SaO_2 is expressed as the oxygen dissociation curve (**Figure 9.5**). It is sigmoid in shape and is due to facilitative binding of oxygen to haemoglobin. Oxygen bound to haemoglobin initially increases its affinity to bind further oxygen. This facilitates further binding. Haemoglobin has the least affinity for the final oxygen molecule. This explains the flattening of the curve with increasing pO_2. The p50 is the partial pressure of oxygen at which 50% of the haemoglobin is saturated. The p50 of adult haemoglobin is about 3.5 kPa.

The affinity of haemoglobin for oxygen is variable. When the affinity reduces, the curve shifts to the right and the p50 increases. When the affinity increases the curve shifts to the left and the p50 is reduced. The curve for haemoglobin in sickle cell anaemia is shifted to the right. The curve for fetal haemoglobin is shifted to the left. Factors reducing the affinity and thus shifting the curve to the right are:

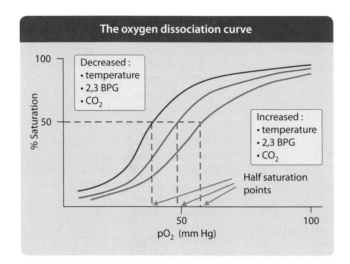

Figure 9.5 The oxygen dissociation curve. 2,3 BPG = 2,3 Biphosphoglycerate

- An increase in pCO_2
- A reduction in pH
- An increase in temperature
- An increase in 2,3-biphosphoglycerate

Similarly, a reduction in these variables results in an increase in the affinity of haemoglobin. Conditions which increase the affinity of haemoglobin for oxygen, exist in the lungs. Therefore, oxygen gets bound to haemoglobin. Conditions which reduce the affinity of haemoglobin for oxygen, exist in peripheral tissues. Therefore, oxygen gets released from haemoglobin. The shift in the dissociation curve due to changes in pCO_2 is known as the Bohr effect.

2,3-biphosphoglycerate

2,3-biphosphoglycerate (2,3-BPG) is a byproduct of anaerobic respiration. It reduces the affinity of haemoglobin for oxygen. Thus it shifts the oxygen dissociation curve to the right. Levels of 2,3-BPG increase in chronic hypoxia and thus more oxygen is delivered to tissues. Levels of 2,3-BPG are reduced in stored blood. Thus oxygen delivery to the tissues is sub-optimal with transfused blood. Fetal haemoglobin is not affected by 2,3-BPG. It has a higher affinity for oxygen than has maternal haemoglobin and ensures transfer of oxygen across the placenta.

Carbon monoxide

The affinity of haemoglobin for carbon monoxide is 250 times more than that towards oxygen. Its binding with haemoglobin is competitive with oxygen. Carboxyhaemoglobin has a hyperbolic oxygen-dissociation curve

Transport of carbon dioxide

Carbon dioxide is 20 times more soluble in plasma than oxygen. It is transported in three forms:

- Dissolved in plasma
- Bound to haemoglobin
- Bicarbonate ion

Haemoglobin combined with carbon dioxide is known as carbaminohaemoglobin. The majority of carbon dioxide produced is transported as bicarbonate. Carbon dioxide diffuses into red cells and reacts with water to produce bicarbonate and carbonic acid. This reaction is catalysed by the enzyme carbonic anhydrase. The bicarbonate produced inside red cells diffuses out into the plasma in exchange with chloride ions. This is known as chloride shift. Chloride moves into red cells and bicarbonate moves out.

Carbon dioxide equilibrium curve

Over the physiological concentrations of carbon dioxide this curve is a straight line.

The curve is shifted to the left in venous blood. This improves carbon dioxide transport and is known as Haldane effect. It occurs because deoxygenated haemoglobin is a weaker acid and allows more carbon dioxide to combine with haemoglobin.

Cardiac disease
Cardiopulmonary bypass

Cardiopulmonary bypass with the use of a pump and oxygenator was first described in the 1950s. The components of a cardiopulmonary bypass circuit are shown in **Figure 9.6**. A cannula is inserted into right atrium to drain the venous return. Venous blood then passes into venous reservoir under gravity. It is oxygenated and CO_2 is removed by the use of a membrane oxygenator. A heat exchanger controls blood temperature. Surgery is often performed with 5–10°C of hypothermia. A 40 μm filter removes air bubbles. A pump returns blood into aorta distal to a cross clamp. Suction is used to remove blood from operative field and this is returned to the patient via the cardiotomy reservoir.

Prolonged bypass induces cytokine activation and an inflammatory response. This results in red cell damage, haemoglobinuria, thrombocytopenia, clotting abnormalities. Reduced pulmonary gas exchange and cerebrovascular accidents.

Coronary artery surgery
Pathology

Coronary artery disease is the commonest cause of death in both men and women in

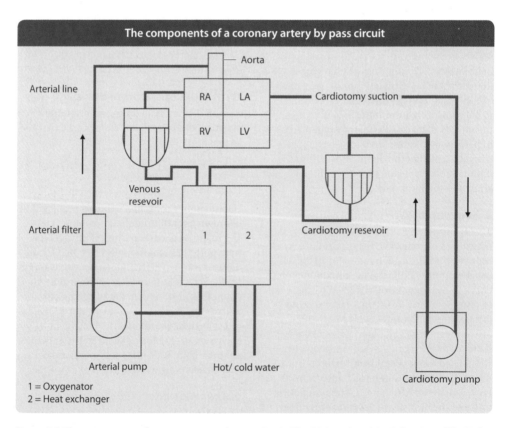

Figure 9.6 The components of a coronary artery bypass circuit. RA = Right atrium, LA = Left atrium, RV = Right ventricle, LV = Left ventricle

the UK. It is progressive, generally begins in childhood but manifests clinically in middle to late adult life. Atherosclerosis occurs in the proximal portions of the three main vessels supplying the heart. The main treatable risk factors for coronary artery disease are:

- Hypercholesterolaemia
- Hypertension
- Diabetes
- Smoking

Depending on the number of vessels involved, the patient is described as having double or triple vessel disease. The prognosis depends on both the number of vessels involved and left ventricular function.

Clinical features

The symptoms of coronary artery disease vary widely. Some patients with mild disease may present with clinically significant symptoms and signs. Some patients with advanced disease may have no symptoms and experience no functional impairment. The spectrum of presentations includes:

- Asymptomatic state
- Stable angina pectoris
- Unstable angina
- Myocardial infarction
- Chronic ischaemic cardiomyopathy
- Congestive heart failure
- Sudden cardiac arrest

Investigation

An ECG will often show evidence of cardiac ischaemia. Left ventricular function can be assessed by measuring the ejection fraction on echocardiography, coronary angiography or multiple-gated acquisition (MUGA) scan. Coronary angiography allows both confirmation of the diagnosis and preoperative planning of the use of stents or the site of a coronary artery graft.

Management

The prevention and treatment of atherosclerosis requires control of the known modifiable risk factors for the disease. This includes lifestyle changes and the medical treatment of hypertension, hyperlipidemia, and diabetes mellitus. The mainstays of pharmacologic therapy of angina includes nitrates, β-blockers, statins and calcium-channel blockers. Revascularisation of the coronary arteries can be by either percutaneous coronary intervention (PCI) or coronary artery bypass surgery (CABG). In the UK, about three times more patients undergo PCI than CABG.

Percutaneous coronary intervention

The use of PCI has increased dramatically over recent years and has become one of the most common medical interventions. PCI describes a range of coronary interventions from angiography to angioplasty and stent insertion. Indications for PCI include:

- Acute ST elevation myocardial infarction (STEMI)
- Non ST elevation acute coronary syndrome
- Stable angina
- Mildly symptomatic patients with evidence of severe ischemia on noninvasive testing

Contraindications to PCI include:

- Left main stem stenosis in a patient who is a surgical candidate
- Diffusely diseased small-caliber artery
- Other coronary anatomy not amenable to percutaneous intervention

Coronary artery bypass surgery

Coronary artery bypass surgery is indicated for severe stenosis (>70%) with left main stem or triple vessel disease. No improved survival has been shown in patients with single or double-vessel disease. Improved survival is also seen in those with poor left ventricular function. Similar survival is seen in patients undergoing angioplasty for multi-vessel disease. Patients at greatest risk have the most to gain from surgical intervention. Mortality risk can be estimated using various scoring tools. Risk can be calculated by summating individual risk factors. The Parsonnet score and Euroscore are the most commonly used validated scoring system (**Table 9.1**).

Choice of conduit The conduits for CABG surgery can be either venous or arterial. Long saphenous vein is easy to harvest by a second surgeon and allows multiple grafts to be fashioned. Venous conduits have a patency rate of 60% at 10 years. The left internal mammary artery is often used to graft the left anterior descending. Arterial conduits have a patency rate of 90% at 10 years.

Surgery For CABG surgery, the chest is entered via a median sternotomy and the left internal mammary artery is dissected. The long saphenous vein can be harvested and prepared by second surgeon. The heart is cannulated and the patient is placed on bypass. The aorta is cross clamped. Injury to heart is reduced by cardioplegic solutions. Cardioplegia can be either warm (37°C) or cold (4°C). Recent advances include off-pump coronary artery surgery and minimally invasive direct coronary artery surgery. Both can avoid either bypass or median sternotomy.

Complications The mortality rate following CABG depends on the risk associated with patient groups but is generally around 2%. The risk is higher in the acute or emergency setting. Complications of coronary artery bypass surgery included bleeding, atrial fibrillation, wound infection, poor cardiac function and stroke. With time restenosis occurs and angina recurs in 20% at 5 years and 40% at 10 years.

Valvular heart disease
Aetiology
The principal causes of valvular heart disease differ between Western and developing countries. Common causes include:

- Congenital valvular abnormalities (e.g. bicuspid aortic valve)
- Infective endocarditis
- Rheumatic fever
- Degenerative valve disease
- Ischaemic heart disease

Pathology
Rheumatic fever results from immune-mediated inflammation of the heart valves. It results from cross reaction between Group A β haemolytic streptococcus and cardiac proteins. Valve disease results in either stenosis or incompetence. Stenosis causes pressure load on the proximal chamber. Incompetence causes volume load on the proximal chamber. Thrombus may form in the dilated left atrium resulting in peripheral embolisation.

Risk changes as assed by the Parsonnet Score and Euroscore

Parsonnet Score	Euroscore
Age greater than 70 years +7%	Age – for each 5 years over 60 years +1%
Age greater than 75 years +12%	Female sex +1%
Age greater than 80 years +20%	Chronic respiratory disease +1%
Female sex +1%	Extracardiac arteriopathy +2%
Hypertension +3%	Neurological dysfunction +2%
Diabetes +3%	Creatinine greater than 200 µmol/L +2%
Obesity +3%	Previous cardiac surgery +3%
Good ejection fraction Nil	Unstable angina +2%
Moderate ejection fraction +2%	Recent myocardial infarction +2%
Poor ejection fraction +4%	Good ejection fraction Nil
	Moderate ejection fraction +1%
	Poor ejection fraction +3%

Table 9.1 Risk changes as assed by the Parsonnet Score and Euroscore

Clinical features

The clinical features of aortic, mitral and tricuspid valve disease as follows:

Aortic stenosis

- Angina pectoris
- Syncopal episodes
- Left ventricular failure
- Slow upstroke to arterial pulse
- Ejection systolic murmur in 2nd right intercostal space

Aortic regurgitation

- Congestive cardiac failure
- Increased pulse pressure
- Water-hammer pulse
- Early diastolic murmur at left sternal edge

Mitral stenosis

- Pulmonary hypertension
- Paroxysmal nocturnal dyspnoea
- Atrial fibrillation
- Loud first heart sound
- Mid diastolic murmur at apex

Mitral regurgitation

- Pulmonary oedema
- Apex beat displace laterally
- Apical pansystolic murmur

Tricuspid stenosis

- Fatigue and peripheral oedema
- Hepatomegaly and ascites
- Increased JVP with prominent a waves
- Diastolic murmur at left sternal edge

Tricuspid regurgitation

- Pulsatile hepatomegaly and ascites
- Right ventricular heave
- Prominent JVP with large v waves
- Pansystolic murmur at left sternal edge

Investigation

Investigation of valvular heart disease will require, an ECG, chest x-ray and echocardiography. Cardiac catheterisation may be necessary to measure the transvalvular pressure gradient.

Management

Few patients with symptomatic aortic stenosis survive 5 years and approximately 20% of symptomatic patients will suffer sudden death. Asymptomatic mitral stenosis is well tolerated with greater than 50% 10-year survival. Medical management consists of treatment of cardiac failure, digitalisation if in atrial fibrillation and anticoagulation if there is evidence of peripheral embolisation.

Surgery

Surgery is usually performed through a median sternotomy. On cardiopulmonary bypass with systemic hypothermia, the heart is arrested and protected with cardioplegic solution. Valves can be either repaired or replaced. Valve repair results in better haemodynamics and does not require long-term anticoagulation. Approximately 7000 patients per year undergo valve replacement in the UK. The aortic valve is the commonest to be replaced.

Indications for aortic valve replacement include:

- Symptomatic aortic stenosis
- Asymptomatic aortic stenosis with pressure gradient more than 50 mmHg
- Symptomatic aortic regurgitation

Indications for mitral valve replacement include:

- Symptomatic mitral stenosis especially if peripheral emboli
- Mitral valve area less than 1 cm^2

Prosthetic heart valves

The principal types of replacement heart valves are:

- Heterografts – stented or unstented (e.g. pig)
- Homografts
- Ball and cage (e.g. Starr–Edwards)
- Tilting disc (e.g. Bjork–Shiley)

Mechanical valves are readily available, have good durability but require life-long anticoagulation. They are also at increased risk of infective endocarditis. Heterografts are readily available but have a limited lifespan. The median survival of aortic and mitral heterografts is 15 and 8 years, respectively. They require a limited duration of anticoagulation. Homografts are not readily available and do not require anticoagulation. The long-term outcome of homografts is uncertain.

Intra-aortic balloon pump

Principles of action

Myocardial ischaemia can cause a fall in cardiac output and the coronary blood flow may subsequently be reduced. Compensatory mechanisms may further reduce cardiac output and coronary blood flow. Cardiac performance can be improved by optimisation of preload, afterload, heart rate, contractility and myocardial oxygenation.

An intra-aortic balloon pump provides haemodynamic support to the failing heart. It works by increasing blood flow in the coronary arteries and reducing the work of the cardiac muscle. The balloon is inflated in diastole which increases diastolic coronary artery perfusion pressure and increases myocardial oxygen delivery. The balloon is deflated in systole which reduces impedance to left ventricular ejection and decreases myocardial oxygen demand.

Indications for the use of an intra-aortic balloon pump include:

- Perioperative myocardial ischaemia
- Acute mitral valve regurgitation
- Postoperative low cardiac output states
- Preoperative use in high-risk coronary artery surgery
- Refractory left ventricular failure
- Cardiogenic shock
- Impending myocardial infarction

Contraindications for the use of an intra-aortic balloon pump include:

- Severe aortic regurgitation
- Severe calcific aorto-iliac disease
- Severe peripheral vascular disease
- Aortic dissection

Mechanics of the pump

A catheter is inserted through the femoral artery using a Seldinger technique. The tip of the balloon is placed about 2 cm distal to left subclavian artery. The balloon pump timing is triggered from the ECG or arterial wave form. Inflation occurs at the peak of the T wave at the end of systole. Deflation occurs just before the R wave. Correct timing of inflation and deflation is essential for optimum diastolic augmentation. Factors that reduce stroke volume also lower diastolic augmentation.

Complications of an intra-aortic balloon pump include:

- Limb ischaemia
- Bleeding at insertion site
- Thromboembolism
- Balloon leak
- Thrombocytopenia
- Infection
- Aortic dissection

Infective endocarditis

Infective endocarditis results from bacterial infection of the endothelial surface of the heart. It produces characteristic vegetations consisting of platelets, fibrin and bacteria. Predisposing factors include:

- Rheumatic valve disease
- Degenerative heart disease
- Mitral valve prolapse
- Congenital heart disease
- Hypertrophic cardiomyopathy
- Intravenous drug abuse
- Prosthetic valve

Native-valve endocarditis often occurs as a complication of central venous catheter infection. Prosthetic-valve endocarditis accounts for 10% cases of infective endocarditis. The greatest risk is during the first 6 months after surgery. MRSA is responsible for most cases seen in the first year.

Microbiology

The relative proportions of infecting organisms depends on the underlying valve disease. Native-valve endocarditis is usually caused by:

- viridans streptococci
- Streptococcus bovis
- Staphylococcus aureus
- enterococci
- Gram-negative coccobacilli

Clinical features

The clinical presentation of endocarditis can be varied. At one extreme there is acute systemic toxicity with rapid progression to cardiac complications. At the other extreme there is an indolent low-grade febrile illness with minimal cardiac dysfunction. About 90% patients have a fever and 85% have a murmur, usually that of underlying cardiac lesion.

About 10–40% have a changing murmur. Peripheral signs are rare.

Investigation

Almost 95% of patients will have positive blood cultures. Echocardiography allows visualisation of vegetations and the detection of cardiac complications. Transthoracic echocardiography has a low sensitivity but high specificity. Transoesophageal echocardiography has a higher sensitivity.

Duke's Clinical Criteria

The diagnosis of infective endocarditis by the Duke's Clinical Criteria (**Table 9.2**) requires the presence of:

- Two major criteria or
- One major and three minor criteria or
- Five minor criteria

Management

The optimal antibiotic therapy for infective endocarditis depends on the infecting organism. Parenteral therapy is required to ensure bactericidal concentrations.

When empirical treatment is necessary, it is important to consider the risk factors for certain organisms and local bacterial resistance patterns. Microbiological investigation needs to determine the antibiotic sensitivities and the minimum inhibitory concentrations. Indications for surgical intervention include:

- Moderate-to-severe heart failure as a result of valvular dysfunction
- Partial dehiscence of a prosthetic valve
- Persistent bacteraemia despite optimal antimicrobial therapy
- Absence of effective bactericidal treatment
- Fungal infective endocarditis
- Relapse of prosthetic-valve endocarditis
- *Staphylococcus aureus* prosthetic-valve endocarditis

Aortic dissection

Aortic dissection is the commonest aortic emergency. The incidence is twice that of ruptured abdominal aortic aneurysm. It is rare less than 40 years of age and is most

Duke's Clinical Criteria for the diagnosis of infective endocarditis	
Major criteria	**Minor criteria**
Positive blood cultures	Predisposing heart condition or intravenous drug abuse
Evidence of endocardial involvement	Fever (more than 38.0°C)
	Vascular phenomenon
	Major arterial emboli
	Septic pulmonary infarcts
	Mycotic aneurysm
	Intracranial haemorrhage
	Conjunctival haemorrhages
	Immunological phenomenon
	Glomerulonephritis
	Osler nodes
	Roth spots
	Microbiological evidence (but less than major criteria)
	Echocardiographic findings (but not meeting major criteria)

Table 9.2 Duke's Clinical Criteria for the diagnosis of infective endocarditis

commonly seen between 50 and 70 years. The male:female ratio is equal and it is associated with hypertension, Marfan's syndrome and bicuspid aortic valves.

Pathology

An intimal tear results in blood splitting the aortic media. This produces a false lumen that can progress in an antegrade or retrograde direction. Rupture can occur back into the lumen or externally in to the pericardium or mediastinum. External rupture often results in fatal pericardial tamponade. The commonest site of the intimal tear is within 2-3 cm of the aortic valve. It is also seen in the descending aorta distal to the left subclavian artery. Dissection can result in occlusion of aortic branches and the most commonly involved are the renal, spinal, coronary or iliac arteries.

Classification

Two classifications systems are in common use (**Figure 9.7**). The Stanford classification divides dissections into Type A and B depending on whether the ascending or descending aorta is involved. The DeBakey divides dissections into Types I to III.

Clinical features

Aortic dissection usually presents with tearing chest pain radiating to the back, often associated with an episode of collapse. Examination may show reduced or absent peripheral pulses and a soft early diastolic murmur. If aortic branches are occluded there may clinical evidence of acute renal failure, paraplegia, acute limb ischaemia, cerebrovascular accident or an inferior myocardial infarction.

Investigation

A chest x-ray usually shows a widened mediastinum. The diagnosis can be confirmed by echocardiogram or CT scanning.

Management

All patients require urgent management of any associated hypertension. Type A dissections usually require surgical intervention. Surgery is performed via a median sternotomy and on cardiopulmonary bypass. The dissection is excised and the aorta replaced with a graft. The aortic valve is preserved if possible. An evolving CVA or established renal

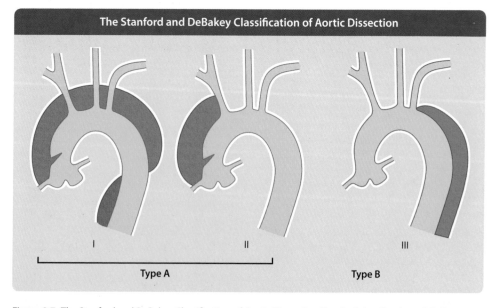

Figure 9.7 The Stanford and DeBakey Classification of Aortic Dissection. Stanford classification = I, II, III. DeBakey Classification = A and B

failure are contraindications to surgery. Without operation the prognosis for Type A dissections is poor with about 40% dying within 24 hours and 80% dying within 2 weeks. Operative mortality is approximately 25%. Type B dissections may be treated without surgery but requires fastidious blood pressure control. Surgery should be considered if there is evidence of aortic expansion. Surgery for Type B dissections is associated with significant risk of paraplegia.

Thoracic disease

Thoracic trauma

Thoracic trauma accounts for only 5% of admissions to a trauma centre but is second only to head injury as the commonest cause of death. The mortality for isolated thoracic trauma is 5% but approaches 35% in those with concomitant abdominal or head injuries.

Chest injuries detected during the primary survey include:

- Airway obstruction
- Tension pneumothorax
- Open pneumothorax
- Massive haemothorax
- Flail chest
- Cardiac tamponade

Chest injuries detected during the secondary survey include:

- Pulmonary contusion
- Myocardial contusion
- Aortic disruption
- Traumatic diaphragmatic hernia
- Tracheobronchial disruption
- Oesophageal disruption

Management of the unstable patient

Indications for an emergency room thoracotomy are:

- Acute pericardial tamponade unresponsive to cardiac massage
- Exsanguinating intra-thoracic haemorrhage
- Intra-abdominal haemorrhage requiring aortic cross clamping
- Need for internal cardiac massage

Indications for urgent thoracotomy are:

- Chest drainage with more than 1500 mL or more than 200 mL per hour
- Large unevacuated clotted haemothorax
- Developing cardiac tamponade
- Chest wall defect
- Massive air leak despite adequate drainage
- Proven great vessel injury on angiography
- Proven oesophageal injury
- Proven diaphragmatic laceration
- Traumatic septal or valvular injury of the heart

Haemothorax

A haemothorax is common after both penetrating and blunt trauma. Each pleural cavity can hold up to 3 litres of blood and 1 litre may easily accumulate before becoming apparent on a chest x-ray. About 90% of cases of haemothorax are due to injury to internal mammary or intercostal vessels. The remaining 10% occur due to bleeding from the pulmonary vasculature. The bleeding usually stops when the lung is re-expanded and most require no more than simple chest drainage.

Pericardial tamponade

Pericardial tamponade is a major complication of penetrating chest trauma. A haemopericardium prevents diastolic filling of the heart. The classic signs of pericardial tamponade are the Beck's triad of:

- Hypotension
- Venous distension
- Muffled heart sounds

Pericardial tamponade may be associated with pulsus paradoxus – an exaggerated drop in systemic blood pressure during inspiration. A chest x-ray shows a globular heart. An unstable patient requires urgent thoracotomy. In a stable patient, the diagnosis can be confirmed by echocardiography or pericardiocentesis. Subxiphoid pericardiotomy is both a diagnostic and therapeutic procedure.

Cardiac stab wounds

With cardiac stab wounds, the right side of the heart is more commonly injured than the left.

Patients with a right ventricular wound are more like to survive than with left-sided injury. The atria, inflow and outflow tracts may also be damaged. Patients usually present with pericardial tamponade and treatment consists of resuscitation and pericardiocentesis. Stab wounds can be accessed via a median sternotomy and can be directly repaired without cardiopulmonary bypass. Teflon-pledgeted prolene sutures are generally used.

Injuries to the great vessels

Injury to the great vessels should be suspected from the mechanism or site of penetrating injury. The patient usually presents with shock or pericardial tamponade. A chest x-ray may show:

- Widening of the mediastinum to greater than 8 cm
- Depression of the left main bronchus to greater than 140 degrees
- Haematoma in the left apical area
- Massive left haemothorax
- Deviation of oesophagus to the right
- Loss of the aortic knob contour
- Loss of the paraspinal pleural stripe

Injury to the great vessels requires an emergency thoracotomy or sternotomy. Injuries to the descending thoracic aorta requires left anterior thoracotomy. Injuries to the proximal aorta and proximal carotid arteries require median sternotomy.

Flail chest

A flail chest is associated with multiple rib fractures on the same side. The flail segment does not have continuity with the remainder of the thoracic cage and results in paradoxical chest wall movement with respiration. It is often associated with an underlying pulmonary contusion. Paradoxical movement results in impaired ventilation and the work of breathing is increased. Ventilation-perfusion mismatch and arterio-venous shunting occurs. A chest x-ray will show:

- Multiple rib fractures
- Underlying lung contusion
- Haemopneumothorax
- Other associated injuries

Treatment of a flail chest requires:

- Adequate ventilation
- Humidified oxygen
- Adequate analgesia

Consideration should be given to intubation and ventilation if:

- Significant other injuries
- Respiratory rate more than 35 per min
- Partial pressure oxygen less than 8.0 kPa
- Partial pressure carbon dioxide greater than 6.6 kPa
- Vital capacity less than 12 mL/kg
- Right to left shunt of more than 15%

Operative fixation is not normally required.

Chest drains

A chest drain is a conduit to remove air or fluid from the pleural cavity. The fluid can be blood, pus or a pleural effusion. It also allows re-expansion of the underlying lung. It must prevent entry of air or drained fluid back into the chest. A chest drain must therefore have three components:

- An unobstructed chest drain
- A collecting container below chest level
- A one-way mechanism such as a water seal or Heimlich valve

Drainage occurs during expiration when the pleural pressure is positive. Fluid from within pleural cavity drains into the water seal. Air also bubbles through water seal to the outside world. The length of drain below the fluid level is important. If greater than 2–3 cm, it increases the resistance to air drainage (**Figure 9.8**).

Indications for chest drain insertion include:

- Pneumothorax
- Malignant pleural effusion
- Empyema and complicated parapneumonic pleural effusion
- Traumatic haemopneumothorax
- Post thoracotomy, oesophagectomy and cardiac surgery

Insertion

Unless performed in an emergency situation, then a pre-procedure chest x-ray should be performed. The drain is usually inserted under local anaesthesia using an aseptic technique.

Principles of a chest drain

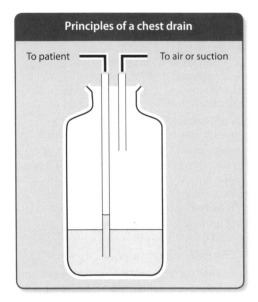

To patient ——— ⎡ ⎤ ——— To air or suction

Figure 9.8 Principles of a chest drain.

It should be inserted in the 5th intercostal space in the mid-axillary line. It should be inserted over the upper border of the rib to avoid the intercostal vessels and nerves. Blunt dissection and insertion of a finger through the wound should ensure that pleural cavity is entered. It used to be taught that to drain fluid it should be inserted towards the base of pleural cavity and to drain air it should be inserted towards the apex of the lung. It probably does not matter provided there is no loculation of fluid within pleural cavity. A large drain (28 Fr or above) should be used to drain blood or pus. The drain should be anchored and a purse-string or Z-stitch inserted in anticipation of removal. Complications of chest drains are shown in **Table 9.3**.

Removal

A chest drain should be removed as soon as it has served it purpose. For a simple pneumothorax it can often be removed within 24 hours. To remove the drain, ask the patient to perform a Valsalva manoeuvre and remove drain at the height of expiration. The pre-inserted purse-string or Z-stitch can then be tied. A post-procedure chest x-ray should be performed to exclude a pneumothorax.

Dos and don'ts of chest drains include:

- Avoid clamping of the drain as it can result in a tension pneumothorax
- The drain should only be clamped when changing the bottle
- Always keep the drain below the level of the patient. If lifted above chest level contents of drain can siphon back into chest
- If disconnection occurs reconnect and ask the patient to cough
- If a persistent air leak occurs consider low pressure suction
- Observe for post-expansion pulmonary oedema

Complications of chest drains

Early	Late
Haemothorax	Blocked drain
Lung laceration	Retained haemothorax
Diaphragm and abdominal cavity penetration	Empyema
Bowel injury in the presence of unrecognised diaphragmatic hernia	Pneumothorax after removal
Tube placed subcutaneously	
Tube inserted too far	
Tube displaced	

Table 9.3 Complications of chest drains

Lung cancer

Epidemiology

Lung cancer is the leading cause of cancer-related deaths in the Western world. About 40,000 cases are diagnosed in the UK each year resulting in 29,000 deaths. It is the commonest malignancy in men and second commonest malignancy in women. In the 1950s, the male:female ratio was 6:1 but with decreasing male and increasing female incidence rates, the ratio is now almost equal. Overall, 5-year survival is about 6%.

Aetiology

Smoking is the primary risk factor and is responsible for 85% cases in UK. The incidence of lung cancer is related to the number of cigarettes smoked. Other risk factors include:

- Passive smoking
- Environmental and occupational hazards
- Diet
- Genetic factors

Pathology

Lung cancers can be classified as either small cell (20%) or non-small cell (80%) carcinomas. The non-small cell tumours can be subdivided into squamous cell carcinomas (30%), adenocarcinomas (35%) and large cell carcinomas (15%). Adenocarcinoma are found peripherally in the lung and lymph node metastases are common. Squamous cell carcinoma are found centrally near the hilum or the major bronchi. They are often locally invasive. Large cell tumours are usually peripherally located. They are poorly differentiated tumours and may cavitate. They spread early to distant sites. Small cell tumours are usually centrally located. They can produce neuroendocrine hormones and may result in paraneoplastic syndromes.

Clinical features

Symptoms that may suggest a diagnosis of lung cancer include:

- Dyspnoea
- Haemoptysis
- Chronic coughing or change in regular coughing pattern
- Wheezing
- Chest pain
- Cachexia, fatigue, and loss of appetite
- Dysphonia
- Clubbing of the fingernails
- Dysphagia

Investigation

Investigation of potential lung cancers include imaging and endoscopy. Useful radiological investigations include a chest x-ray, high-resolution thoracic CT, positron emission tomography and MRI. Endoscopic and invasive procedures include bronchoscopy, CT-guided percutaneous needle biopsy, mediastinoscopy and endoscopic ultrasound.

Staging of lung cancer:

- **Stage 1** – Tumour is found only in one lung and has not spread to the lymph nodes
- **Stage 2** – Tumour is found only in one lung and has spread to the lymph nodes
- **Stage 3a** – The tumour has spread to the lymph nodes outside of the lung, including the chest wall and diaphragm on the same side as the cancer
- **Stage 3b** – The tumour has spread to the lymph nodes on the opposite lung or in the neck
- **Stage 4** – The tumour has spread to other parts of the lungs or distant metastases present

Management

The aims of evaluating a patient with suspected lung cancer are to determine:

- Cell type of the tumour
- Anatomical extent of the disease
- Functional status of the patient

Only surgery can cure non-small cell lung cancer but only 25% patients have potentially resectable disease at presentation. If a patient is considered for surgical intervention, preoperative assessment requires assessment of:

- Pulmonary function
- Cardiac status
- Nutritional and performance status

Pulmonary complications are the commonest cause of postoperative morbidity and mortality and assessment of respiratory reserve is important. Pulmonary function tests are essential before surgery. Full respiratory assessment includes:

- Spirometry and peak flows
- Estimation of transfer factor
- Postoperative lung function prediction using anatomical equations
- Quantitative isotope perfusions scans

An FEV_1 and transfer factor less than 40% places a patient in the high-risk group

Surgery

Lung resection is the best treatment for Stage 1 and 2 disease. Most patients with small-cell cancer are not suitable for surgery. Five-year survival decreases with the extent of the disease. The aims of surgery are complete resection of the tumour and intrapulmonary lymphatics. This can be achieved with:

- Pulmonary lobectomy
- Pneumonectomy
- Sublobar resections
- Bronchoplastic resections

The mortality from a lobectomy is 2–4%. The mortality from pneumonectomy is 6–8%

Thoracotomy

Thoracotomy allows access to the chest cavity. The position of the incision depends on the intended operation or procedure. Two different approaches exist – lateral thoracotomy or median sternotomy. Lateral thoracotomy can be carried out in three different positions – posterolateral, anterolateral or lateral/axillary. Median sternotomy allows access to the anterior and superior mediastinum. The sternum is divided with an oscillating or Gigli saw or Lebsche knife. Ooze from the bone marrow may be stopped with bone wax. The sternum is usually closed with steel wire.

Complications of thoracic operations

Intrathoracic bleeding

Intrathoracic bleeding usually occurs from the lung parenchyma or bronchial vessels. It may present with clinical features of hypovolaemia but is usually apparent from mediastinal or pleural drains. Drains may however block and a haemothorax may only be detected on a chest x-ray. It can often be treated conservatively with transfusion. Reoperation is required if:

- Rapid blood loss via chest drain
- Significant intrapleural collection on a chest x-ray
- Persistent hypovolaemia despite transfusion
- Hypoxia due to compression of the underlying lung

Sputum retention and atelectasis

Failure to clear bronchial secretions can result in bronchial obstruction, atelectasis, lobar collapse and secondary pulmonary infection. It usually presents with tachypnoea and hypoxia. Examination usually shows reduced bilateral basal air entry. Prevention is preferred to treatment. The risk of sputum retention can be reduced by:

- Preoperative cessation of smoking
- Adequate postoperative pain relief
- Chest physiotherapy
- Humidification of inspired oxygen
- Bronchodilator therapy
- Early mobilisation after surgery

Treatment requires formal chest physiotherapy. Mini-tracheostomy and suction may be required. Antibiotics should be reserved for those with proven pneumonia.

Air leak

Following lung resection, the residual lung tissue usually expands to fill the pleural cavity. A raw area can result in an air leak into the pleural cavity which presents as persist air leak or bubbling of a chest drain. It usually settles spontaneously over 2–3 days but may require suction to be applied to pleural drains. Apposition of the lung to the parietal pleura encourages efficient healing.

Bronchopleural fistula

A bronchopleural fistula results from major air leak from a post-pneumonectomy bronchial stump. It is seen in about 2% of patients undergoing pneumonectomy. The airway directly communicates with pleural space. It usually occurs as a result of a leak from a suture line and is particularly seen in those with factors impairing wound healing. It most commonly occurs 7–10 days after surgery. It presents with sudden breathlessness and expectoration of bloodstained fluid. The fluid is that which normally fills the postpneumonectomy space. Emergency treatment consists of lying the patient with the operated side downwards. Oxygen should be administered and a pleural drain inserted. Thoracotomy and repair of the fistula may be required. The repair may be reinforced with an omental or intercostal muscle patch. A thoracoplasty may be necessary to obliterate the postpneumonectomy space.

Pneumothorax

Pneumothorax is the presence of air within the pleural space usually due to disruption of the parietal, visceral or mediastinal pleura. The classification of pneumothoraces is shown in **Table 9.4**. A tension pneumothorax occurs when the pleura forms a 'one-way' flap valve. Tension pneumothorax is a medical emergency.

Primary spontaneous pneumothorax

Primary spontaneous pneumothorax usually occurs in healthy young adult men. Approximately 85% of patients are less than 40 years of age. The male:female ratio is 6:1 and in 10% of cases they are bilateral. It usually occurs as result of rupture of an acquired subpleural bleb. Blebs have no epithelial lining and arise from rupture of the alveolar wall. Apical blebs are found in 85% of patients undergoing thoracotomy. The frequency of spontaneous pneumothorax increases after each episode and most recurrences occur within 2 years of the initial event.

Secondary spontaneous pneumothorax

Secondary spontaneous pneumothorax accounts for 10–20% of spontaneous pneumothoraces due to:

- Chronic obstructive pulmonary disease with bulla formation
- Interstitial lung disease
- Primary and metastatic neoplasms
- Ehlers–Danlos syndrome
- Marfan's syndrome

Traumatic pneumothorax

Traumatic pneumothorax results from either blunt or penetrating trauma. Tracheobronchial and oesophageal injuries can cause both mediastinal emphysema and a pneumothorax. Iatrogenic pneumothorax is common and occurs after:

- Pneumonectomy
- Thoracocentesis
- High-pressure mechanical ventilation
- Subclavian venous cannulation

Clinical features of pneumothorax

The predominant symptom is acute pleuritic chest pain. Dyspnoea results from pulmonary

Classification of a pneumothorax	
Spontaneous	**Traumatic**
Primary – no identifiable pathology	Blunt or penetrating thoracic trauma
Secondary – underlying pulmonary disorder	Iatrogenic
	Postoperative
	Mechanical ventilation
	Thoracocentesis
	Central venous cannulation

Table 9.4 Classification of a pneumothorax

compression. Symptoms are proportional to the size of the pneumothorax and also depends on the degree of pulmonary reserve. Physical signs include tachypnoea with increased resonance and absent breath sounds on the affected side. In a tension pneumothorax, the patient may be hypotensive with acute respiratory distress, the trachea may be shifted away from the affected side and the neck veins may be engorged. Tension pneumothorax is a clinical diagnosis. In other cases the diagnosis can be confirmed with a chest x-ray.

Investigation

A chest x-ray will confirm the diagnosis (**Figure 9.9**). This usually shows radiolucency and absence of the lung vascular markings on the affected side. There may be mediastinal shift and the percentage volume of the pneumothorax can be calculated. The cause of the pneumothorax, such as fractured ribs, may also be visible.

Management

Spontaneous pneumothorax

The management of a spontaneous pneumothorax depends the symptoms and the radiological size of the pneumothorax. Small asymptomatic pneumothoraces may simply be followed up with serial chest x-rays. If drainage is required, a chest drain should be inserted through the 5th intercostal space, just above the upper border of the rib. Blunt insertion should be used and the position of the drain should be checked with a chest x-ray. It should be connected to an underwater seal, placed below the level of the patient.

Tension pneumothorax

Prophylactic chest drains should be inserted in patients with rib fractures prior to ventilation to reduce the risk of a tension pneumothorax. Tension pneumothorax requires immediate needle aspiration. A canula should be inserted anteriorly through the 2nd intercostal space prior to chest drain placement.

Surgery

Surgery is required for a pneumothorax if an air leak persists for more than 10 days, there is failure of lung re-expansion, or for a recurrent spontaneous pneumothorax. The surgical options include:

- Partial pleurectomy
- Operative abrasion of pleural lining
- Resection of pulmonary bullae

Figure 9.9 Chest x-ray showing a right spontaneous pneumothorax

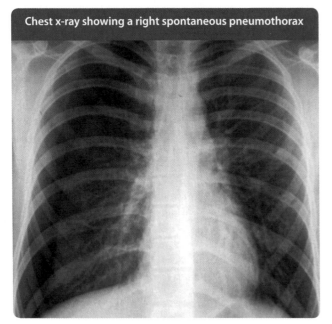

Chest x-ray showing a right spontaneous pneumothorax

Poor-risk patients may benefit from chemical pleurodesis with tetracycline.

Pneumonia, lung abscess and empyema

Lung abscess

Some patients with pneumonia develop focal necrosis and a lung abscess. This particularly occurs in patients with malignancy and malnutrition. It can also occur following aspiration or inhalation of a foreign body. The diagnosis can be difficult.

Clinical features

Patients usually present with clinical features of a pneumonia that fails to improve with antibiotics. They can develop pleuritic chest pain and haemoptysis. The volume of sputum produced may increase. Patients are usually systemically unwell with a swinging pyrexia. Examination usually shows signs of pneumonia. The commonest complication is an empyema. The differential diagnosis includes:

- Primary lung neoplasm
- Tuberculosis
- Aspergillosis
- Lung cyst

Investigation

A chest x-ray may show a pulmonary cavity with air/fluid level. CT scanning will confirm the diagnosis if a chest x-ray is inconclusive. Bronchoscopy should be considered to exclude a foreign body.

Management

Initial management should include appropriate antibiotic therapy based on sputum culture results. Percutaneous aspiration should be considered if the abscess fails to improve with antibiotic therapy. For abscesses greater than 5 cm diameter, open drainage may be required. Thoracotomy and lung resection should be considered in complicated cases.

Empyema

Empyema is defined as pus within a body cavity. A lung empyema usually occurs secondary to pneumonia. The collection is often multiloculated. Lung empyemas are also seen following oesophageal perforation or rupture, blunt or penetrating thoracic trauma, nasopharyngeal sepsis that has spread to the chest and thoracic surgical procedures. If the diagnosis is delayed, the empyema will develop a thick, fibrous wall making future management more difficult.

Clinical features

An empyema usually presents with features of pneumonia that fails to improve with antibiotics. There is often pleuritic chest pain and breathlessness. Examination may show features of pleural effusion.

Investigation

A chest x-ray will show fluid within the pleural cavity and a CT scan will confirm the diagnosis. Percutaneous aspiration will provide microbiological samples for culture.

Management

Appropriate antibiotic therapy should be given based on sputum culture results. Pleural drainage should be with adequate (28 Fr) chest drain. Thoracoscopy may be required to break down loculi. Decortication of the visceral and parietal pleura may be required to allow lung expansion. Following surgery, adequate drainage is required. Pneumothorax is not a risk due to the resulting pleural scarring.

Bronchiectasis

Bronchiectasis is chronic bronchial dilatation with parenchymal infection and an inflammatory reaction. It typically affects the basal segments of the lower lobes. Acquired infections are the most common cause, typically when occurring in childhood. Congenital causes include:

- Cystic fibrosis
- Kartagener syndrome
- Various immunodeficiency disorders
- Bronchopulmonary sequestration

Clinical features

The clinical features of bronchiectasis are recurrent pneumonia, a persistent cough and copious foul smelling sputum. Haemoptysis is common in adults but rare in children.

Investigation

A chest x-ray may show a typical 'honeycomb' pattern. Microbiological studies typically show *Haemophilus influenza*, *Escherichia coli* or *Klebsiella* as the causative agents. High resolution thoracic CT has replaced bronchography as the investigation of choice. Bronchoscopy may be required to rule out an obstruction lesion and allow pulmonary lavage.

Management

Medical therapy is the primary approach, using antibiotics, humidification and bronchodilators. Surgical intervention is indicated for:

- Failure of medical management
- Persistent symptoms
- Recurrent pneumonias
- Haemoptysis

The ideal surgical candidate has unilateral disease confined to one lobe. Most patients have bilateral disease. Surgery should be reserved for localised disease, operating on the worst side first.

Thymoma

The thymus is a lymphoid organ located in the anterior mediastinum composed of epithelial cells and lymphocytes. It is responsible for maturation of cell-mediated immunity and reaches maximum size at puberty. It regresses in later life.

Pathology

Thymoma is the most common neoplasm of the anterior mediastinum and accounts for 25% of all mediastinal tumours. The peak incidence is between 40 and 50 years of age. It originates from epithelial cells of the thymus gland. No clear aetiological factors have been defined. It is associated with the development of myaesthenia gravis. No clear distinction between benign and malignant tumours exist. Malignant tumours can invade the vasculature and adjacent structures. Death often occurs from cardiac tamponade or cardiorespiratory complications.

Clinical features

Almost 50% of thymomas are asymptomatic but 30% present with local symptoms related to encroachment on adjacent structures. It may present with a cough, chest pain or superior vena cava compression. About 20% are identified during the investigation of myaesthenia gravis.

Investigation

Most thymomas are visible on chest x-ray and CT may be used to delineate the mass further. Contrast-enhancement is useful in defining vascularity and the extent of invasion. The diagnosis can be confirmed by biopsy taken at anterior mediastinoscopy. The Masaoka staging system is as follows:

- Stage 1 – Encapsulated tumour with no gross or microscopic invasion
- Stage 2 – Macroscopic invasion into mediastinal fat or pleura
- Stage 3 – Invasion of pericardium, great vessels or lung
- Stage 4 – Pleural or pericardial metastatic spread
- Stage 5 – Lymphatic or haematogenous spread

Management

Treatment depends on the stage of the disease. Stage 1 disease can be managed by complete surgical excision. Stages 2 and 3 disease requires surgical excision and postoperative radiotherapy. Stages 4 and 5 disease requires surgical debulking, radiotherapy and chemotherapy.

Thymectomy

The initial management of most thymomas is by surgery, usually performed via a median sternotomy. Resection may require excision *en-bloc* of any involved pericardium, pleura and phrenic nerves. If possible, damage to the phrenic nerves should be avoided. Clips should be placed to aide subsequent radiotherapy planning. Prognosis is worse for symptomatic thymomas. The most important factor that determines prognosis is invasion of adjacent structures. Stage 1 disease is associated with greater than 90% 5-year survival. Stage 4 disease is associated with less than 25% 5-year survival.

Abdominal trauma

Assessment of abdominal trauma

Assessment of patients with abdominal trauma can be difficult due to altered sensorium (head injury, alcohol), altered sensation (spinal cord injury) and injury to adjacent structures (pelvis, chest). The pattern of injury will be different between penetrating and blunt trauma. Indications for laparotomy without extensive investigation include:

- Unexplained shock
- Rigid silent abdomen
- Evisceration
- Radiological evidence of intraperitoneal gas
- Radiological evidence of ruptured diaphragm
- Gunshot wounds
- Positive result on peritoneal lavage

Imaging

Either CT or ultrasound can be used for the assessment of abdominal trauma. CT scanning is the preferred method but does require the patient to be cardiovascularly stable. Ultrasound has high specificity but low sensitivity for the detection of free fluid or visceral damage. Focused assessment for the sonographic assessment of trauma (FAST) is the use of ultrasound to rapidly assess for intraperitoneal fluid. The ultrasound probe is placed on the right upper quadrant, left upper quadrant and suprapubic region to detect fluid in the subphrenic or subhepatic spaces or pouch of Douglas in a hypotensive patient. It can be used to confirm the likely need for an emergency laparotomy.

Peritoneal lavage

With the more ready availability of abdominal CT scanning, then the use of peritoneal lavage is falling. Indications for peritoneal lavage include:

- Equivocal clinical examination
- Difficulty in assessing patient – alcohol, drugs, head injury etc
- Persistent hypotension despite adequate fluid resuscitation
- Multiple injuries
- Stab wounds where the peritoneum is breached

Prior to the procedure, it is important to ensure that a urinary catheter and nasogastric tube are in place. Under local anaesthesia, a sub-umbilical incision is made down to the linea alba. The peritoneum is incised and a peritoneal dialysis catheter is inserted. The catheter is aspirated and any free blood or enteric contents is noted. If no blood is aspirated, then 1 L of normal saline is infused and left in the peritoneal cavity for 3 minutes. A drainage bag is attached to the catheter and the bag placed on the floor and allowed to drain. A 20 mL sample of the fluid is sent to the laboratory for measurement of RBC, WCC and microbiological examination. A positive result is regarded as:

- Red cell count more than $100,000/\text{mm}^3$
- White cell count more than $500/\text{mm}^3$
- The presence of bile, bacteria or faecal material

Damage control surgery

Following multiple trauma, a poor outcome is seen in those with hypothermia, coagulopathy and severe acidosis. Prolonged surgery can exacerbate these factors. As a result the concept of 'damage control' surgery has been developed. Damage control surgery should be considered if a patient with multiple trauma has an Injury Severity Score greater than 25, core temperature less than 34 degree or an arterial gas pH less than 7.1

Initial operation

The early surgical management of major abdominal trauma should aim to:

- Control haemorrhage with ligation of vessels and packing

- Remove dead tissue
- Control contamination with clamps and stapling devices
- Lavage the abdominal cavity
- Close the abdomen without tension

Options for temporary abdominal wound closure include:

- Skin-closure only
- Plastic sheet or 'Bogota bag'
- Absorbable mesh
- Non-absorbable mesh with protection of the underlying viscera

Intensive care unit

Early surgery should be followed by a period of stabilisation on the intensive care unit. During this period the following should be addressed:

- Rewarming
- Ventilation
- Restoration of perfusion
- Correction of deranged biochemistry
- Commence enteral or parenteral nutrition

Second look laparotomy

A further planned re-laparotomy should take place at 24–48 hours to allow:

- Removal of packs
- Removal of dead tissue
- Definitive treatment of injuries
- Restoration of intestinal continuity
- Closure of the musculofascial layers of the abdominal wall

This approach has been shown to be associated with a reduced mortality.

Gastrointestinal injury

Small bowel perforations can invariably be primarily closed. The management of colonic perforations is more controversial. It used to be common practice to excise the damaged segment and fashion a proximal stoma. The perforation could also be exteriorised as a stoma. It is increasingly recognised that primary repair of colonic injuries is safe and it is now the recommended method, especially in the absence of significant contamination.

Splenic injury

Splenic injury can be either accidental or iatrogenic. It is most commonly associated with blunt abdominal trauma and often occurs in the presence of lower rib fractures. It may become clinically apparent either early or late after injury. Delayed presentation is usually due to rupture of a subcapsular haematoma. About 20% of splenic injuries occur inadvertently during other abdominal operations. In some patients spontaneous rupture can occur following trivial trauma. In these situations, the spleen is invariably abnormal due to other pathology such as malaria or infectious mononucleosis.

Clinical features

The clinical features of splenic injury depend on the extent of the blood loss and the presence of associated injuries. The clinical presentation ranges from left upper quadrant pain with few clinical signs to shock and generalised peritonitis. About 30–60% of patients have other associated intraperitoneal injuries.

Investigation

Abdominal ultrasound will often show blood in the peritoneal cavity or a splenic haematoma. Accurate definition of the extent of splenic trauma requires a CT scan. The grading of splenic injuries is as follows:

- Grade 1 – Minor subcapsular tear or haematoma
- Grade 2 – Parenchymal injury not extending to the hilum
- Grade 3 – Major parenchymal injury involving vessels and the hilum
- Grade 4 – Shattered spleen

Management

If the patient is cardiovascularly unstable, they require resuscitation and early surgery. If the patient is cardiovascularly stable, then consideration can be given to CT scan and if an isolated Grade 1 or 2 splenic injury is identified, then consideration should be given to conservative management.

Surgical options

The surgical management of splenic injuries can involve either splenectomy or splenic repair. The main benefit of retaining the spleen is the prevention of overwhelming post-splenectomy infection (OPSI). If splenic conservation is attempted, it is necessary to preserve more than 20% of the spleen.

Conservative management

Overall 20–40% of patients are suitable for conservative management. In particular, children can often be managed conservatively as they have more low grade injuries and fewer multiple injuries. Patients require close cardiovascular and haematological monitoring preferably in a high dependency unit. Surgery is necessary if the patient becomes hypovolaemic or they have a falling haematocrit. Approximately 30% of patients fail conservative management. Failure usually occurs within the first 72 hours of injury. Failed conservative management often results in splenectomy and it has been argued that, overall, more spleens can often be conserved by early surgical intervention. If splenic conservation is successful, patients should remain on bed rest for 72 hours, have limited physical activity for 6 weeks and no contact sports for 6 months.

Liver injury

The liver is the second most commonly injured organ in abdominal trauma, but damage to the liver is the most common cause of death after abdominal injury. It is often associated with splenic injury and rib fractures. CT is the investigation of choice allowing grading of the extent of injury and detection of associated injuries. In the past, most of these injuries were treated surgically. However, as many as 90% of liver injuries have stopped bleeding by the time of operation. Angiography and embolisation may allow conservative management that previously would have come to operation.

Abdominal emergencies
Peritonitis

Intra-abdominal infection results in two major clinical manifestations. Early or diffuse infection results in localised or generalised peritonitis. Late and localised infections produce an intra-abdominal abscess. The pathophysiology depends on the competing factors of bacterial virulence and host defences. Bacterial peritonitis is classified as primary or secondary.

Primary peritonitis is diffuse bacterial infection without loss of integrity of gastrointestinal tract. It often occurs in adolescent girls. *Streptococcus pneumonia* is the commonest organism involved. Secondary peritonitis is acute peritoneal infection resulting from gastrointestinal perforation, anastomotic dehiscence or infected pancreatic necrosis. It often involves multiple organisms – both aerobes and anaerobes. The commonest responsible organisms are *Escherichia coli* and *Bacteroides fragilis*.

Management
The management of secondary peritonitis involves:

- Elimination of the source of infection
- Reduction of bacterial contamination of the peritoneal cavity
- Prevention of persistent or recurrent intra-abdominal infection

These should be combined with fluid resuscitation, antibiotics and intensive care management. Source control can achieved by closure or exteriorisation of perforation. Bacterial contamination can be reduced by aspiration of faecal matter and pus. Recurrent infection may be prevented by the used of drains, planned re-operations or leaving the wound open.

Peritoneal lavage
Peritoneal lavage with saline is often used during abdominal surgery, but its benefit is unproven. Simple swabbing of pus from the peritoneal cavity may be of similar value. It has been suggested that lavage may spread infection or damage the peritoneal surface. There is no benefit of adding antibiotics to lavage fluid. There is no benefit of adding chlorhexidine or iodine to lavage fluid. If used, lavage with large volume of crystalloid solution probably has the best outcome.

Intra-abdominal abscesses

An intra-abdominal abscess may arise following localisation of peritonitis, gastrointestinal perforation, an anastomotic leak or following haematogenous spread. They develop in sites of gravitational drainage such as the pelvis, subhepatic spaces, subphrenic spaces and paracolic gutters.

Clinical features

Postoperative abscesses usually present at between 5 and 10 days after surgery. Following gastrointestinal surgery, an intra-abdominal abscess should be suspected if there is an unexplained persistent or swinging pyrexia. It may also cause abdominal pain and diarrhoea. A mass may be present with overlying erythema and tenderness. A pelvic abscess may be palpable only on rectal examination.

Management

A contrast-enhanced CT is probably the investigation of choice. It will confirm the presence of an abscess or collection and may delineate a gastrointestinal or anastomotic leak. It may determine the possibility of percutaneous drainage. Operative drainage may be required if the there is a multi-locular abscess, there is no safe route for percutaneous drainage or if an abscess recollects after percutaneous drainage. Patients should receive antibiotic therapy guided by organism sensitivities.

Appendicitis

About 10% of the population will develop acute appendicitis at some stage in their lives. The incidence of appendicitis is falling but 70,000 appendicectomies are still performed each year in the UK. The peak incidence is between 10 and 15 years of age. Appendicitis is more common in men but appendicectomy is performed more often in women. In about 10% of operations a normal appendix is removed. A woman is more likely to have a normal appendix removed. The risk of perforation is highest at the extremes of age.

Anatomy

The appendix is about 5 cm long and arises from the caecum. Although the base has a fairly constant position, the tip can be located in the pelvis, behind the caecum or in the paracolic gutter. The anatomical position of the appendix determines the clinical presentation of acute appendicitis. The appendix is lined by colonic epithelium and the submucosa contains lymphoid follicles. These increase in number to a peak at 1–20 years of age and then subsequently decline.

Pathology

Acute appendicitis usually arises secondary to obstruction of the appendicular lumen. Obstruction is usually caused by lymphoid hyperplasia or faecoliths. It can also occur as a result of tumours or worms. Obstruction causes stasis and infection of the luminal contents. Increased pressure within the lumen causes venous congestion and thrombosis. Ischaemia can cause ulceration, necrosis and eventual perforation. The progression from obstruction to perforation usually takes about 72 hours. The degree of peritonitis depends on the ability of the omentum and adjacent bowel loops to contain the infection.

Clinical features

The typical clinical features of appendicitis are well described but the presentation can be atypical. Patients often have central abdominal pain that migrates to right iliac fossa. This may be associated with nausea, vomiting and anorexia. A low-grade pyrexia and tachycardia may be present. Patients appear flushed with fetor oris. Abdominal examination may show localised tenderness in the right iliac fossa with signs of right iliac fossa peritonism. Percussion tenderness is a kinder sign of peritonism to elicit than rebound tenderness. Rovsing's sign is pain in right iliac fossa during palpation in the left iliac fossa. At the time of diagnosis, the rate of perforation is about 20%. These patients usually present with signs of generalised peritonitis.

Causes of right iliac fossa pain include:

- Appendicitis
- Urinary tract infection
- Non-specific abdominal pain
- Pelvic inflammatory disease
- Renal colic
- Ectopic pregnancy
- Constipation

Causes of a right iliac fossa mass include:

- Appendix mass
- Crohn's disease
- Caecal carcinoma
- Mucocele of the gallbladder
- Psoas abscess
- Pelvic kidney
- Ovarian cyst

Investigation

Appendicitis is essentially a clinical diagnosis. Investigations are primarily used to exclude an alternative diagnosis. Urinalysis may exclude a urinary tract infection. A pregnancy test may be necessary to exclude an ectopic pregnancy. The serum white cell count and CRP may be increased. A normal white cell count does not exclude a diagnosis of acute appendicitis. A plain abdominal x-ray is of little value. An ultrasound may be helpful in the assessment of an appendix mass or abscess. An abdominal CT scan should be considered in adults if the diagnosis is unclear or if there is clinical suspicion of an appendix mass. Laparoscopy may be used as a diagnostic procedure as well as offering the opportunity to proceed to treatment.

Scoring systems

Scoring systems and computer-aided diagnosis have been developed and may be helpful. The Alvarado Scoring system is based on eight variables:

- Migration of pain to right iliac fossa
- Anorexia
- Nausea/vomiting
- Tenderness in the right iliac fossa
- Rebound pain
- Elevated temperature (more than 37.3°C)
- Leukocytosis (more than 10,000/µL)
- Left shift

A score of more than seven has both a sensitivity and specificity of 80% for the diagnosis of acute appendicitis. Meta-analysis has suggested that raised inflammatory markers, clinical signs of peritoneal irritation and migration of abdominal pain may be the most useful predictors of a diagnosis of acute appendicitis in patients with abdominal pain.

Management

In cases of diagnostic doubt, a period of 'active observation' is useful. Active observation reduces the negative appendicectomy rate without increasing the risk of perforation. Intravenous fluids and analgesia should be given. Opiate analgesia does not mask the signs of peritonism. Antibiotics should not be given until a decision to operate has been made.

Diagnostic laparoscopy may be considered particularly in young women.

Appendicectomy

Early appendicectomy for non-perforated appendicitis was first performed in the 1880s. Open appendicectomy is usually performed via a Lanz incision with a muscle splitting approach. Any pus found should be sent for microbiological assessment. Vessels in the mesoappendix should be ligated. The base of the appendix should then be ligated and the appendix excised. There is no evidence that burying the stump reduces the infection rate. A drain is not necessary unless there has been an appendicular abscess. Consideration should be given to a midline incision in elderly patients, particularly if the diagnosis is uncertain. Laparoscopic appendicectomy may be associated with reduced hospital stay and more rapid return to normal activity.

Appendix mass

An appendix mass, usually presents with a several day history of right iliac fossa pain. Inflammation is localised to the right iliac fossa by the omentum. The patient is usually pyrexial with a palpable mass. Initial treatment should be conservative with fluids, analgesia and antibiotics. The general condition of the patient and the size of the mass should be observed. Conservative management can continue whilst there is evidence of clinical improvement.

Appendix abscess

An appendix abscess results from localised perforation. The abscess should be surgically or percutaneously drained. Appendicectomy at initial operation can be difficult. The need for interval appendicectomy after an appendix abscess drainage is unclear. Often the appendix is destroyed when the abscess forms.

Perforated peptic ulcer

Several decades ago, perforated peptic ulcer was a common disease of young men but today it is mainly seen in elderly women. Overall, the number of admissions with peptic ulceration is falling. However, the number of perforated ulcers remains unchanged. The sustained incidence of perforation is possibly due to increased anti-inflammatory use in the elderly. About 80% of perforated duodenal ulcers are *Helicobacter pylori* positive.

Clinical features

Most perforated peptic ulcers occur in patients with pre-existing dyspepsia. Only about 10% of patients have no previous symptoms. The classic presentation is with sudden onset of epigastric pain with rapid generalisation. Examination shows generalised peritonitis with absent bowel sounds. About 10% patients have an associated episode of melaena.

Investigation

Free gas under the diaphragm on an erect chest x-ray is a classical radiological sign (**Figure 10.1**). However, 10% of patients have no demonstrable gas on a chest x-ray. If diagnostic doubt exists, then a CT scan will confirm a perforation even if it can not always show the site. Perforated peptic ulceration can be associated with elevated serum amylase but not to same level as in pancreatitis.

Management

Most patients require surgery after appropriate resuscitation. Conservative management may be considered if there is significant co-morbidity but this is more likely to fail if perforation is of a gastric ulcer. Fluid resuscitation with monitoring of the urine output is required. Analgesia and antibiotics should be administered and a nasogastric tube placed.

Following adequate resuscitation, the perforation should be oversewn with an

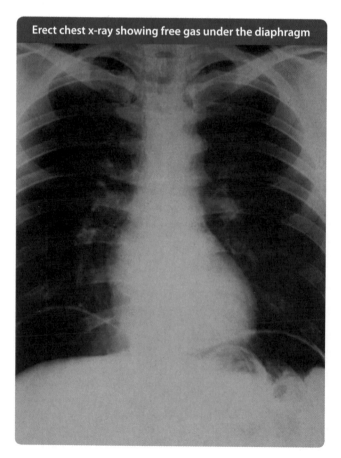

Erect chest x-ray showing free gas under the diaphragm

Figure 10.1 Erect chest x-ray showing free gas under the diaphragm.

omental patch. If the surgeon is unable to find the perforation, it is important to open the lesser sac. It should also be remembered that multiple perforations can occur. If closure is secure and adequate peritoneal lavage has been performed then a drain is not required.

Pre-pyloric gastric ulcers behave as duodenal ulcers. All gastric ulcers require biopsy to exclude malignancy. Definitive ulcer surgery is probably not required as 50% patients develop no ulcer recurrence. Postoperatively, patients should receive *Helicobacter pylori* eradication therapy. Surgery is increasingly performed laparoscopically and is associated with no increased morbidity and reduced hospital stay. The operative mortality depends on the time from perforation to admission, age, co-morbidity and the presence of hypovolaemia on admission.

Acute mesenteric ischaemia

Acute mesenteric ischaemia was first recognised by Virchow in 1852. It occurs as result of either superior mesenteric arterial or venous occlusion and can affect the bowel from the 2nd part of duodenum to the transverse colon. Embolic arterial occlusion, atheromatous arterial occlusion and venous thrombosis account for 50%, 25% and 10% of cases, respectively. Whatever the underlining aetiology, reduced capillary flow causes intestinal necrosis. Overall mortality is approximately 90%.

Clinical features
No single clinical feature provides conclusive evidence of the diagnosis. As a result, the diagnosis is difficult and often delayed. Early diagnosis requires a high index of suspicion. Severe central abdominal pain is a common presentation. The pain is often out of proportion to the apparent clinical signs. Vomiting and rectal bleeding may also occur. Features of chronic mesenteric ischaemia such a postprandial abdominal pain and weight loss may also be present. There may be evidence of an embolic source (e.g. recent myocardial infarct, cardiac arrhythmia) and there may be features of atherosclerotic disease with 75%, 25% and 10% of patients

having ischaemic heart, cerebrovascular and peripheral vascular disease respectively.

Investigation
No single investigation provides pathognomic evidence of mesenteric ischaemia. The serum white cell count is often raised. Arterial blood gases may show a metabolic acidosis. The serum amylase is raised in 50% of patients. An abdominal x-ray may be normal early in the disease process. Late radiological features include dilated small bowel and 'thumb printing' of the bowel wall due to mucosal oedema. Mesenteric angiography may confirm the diagnosis.

Management
Following angiography, a papaverine infusion into the superior mesenteric artery (SMA) may be beneficial. If this fails to rapidly improve symptoms, then laparotomy may be indicated. Surgery allows confirmation of diagnosis and assessment of the extent of ischaemia, the opportunity to revascularise the SMA if appropriate and to resect necrotic bowel. Revascularisation may be achieved by embolectomy, bypass or endarterectomy. Resection and primary anastomosis may be possible. If doubt exists over the bowel viability then a 'second-look' laparotomy may be considered. If there is extensive necrosis in an elderly patient, then palliative care may be the preferred option.

Upper gastrointestinal haemorrhage

Clinical features
The presentation of an upper gastrointestinal haemorrhage depends on the amount and location of bleeding but invariably it causes haematemesis, coffee ground vomiting or melaena. Patients may also present with complications of anaemia, including chest pain, syncope, fatigue and shortness of breath. Examination should assess the vital signs in order to determine the severity of the bleeding and the timing of intervention. Abdominal examination may be normal but there may be stigmata of chronic liver disease. Causes of upper gastrointestinal haemorrhage include:

- Peptic ulcer (50%)
- Gastric erosions
- Oesophageal or gastric varices
- Mallory–Weiss tear
- Angiodysplasia
- Dieulafoy malformation
- Gastric neoplasia

Initial management

Patients should be managed according to agreed multidisciplinary protocols. Close collaboration is required between physicians and surgeons. Aggressive fluid resuscitation is important. Circulating blood volume should be restored with colloid or crystalloid. Cross-matched blood should be given when available. All patients require closed monitoring, possibly in an intensive care environment with central and arterial pressure monitoring.

Bleeding peptic ulcer

Of all patients with a bleeding peptic ulcer, in about 80% the bleeding stops spontaneously. However, about 25% will require intervention for recurrent bleeding within 48 hours. It is difficult to predict those that will continue to bleed.

Management

All patients require early endoscopy to determine the site of bleeding and any continuing blood loss. Features of recent bleeding include:

- Ooze from ulcer base
- Clot covering ulcer base
- Black spot in ulcer base
- Visible vessel

Proton pump inhibitors may improve the outcome in acute non-variceal upper gastrointestinal haemorrhage. Endoscopic techniques to stop bleeding include:

- Laser photocoagulation using the Nd-YAG laser
- Bipolar diathermy
- Heat probes
- Adrenaline or sclerosant injection

No technique is superior.

Surgery

Indications for surgical intervention include:

- Continued bleeding that fails to respond to endoscopic measures
- Recurrent bleeding
- Patients more than 60 years
- Gastric ulcer bleeding
- Cardiovascular disease with predictive poor response to hypotension

For a bleeding duodenal ulcer, the surgical approach should involve the creation of a gastroduodenotomy between stay sutures. Bleeding is usually from the gastroduodenal artery which should be underun with a nonabsorbable suture on round-bodied needle. It is essential to avoid picking up common bile duct in the suture. The gastroduodenotomy can then be closed as a pyloroplasty. All patients should be given *Helicobacter pylori* eradication therapy postoperatively. If a pyloroplasty will be difficult because of large ulcer, consideration should be given to a Polya gastrectomy. For a bleeding gastric ulcer, either local resection of the ulcer or a partial gastrectomy may be appropriate.

Variceal upper gastrointestinal haemorrhage

Approximately 90% of patients with portal hypertension have oesophageal varices and 30% of patients with varices will have an upper gastrointestinal bleed at some time. About 80% of upper gastrointestinal bleeds in patients with portal hypertension are from varices but other causes do occur. The mortality following a variceal bleed is approximately 50% and of those who survive, 70% patients will have a rebleed. Survival is dependent on the degree of hepatic impairment.

Primary prevention

Bleeding from oesophageal varices is more likely if there is poor hepatic function or large varices. Primary prevention of bleeding is possible with β blockers which reduce the risk of haemorrhage by 40–50%. Band ligation may also be considered. Sclerotherapy or shunting is ineffective.

Active bleeding

In patients with presumed bleeding from oesophageal varices, resuscitation should be as for any other cause of upper gastrointestinal haemorrhage. Endoscopy should be performed to confirm the site of haemorrhage. Vasopressin and octreotide can be used to decrease both the splanchnic blood flow and portal pressure. Lactulose may also be used to decrease gastrointestinal transit and reduce ammonia absorption. Metronidazole and neomycin may be used to reduce gut flora.

Temporary tamponade can be achieved with a Sengstaken–Blakemore tube. It has three channels:

- One to inflate the gastric balloon
- One to inflate the oesophageal balloon
- One to aspirate the stomach

The use of a Sengstaken–Blakemore tube should be considered as a salvage procedure. Tamponade is 90% successful at stopping haemorrhage. Unfortunately, 50% patients rebleed within 24 hours of removal of the balloon.

Emergency endoscopic therapy is by either endoscopic banding of varices or intravariceal or paravariceal sclerotherapy. The sclerosants used include ethanolamine and sodium tetradecyl sulphate. If endoscopic methods fail, consideration needs to be given to oesophageal transection, devascularisation or porto-caval or mesenterico-caval shunting. Emergency shunting is associated with a 20% operative mortality and 50% risk of encephalopathy. Shunting can also be performed non-surgically by transjugular intrahepatic portosystemic shunting (TIPPS). It has a reduced risk of rebleeding but increases the risk of encephalopathy.

Secondary prevention

About 70% of patients with a variceal haemorrhage will rebleed. The following have been shown to be effective in the prevention of rebleeding:

- β-blockers possibly combined with isosorbide mononitrate
- Endoscopic ligation
- Sclerotherapy
- TIPSS
- Surgical shunting

Lower gastrointestinal haemorrhage

Lower gastrointestinal haemorrhage accounts for 20% cases of acute gastrointestinal bleeding. Most patients are elderly. Most cases settle spontaneously without the need for emergency surgery. Following investigation a cause of bleeding is often not found. Causes of lower gastrointestinal haemorrhage include:

- Diverticular disease
- Angiodysplasia
- Inflammatory bowel disease
- Ischaemic colitis
- Infective colitis
- Colorectal carcinoma

Angiodysplasia

Angiodysplasia is an acquired malformation of intestinal blood vessels seen in up to 25% of asymptomatic patients over the age of 75 years. It is an incidental finding during 5% of colonoscopies. About 80% lesions occur in the right side of the colon and are often associated with cardiac valvular disease. Dilated vessels or a 'cherry red' areas may be seen at colonoscopy. Early filling of the vessels is seen at angiography. Bleeding may be visible during the capillary phase of an angiogram.

Investigation

Most patients with lower gastrointestinal haemorrhage are cardiovascularly stable and can be investigated once the bleeding has stopped. In the actively bleeding patient, colonoscopy can be difficult and often incomplete examinations are performed. Selective mesenteric angiography may be helpful but to see active bleeding it requires continued blood loss of more than 1 mL/ minute. It may show angiodysplastic lesions even once the bleeding has ceased. Radionuclide scanning can be considered using technetium-99m labelled red blood cells.

Management

Acute bleeding tends to be self-limiting and most patients can be managed conservatively with intravenous fluids and blood transfusion, if required. If bleeding persists, an upper gastrointestinal endoscopy should be performed to exclude an upper gastrointestinal cause. In those patients with significant or ongoing bleeding, consideration should be given to a laparotomy and on-table lavage and panendoscopy. If right-sided angiodysplasia is confirmed, a right hemicolectomy is the operation of choice. If bleeding diverticular disease is likely, a sigmoid colectomy is the operation of choice. If the source of colonic bleeding is unclear a subtotal colectomy and end-ileostomy may be required.

Small bowel obstruction

Aetiology

Small bowel obstruction accounts for 5% of all acute surgical admissions. In the UK, the commonest causes of small bowel obstruction are:

- Adhesions (60%)
- Strangulated hernia (20%)
- Malignancy (5%)
- Volvulus (5%)

Pathophysiology

Dilatation of the bowel occurs above the level of the obstructing lesion. This results in the accumulation of gas and fluid and reduced fluid reabsorption. Dilation of the gut wall produces mucosal oedema. This initially impairs the venous and subsequently the arterial blood flow. Intestinal ischaemia eventually results in infarction and perforation of that segment of bowel. Ischaemia also results in bacterial and endotoxin translocation. The overall effect is progressive dehydration, electrolyte imbalance and systemic toxicity.

Clinical features

The cardinal clinical features of intestinal obstruction are:

- Colicky central abdominal pain
- Vomiting
- Abdominal distension
- Absolute constipation

Vomiting is an early feature of high obstruction. The degree of abdominal distension depends on the level of the obstruction. Distension may be minimal in high obstruction. Absolute constipation is a late feature of small bowel obstruction. Dehydration is associated with tachycardia, hypotension and oliguria. Features of peritonism indicate strangulation or perforation. Auscultation may show high-pitched or tinkling bowel sounds.

Investigation

A supine abdominal x-ray may show dilated small bowel. The valvulae coniventes differentiate the small from large intestine. An x-ray may be normal if there is no air–fluid interface. An erect abdominal film rarely provides additional information. A CT scan will confirm the diagnosis and may show the level and cause of the obstruction.

Management

Adequate resuscitation prior to surgery is vital. Patients may have severe dehydration and may require several litres of intravenous crystalloid. Adequacy of resuscitation should be judged by measurement of the urine output or assessment of the central venous pressure. Surgery in under-resuscitated patients is associated with increased mortality. If the cause of obstruction is presumed to be due to adhesions and there are no features of peritonism, then conservative management for up to 48 hours is often safe. Patients undergoing conservative management requires regular clinical review and the willingness to consider surgical intervention if conservative management fails. If there are features of peritonism or systemic toxicity present, then it is necessary to consider early operation. The exact procedure will depend on the underlying cause. Absolute indications for surgery include generalised or localised peritonitis, visceral perforation or the presence of an irreducible hernia. Relative indications include a palpable mass lesion, a 'virgin' abdomen or failure to improve with conservative management.

Paralytic ileus

Paralytic ileus is a functional obstruction most commonly seen after abdominal surgery. It is also associated with trauma, intestinal ischaemia and sepsis. The small bowel is distended throughout its length. Absorption of fluid, electrolytes and nutrients is impaired. Significant amounts of fluid may be lost from the extracellular compartment.

Clinical features

There is usually a history of recent operation or trauma. Abdominal distension is often apparent. Pain is often not a prominent feature. If no nasogastric tube is in situ, vomiting may occur. Large volume aspirates my occur via a nasogastric tube. Flatus will not be passed until resolution of the ileus. Auscultation will reveal absence of bowel sounds.

Investigation

A plain abdominal x-ray may show dilated loops of small bowel. Gas may be present in the colon. If doubt exists as to whether there is a mechanical or functional obstruction, then an abdominal CT scan or water soluble contrast study may be helpful.

Management

Prevention is better than cure. The bowel should be handled as little as possible at the time of surgery. Sources of sepsis should be eradicated. For an established ileus, then a nasogastric tube and fluid and electrolyte replacement are required. No drugs are available to reverse the condition. Paralytic ileus usually resolves spontaneously after 4 or 5 days.

Large bowel obstruction

In the UK, about of 15% colorectal cancers present with intestinal obstruction. Most patients are over 70 years of age. The risk of obstruction is greatest with left-sided colonic lesions. Obstructing tumours usually present at a more advanced stage and 25% have distant metastases at presentation. Intestinal perforation can occur at the site of the tumour or in a dilated caecum if there is closed-loop obstruction.

Clinical features

Caecal tumours present with small bowel obstruction

- Colicky central abdominal pain
- Early vomiting
- Late absolute constipation
- Variable extent of distension

Left-sided tumours present with large bowel obstruction

- Change in bowel habit
- Absolute constipation
- Abdominal distension
- Late vomiting

Investigation

A plain supine abdominal x-ray may show dilated large bowel. The small bowel may also be dilated depending on the competence of the ileocaecal valve. The additional value of erect film is debatable. If doubt exists over either the diagnosis or the site of obstruction, then an abdominal CT scan or a water soluble contrast enema may provide additional information.

Management

All patients with large bowel obstruction require adequate resuscitation and prophylactic antibiotics. They should be consented and marked for a potential stoma. At operation, a full laparotomy should be performed. The liver should be palpated for metastases and the colon should be inspected for synchronous tumours. The appropriate operation depends on the level of the obstruction. For right-sided lesions, a right hemicolectomy is the procedure of choice. For transverse colonic lesion, an extended right hemicolectomy is often the most appropriate operation. In both cases a stoma can be avoided. For left-sided lesions, there are various options depending on the age and fitness of the patient, the pathology and the experience of the surgeon.

A 'three-staged' procedure involves an initial defunctioning colostomy, followed by a resection and anastomosis and finally closure of colostomy. A 'two-staged' procedure involves an initial sigmoid resection and end colostomy (Hartmann's procedure) followed by closure of colostomy. A 'single-staged' procedure involves resection, on-table lavage and primary anastomosis. With a two-staged procedure, only 60% of stomas are ever reversed. With a single stage procedure, a stoma is avoided. Anastomotic leak rates of less than 4% have been reported following on-table lavage and primary anastomosis. Despite this, the total perioperative mortality of malignant large bowel obstruction remains at about 20%.

Sigmoid and caecal volvulus

A volvulus is defined as rotation of the gut on its own mesenteric axis. It produces partial or complete intestinal obstruction. The blood supply to the segment of intestine is compromised resulting in intestinal ischaemia. Venous congestion leading to infarction can occur. The arterial supply is rarely compromised. A long narrow-based mesentery predisposes to a volvulus.

Sigmoid volvulus

The sigmoid colon is the commonest site of a colonic volvulus. A sigmoid volvulus accounts for 5% of cases of large bowel obstruction in the UK. It is usually seen in the elderly or in those with psychiatric disorders. It is a more common cause of obstruction in Africa or Asia. The incidence is 10 times higher than in Europe or USA.

Clinical features and investigation

The clinical presentation is that of large bowel obstruction. Pain may be minimal and the abdominal distension disproportionate. About 50% patients have had a previous episode. Severe pain and abdominal tenderness suggests ischaemia. A plain abdominal x-ray may show large 'bean' shaped loop of large bowel arising from pelvis. If diagnostic doubt exists, consideration should be given to a CT scan or water-soluble contrast enema. Either investigation should demonstrate the site of obstruction.

Management

Resuscitation with intravenous fluids is essential. Conservative management can be attempted if there are no clinical features of ischaemia or perforation. A rigid or flexible sigmoidoscopy can be both diagnostic and therapeutic. The obstruction is encountered at about 15 cm from the anal margin. When

the scope is advanced beyond this point there is often a dramatic release of flatus and liquid stool. A flatus tube can be inserted and left *in situ* for 2 or 3 days. Overall, 80% of patients will settle with conservative management and if adequate decompression is achieved, no emergency surgical treatment is required. Unfortunately, about 50% patients will have a further episode of volvulus within 2 years. If decompression fails or there are clinical features of peritonitis, the various surgical options are:

- Sigmoid colectomy and primary anastomosis
- Hartmann's procedure
- Paul Mikulicz colostomy

Caecal volvulus

The incidence of caecal volvulus is less than that of sigmoid volvulus. It accounts for about 25% cases of colonic volvulus. Incomplete midgut rotation is a predisposing factor. Incomplete rotation results in inadequate fixation of the caecum to the posterior abdominal wall and the volvulus usually occurs clockwise around the ileocolic vessels. It usually also involves the terminal ileum ileum and ascending colon.

Clinical features and investigation

A caecal volvulus usually presents with clinical features of proximal large bowel obstruction. Colicky abdominal pain and vomiting are common and abdominal distension may occur. A plain abdominal x-ray shows a 'comma-shaped' caecal shadow in the mid-abdomen. Small bowel loops may lie to the right of the caecum. If diagnostic doubt exists, consideration should be given to a CT scan or water-soluble contrast enema. A contrast enema will show a 'beaked' appearance in the ascending colon.

Management

Colonoscopic decompression may be appropriate if the patient is unfit for surgery. It is successful in only about 30% of patients. A laparotomy is normally required. If colonic ischaemia is present, then a right hemicolectomy should be performed though a primary anastomosis may be inappropriate. Exteriorisation of both ends of the bowel may be the safest option. If the caecum is viable and the volvulus reduced, the following can be considered:

- Right hemicolectomy
- Caecostomy
- Caecopexy

Reduction alone is often associated with a high recurrence rate.

Colonic pseudo-obstruction

Colonic pseudo-obstruction is often referred to as Ogilvie's syndrome. It is a condition characterised by reduced colonic mobility and dilatation. It presents with symptoms and signs of large bowel obstruction but in the absence of a mechanical obstructing lesion. The diagnosis is confirmed by CT scan or single contrast enema. Either investigation will exclude an obstructing lesion. Several medical or surgical predisposing conditions have been identified including:

- Chest infection
- Myocardial infarction
- Cerebrovascular accident
- Renal failure
- Puerperium
- Abdominal malignancy
- Orthopaedic trauma
- Myxoedema
- Electrolyte disturbances

Management

The management of colonic pseudo-obstruction involves removing the precipitating causes and decompressing the colon. Drugs with anticholinergic side effects should be stopped, electrolyte disturbances corrected and the use of opiates limited. The colon can be decompressed with a flexible sigmoidoscope or a flatus tube. The cautious use of enemas or intravenous neostigmine may be considered. Surgery is rarely required but should be considered if there is failure of conservative management. The surgical options include tube caecostomy or resection with end ileostomy and mucus fistula formation.

Applied basic sciences
Anatomy of the anterior abdominal wall

The anterior abdominal wall has several layers including skin, superficial fascia and muscles.

Skin

The cutaneous nerve supply to the skin of the anterior abdominal wall is from the anterior rami of the lower six thoracic and the first lumbar nerves. The dermatomes supplied are as follows:

- T7 – epigastrium
- T10 – umbilicus
- L1 – inguinal ligament

Cutaneous arteries are branches of the superior and inferior epigastric arteries and the intercostal and lumbar arteries. The venous drainage is into the axillary and femoral veins. A few small paraumbilical veins drain into the portal vein. The lymphatic drainage is into the axillary and superficial inguinal nodes.

Superficial fascia

The superficial fascia is divided into two layers. The superficial fatty layer is known as Camper's fascia and the deep membranous layer is known as Scarpa's fascia. The fatty layer is continuous with superficial fat of the rest of the body. The deep fascia is continuous with deep fascia of the thigh. The deep layer also invests the perineum and is known as Colles fascia.

Muscles

The muscles of the anterior and lateral abdominal walls are the:

- External oblique
- Internal oblique
- Transversus abdominis
- Rectus abdominis
- Pyramidalis

Rectus sheath

The rectus sheath encloses the rectus abdominis and pyramidalis muscles. It contains the anterior rami of the lower six thoracic nerves and the superior and inferior epigastric vessels. It is formed by the aponeurosis of the three lateral abdominal muscles. Between the costal margin and anterior superior iliac spine the aponeurosis of the internal oblique splits to enclose the rectus muscle, the external oblique aponeurosis passes in front of muscle and the transversus aponeurosis passes behind muscle. Between the anterior superior iliac spine and the pubis, the aponeurosis of all three muscles form the anterior wall and the posterior wall is absent. The curved lower posterior border of the rectus sheath is known as the arcuate line. At this level the inferior epigastric vessels enter the rectus sheath. The rectus sheath is separated from its fellow on the opposite side by the linea alba.

The inguinal canal
Boundaries of the inguinal canal

The deep inguinal ring is the lateral boundary of the inguinal canal. It is an opening in the fascia transversalis about 1 cm above the inguinal ligament, midway between the anterior superior iliac spine and the symphysis pubis. It lies just lateral to the inferior epigastric vessels. The medial boundary is the superficial inguinal ring. This a triangular defect in the external oblique aponeurosis which overlies the pubic crest which forms the base of the opening. The anterior wall is the external oblique aponeurosis, reinforced in the lateral third by the internal oblique muscle. The posterior wall is the fascia transversalis, reinforced in medial third by the conjoint tendon. The floor of the inguinal canal is the inguinal ligament which is the lower border of the external oblique aponeurosis. Medially it is continuous with lacunar ligament which gives attachment to fascia lata of the thigh on the inferior border. The roof of the inguinal canal is formed by the arched fibres of the conjoint tendon.

Contents of the inguinal canal

The inguinal canal contains the spermatic cord in males and the round ligament of the uterus in females. In both, the inguinal canal contains the ilioinguinal nerve. Each anterior abdominal wall layer gives rise to a layer of the spermatic cord. From within outwards the coverings are derived as follows:

- Internal spermatic fascia from fascia transversalis
- Cremaster fascia from internal oblique muscle
- External spermatic fascia from external oblique muscle

The spermatic cord contains the:

- Vas deferens
- Artery to vas deferens (branch of the inferior vesical artery)
- Testicular artery (branch of the abdominal aorta)
- Testicular vein
- Testicular lymphatics
- Testicular nerve fibres
- Processus vaginalis
- Cremasteric artery (branch of the inferior epigastric artery)
- Nerve to cremaster (genital branch of genitofemoral nerve)

Boundaries of the femoral canal

The anatomical boundaries of the femoral canal are:

- Anterior – inguinal ligament
- Posterior – pectineal ligament
- Medial – lacunar ligament
- Lateral – femoral vein

Incisions and laparoscopic access

Abdominal incisions are based on anatomical principles. They must allow adequate assess to the abdomen and should be capable of being extended if required. Ideally muscle fibres should be split rather than cut and nerves should not be divided. The rectus muscle has a segmental nerve supply and, as a result, it can be cut transversely without weakening a denervated segment of muscle. Above the umbilicus, tendinous intersections prevent retraction of the muscles. Commonly used incisions are shown in **Figure 11.1**.

Figure midline incision

A midline incision (**Figure 11.2**) is the commonest approach to the abdomen and the following structures are divided:

- Skin
- Linea alba
- Transversalis fascia
- Extraperitoneal fat
- Peritoneum

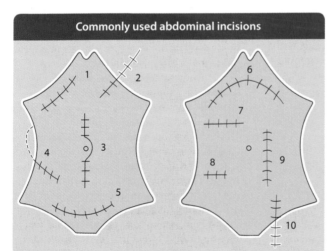

Commonly used abdominal incisions

Figure 11.1 Commonly used abdominal incisions. 1 = Kocher; 2 = Thoracoabdominal; 3 = Midline; 4 = Muscle splitting loin; 5 = Pfannenstiel; 6 = Gable; 7 = Transverse muscle splitting; 8 = Lanz; 9 = Paramedian; 10 = McEvedy

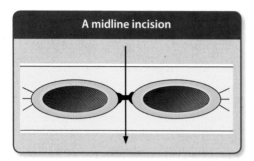

Figure 11.2 A midline incision

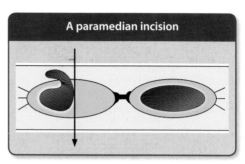

Figure 11.3 A paramedian incision

The incision can be extended by cutting through or around the umbilicus. Above the umbilicus, the falciform ligament should be avoided. The bladder can be accessed via an extraperitoneal approach through the space of Retzius. The wound can be closed using a mass closure technique.

Paramedian incision

A paramedian incision (**Figure 11.3**) is made parallel to and approximately 3 cm from the midline. The incision transverses the:

- Skin
- Anterior rectus sheath
- Rectus – retracted laterally
- Posterior rectus sheath – above the arcuate line
- Transversalis fascia
- Extraperitoneal fat
- Peritoneum

The potential advantages of this incision are that the rectus muscle is not divided and the incisions in the anterior and posterior rectus sheath are separated by muscle. The incision is closed in layers and takes longer to make and close. In the past, it was reported that paramedian incisions has a lower incidence of incisional hernias.

Abdominal hernias

A hernia is a protrusion of an organ through the wall that normally contains it. The wall can be the abdomen, muscle fascia or the diaphragm. Hernias can be congenital or acquired. Abdominal wall hernias are common and account for approximately 10% of the general surgical workload. A hernia consists of a sac, its coverings and contents. Hernias can be:

- Reducible
- Irreducible
- Obstructed or incarcerated
- Strangulated

Irreducible hernias have either a narrow neck or the contents of the hernia are adherent to the sac wall. Obstructed or incarcerated hernias contain compromised but viable intestine. Strangulation occurs when the venous drainage from the contents of the sac is compromised.

Inguinal hernias

About 3% of adults will require an operation for inguinal hernia at some stage in their lives and 80,000 operations are performed each year in UK. The male:female ratio is 12:1 and the ratio of elective to emergency operation is also about 12:1. The peak incidence is in the 6th decade.

Direct inguinal hernia

A direct inguinal hernia is due to weakness in the abdominal wall musculature. It is more common in older patients. The sac is found medial to inferior epigastric artery. Complications are unlikely due to the wide neck of the hernial sac. In adult males, 35% of inguinal hernias are direct. Predisposing factors include smoking, ilioinguinal nerve damage and abdominal straining. A pantaloon hernia is a special type of direct inguinal hernia. The sac has two parts, one is medial and the other is lateral to inferior epigastric artery.

Indirect inguinal hernia

Indirect hernias pass through the inguinal canal. They can occur in children. The sac is found lateral to inferior epigastric artery. Complications are more common than with direct hernias. In adult males, 65% of inguinal hernias are indirect. They are more common on the right side, especially in children

Clinical features

A reducible hernia usually present with a lump at the appropriate anatomical site (**Figure 11.4**). It increases in size on coughing or straining and reduces in size or disappears when relaxed or supine. With an inguinal hernia, the lump is often above and medial to the public tubercle. Examination may show it to have a cough impulse. Irreducible but non-obstructed hernias may cause little pain. If obstruction occurs, colicky abdominal pain, distension and vomiting may occur.

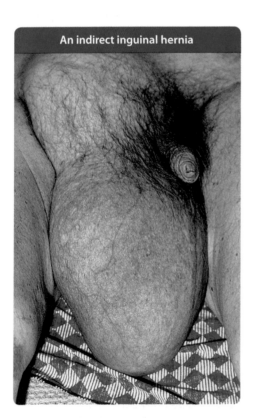

An indirect inguinal hernia

Figure 11.4 An indirect inguinal hernia

The hernia may be tense tender and irreducible. If strangulation occurs, the lump will become red and tender and the patient may be systemically unwell.

Investigation

The diagnosis is usually based on clinical features alone. The differential diagnosis is shown in **Table 11.1**. A herniogram may help in the investigation of chronic groin pain. Ultrasound, CT or MRI may be useful if a clinically occult hernia is suspected.

Management

Herniotomy involves removal of the sac and closure of the neck. This is the treatment of choice in children and adolescents. Herniorrhaphy involves a form of reconstruction to restore the disturbed anatomy, increase the strength of the abdominal wall and construct a barrier to recurrence. Herniorrhaphy can be achieved with the following techniques:

- Bassini +/– Tanner Slide
- Nylon darn
- Shouldice
- Lichtenstein
- Other mesh – Stoppa
- Laparoscopic

A Liechtenstein mesh repair is now regarded as the 'gold standard' technique for inguinal hernia repair as judged by the low-risk of recurrence. Reducible asymptomatic direct hernias in adults do not require surgical intervention. Laparoscopic hernia repair should be reserved for bilateral or recurrent hernia. Complications of hernia repairs include:

- Urinary retention
- Scrotal haematoma
- Damage to the ileoinguinal nerve
- Ischaemic orchitis
- Recurrent hernia

Trusses

About 40,000 trusses are sold annually in UK of which 20% are purchased prior to seeing a doctor. About 45% of patients have had no instruction on correct fitting and 75% of trusses are reported to be fitted whilst the patient is standing and the hernia still apparent.

The differential diagnosis of an inguinal and femoral hernia	
Inguinal hernia	**Femoral hernia**
Femoral hernia	Inguinal hernia
Vaginal hydrocele	Lymphadenopathy
Hydrocele of cord	Saphena varix
Undescended testis	Ectopic testis
Lipoma of cord	Psoas abscess
	Psoas bursa
	Lipoma

Table 11.1 The differential diagnosis of an inguinal and femoral hernia

Surgery for strangulated hernias

The peak incidence of inguinal hernia strangulation is approximately 80 years of age. About 10% of patients presenting with a strangulated hernia give no previous history of a reducible lump. In those with the acute onset of a hernia, the greatest risk of strangulation is in the first 3 months. The risk of strangulation depends on the type of hernia and is more common with indirect hernias. The mortality of surgery for strangulated hernias has changed little over the past 50 years and remains at approximately 10%. The mortality is ten times greater than that following an elective repair.

Recurrent inguinal hernia

The recurrence rate following primary inguinal hernia repair varies with the herniorrhaphy technique and duration of follow-up. With Bassini and darn repairs, the recurrence rate may be as high as 20%. With Shouldice and Lichtenstein repairs, recurrence rates less than 1% have been reported. Factors important in recurrence include the type of hernia, type of operation and postoperative wound infection. Recurrent hernias should be repaired using a mesh technique and this can be performed as either an open or a laparoscopic procedure. Patients should be consented for a possible orchidectomy.

Femoral hernias

Femoral hernias account for 7% of all abdominal wall hernias. The female:male ratio is 4:1. They are more commonly seen in middle-aged and elderly women and are rare in children. They are less common than inguinal hernias but as common as inguinal hernias in older women.

Clinical features

Femoral hernias present with a groin lump below and lateral to the public tubercle. Unlike inguinal hernias, the lump is often irreducible. The differential diagnosis is shown in **Table 11.1**. Femoral hernias are more likely than inguinal hernias to present with complications such as obstruction and strangulation. All patients presenting with small bowel obstruction should be examined for a possible femoral hernia.

Management

All uncomplicated femoral hernias should be repaired as an urgent elective procedure. Three classical approaches to the femoral canal have been described:

- Low (Lockwood)
- Transinguinal (Lotheissen)
- High (McEvedy)

Irrespective of the approach, surgery involves dissection of the sac, reduction of the contents, ligation of the sac and approximation of the inguinal and pectineal ligaments. It is important to avoid compromising the femoral vein which forms the lateral border of the femoral canal.

Special types of hernia

Some hernia types have eponymous names (**Figure 11.5**) attached to them. A Richter hernia is a partial enterocele. It may present with strangulation and obstruction but no clinically apparent hernia. A Maydl hernia contains a 'W-loop' of bowel. Obstruction with the strangulated bowel within the abdominal cavity occurs. A Littre hernia is a strangulated Meckel diverticulum and may present as a small bowel fistula.

Other abdominal wall hernias

Umbilical hernias

Clinical features

Two types of umbilical hernia occur in adults. True umbilical hernias are rare. They occur with abdominal distension (e.g. ascites). Para-umbilical hernias are more common. These occur through the superior aspect of the umbilical scar. They are more common in women. They usually contain omentum and only rarely contain bowel. The neck is often tight and the hernia is often irreducible. The differential diagnosis of an umbilical hernia includes:

- Cyst of the vitello-intestinal duct
- Urachal cyst
- Metastatic tumour deposit (Sister Joseph nodule)

Management

The management of true and para-umbilical hernias is similar. Surgery is usually performed through a infra-umbilical incision. Occasionally the umbilicus needs to be excised. The contents of the hernia are reduced. The defect in the linea alba can be repaired with an overlapping Mayo repair or with the use of a prosthetic mesh.

Epigastric hernia

Epigastric hernias arise through a congenital weakness if the linea alba. The hernia usually consists of extra-peritoneal fat from near to the falciform ligament. They are more common in men. Many are asymptomatic or produce only local symptoms. Strangulation is rare. They can be repaired with either sutures or the use of a prosthetic mesh.

Incisional hernia

Incisional hernias occur through the scar from a previous operation. Approximately 1% of all abdominal incisions result in an incisional hernia. They account for 10% of all abdominal wall hernias. They arise when there is partial dehiscence of the deep fascial layers but the overlying skin remains intact. Most develop within a year of surgery. Symptoms are often minimal with the cosmetic appearance often the main concern. Most are wide-necked but strangulation can occur. Preoperative, operative or postoperative factors may be important in the aetiology.

Preoperative factors include:

- Increasing age
- Malnutrition
- Sepsis
- Uraemia
- Jaundice
- Obesity

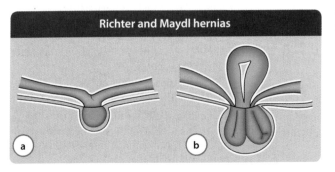

Richter and Maydl hernias

a   b

Figure 11.5 (a) Richter and (b) Maydl hernias

- Diabetes
- Steroids

Operative factors include:

- Type of incision
- Technique and materials used
- Type of operations
- Use of abdominal drains

Postoperative factors include:

- Wound infection
- Abdominal distension
- Chest infection or cough

Management

A CT or ultrasound may help clarify the site of the muscular defect, the hernial sac and its contents. Surgical repair can be challenging and may not always be appropriate. The elderly or infirm may be helped by an abdominal wall support. If surgery is required, the following should be considered:

- Fascial closure or mayo-type repair using sutures
- A 'keel repair' using sutures
- A mesh repair using polypropylene or PTFE
- Laparoscopic mesh repair

The results of surgery for incisional hernias are variable. Re-recurrence rate of 20% have been reported. The results with mesh are superior to suture repairs. Composite meshes may offer a reduced risk of complications. A sublay technique, with the mesh placed deep to the abdominal muscles, may have the lowest recurrence rate.

Spigelian hernia

A Spigelian hernia occurs at the lateral edge of the rectus sheath. It is an interparietal hernia in the line of the linea semilunaris. It usually occurs at the level of the arcuate line.

Obturator hernia

An obturator hernia occurs in the obturator canal. It is usually asymptomatic until strangulation occurs. Patients present with small bowel obstruction and may complain of pain on the medial aspect of the thigh. A vaginal examination may allow identification of a lump in the region of the obturator foramen.

Intestinal fistulas
Enterocutaneous fistulas

A fistula is an abnormal connection between a hollow viscus and an adjacent organ or the skin. A simple fistula is a direct communication between the gut and skin. A complex fistula has multiple tracks and is usually associated an abscess cavity. Fistulae, particularly if high output (more than 500 mL/day), can result in dehydration, electrolyte and acid–base imbalance, malnutrition and sepsis. Fistulae can arise as a result of:

- Anastomotic leaks
- Trauma – often iatrogenic post surgery
- Inflammatory bowel disease
- Malignancy
- Radiotherapy

In the investigation of a fistula it is important to determine the anatomy of the tract. Fistulography will define the tract. A small bowel or barium enema will define the state of the intestine or the presence of distal obstruction. A CT or MRI can define abscess cavities.

Management

The management of a fistula, at least initially, is conservative. This involves skin protection from corrosive gastrointestinal contents. It is also necessary to maintain careful fluid balance, restore blood volume and correct any acid–base imbalance. A proton pump inhibitor may be used to reduce gastric secretions. Somatostatin analogues (e.g. octreotide) may be considered to reduce gastrointestinal and pancreatic secretions. Nutritional support is important. There may be the need to restrict oral intake. A nasogastric tube should be the considered. Malnutrition can be corrected by either parenteral or enteral nutrition. Enteral nutrition can be given distal to fistula. Any associated abscess cavities should be drained.

Surgery

An enterocutaneous fistula will not close if:

- There is total discontinuity of bowel ends
- There is distal obstruction
- Chronic abscess cavity exists around the site of the leak

- Mucocutaneous continuity has occurred

Fistulas are less likely to close if:

- They arise from disease intestine (e.g. Crohn's disease)
- They are end fistulae
- The patient is malnourished
- They are internal fistulas

Large bowel fistulas are more likely than small bowel fistulas to close spontaneously. About 60% of small bowel fistulas will close with conservative treatment in 1 month once sepsis has been controlled. Surgery should be considered if fistula does not close by 30–40 days. The mortality associated with fistula is still at least 10%.

Gastrointestinal stomas

Abdominal stomas

A stoma is a surgically created communication between a hole viscus and the skin. Types of stomas includes a:

- Colostomy
- Ileostomy
- Urostomy
- Caecostomy
- Jejunostomy
- Gastrostomy

Functionally they can be an end, loop or continent stoma. They should be positioned away from the umbilicus, scars, costal margin and the anterior superior iliac spine. Positioning should be compatible with the clothing normally worn by the patient. A loop stoma is usually required to divert bowel contents away from a distal anastomosis or to rest distal bowel affected by disease.

Ileostomy output is small bowel contents and is normally between 500–1000 mL per day. Output greater than this can result in electrolyte imbalance. The high bile content can damage the skin, hence the need for fashioning a spout on an ileostomy. If the output from an ileostomy is excessive consideration should be given to the presence of inflammatory bowel disease, para-intestinal sepsis or subacute obstruction. Colostomy output is normal stool and is usually less than 500 mL per day. It is not corrosive to the skin. Complications of stomas can be either physical or functional.

Physical complications include:

- Necrosis
- Detachment
- Recession
- Stenosis
- Prolapse
- Ulceration
- Parastomal herniation
- Fistula formation

Functional disorders include:

- Excess action
- Reduced action

Chapter 12

Upper gastrointestinal surgery

Applied basic sciences

Embryology of the gastrointestinal tract

Embryologically, the gastrointestinal tract is divided into three sections. The foregut extends from the oesophagus to the Ampulla of Vater in the second part of the duodenum. The midgut starts at the Ampulla of Vater and continues to the junction of mid and distal transverse colon. The hindgut consists of the distal colon and upper rectum. The blood supply of the three sections arise form the coeliac axis, superior mesenteric artery and inferior mesenteric artery, respectively.

Anatomy of gastrointestinal tract

From the oesophagus to the anal canal the wall of the tract has the same basic four layers (**Figure 12.1**):

- Mucosa
- Submucosa
- Muscularis mucosa
- Serosa

The mucosa is the innermost layer, which lines the lumen. Its functions include:

- The secretion of mucus and enzymes
- The release of hormones into the plasma
- Protection against infectious disease
- Absorption of digestive end products

The mucosa consists of three layers. The epithelium lines the lumen and is typically simple columnar in type. The lamina propria is loose connective tissue under the epithelium and contains capillaries and lymphoid tissue. A thin layer of smooth muscle underlies the lamina propria. The submucosa lies deep to the mucosa. It is made up of connective tissue containing blood and lymphatic vessels and nerve fibres. The muscularis mucosa lies deep to

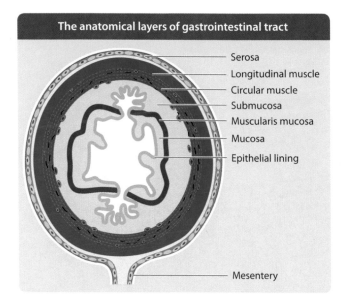

The anatomical layers of gastrointestinal tract

- Serosa
- Longitudinal muscle
- Circular muscle
- Submucosa
- Muscularis mucosa
- Mucosa
- Epithelial lining
- Mesentery

Figure 12.1 The anatomical layers of gastrointestinal tract

the submucosa. It is the smooth muscle layer responsible for peristalsis and segmentation. It is divided into two layers, an inner circular layer and an outer longitudinal layer. In several sites the circular layer is thickened to form a sphincter. These regulate the passage of materials through the gut. The serosa is the outermost layer of the intraperitoneal organs. It is also known as the visceral peritoneum. It consists of a simple squamous epithelium overlying thin areolar connective tissue. The oesophagus has an adventitia rather than a serosa. This is a layer of fibrous connective tissue that firmly supports the organ. Retroperitoneal digestive organs have both a serosa and an adventitia.

Anatomy of the oesophagus

The oesophagus is approximately 25 cm in length and is divided into cervical, thoracic and intra-abdominal parts. It extends from the pharynx, at the level of C6 vertebra, to the cardia of the stomach in the abdomen. It traverses the diaphragm at the level of T10 vertebra. It is lined throughout by a stratified squamous mucosa. It has a rich blood supply from the inferior thyroid artery, branches directly from the aorta and from the oesophageal branch of the left gastric artery. At the lower end there is a porto-systemic anastomosis between the oesophageal branch

of the left gastric vein and the tributaries of the azygos vein. Although no anatomical sphincter can be demonstrated, at the lower end of the oesophagus, a multifactorial 'physiological' sphincter mechanism is present. The lower oesophageal sphincter functions by:

- Basal tone
- Adaptive pressure changes
- Transient lower oesophageal sphincter relaxation

External mechanical factors in preventing gastro-oesophageal reflux include:

- Flap valve mechanism
- Cardio-oesophageal angle
- Diaphragmatic pinchcock
- Mucosal rosette
- Distal oesophageal compression
- Phreno-oesophageal ligament
- Transmitted abdominal pressure

Anatomy of the stomach

For descriptive purposes the stomach has two curvatures and is divided into various regions (**Figure 12.2**) as follows:

- Lesser curve
- Greater curve
- Fundus
- Incisura angularis
- Body
- Pylorus

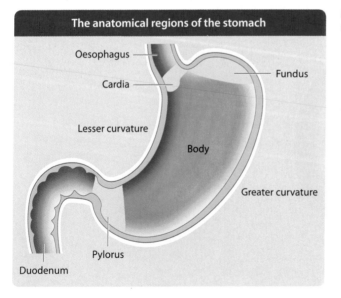

The anatomical regions of the stomach

Oesophagus

Cardia

Fundus

Lesser curvature

Body

Greater curvature

Pylorus

Duodenum

Figure 12.2 The anatomical regions of the stomach

The lesser omentum connects the lesser curve of the stomach to the liver. The greater omentum is connected to the greater curve of the stomach.

Blood supply

The five main arteries that supply the stomach (**Figure 12.3**) are as follows:

- Left gastric
- Right gastric
- Right gastro-epiploic
- Left gastro-epiploic
- Short gastric

The left gastric artery arises from the coeliac access. The right gastric artery arises from the common hepatic artery. The right gastro-epiploic artery arises from the gastroduodenal artery. The left gastro-epiploic artery arises from the splenic artery. The short gastric arteries are branches of the splenic artery.

Lymphatic drainage

The stomach drains into four groups of nodes as follows:

- Hepatic group
- Sub-pyloric group
- Gastric group
- Pancreatico-lienal group

Histology

The gastric mucosa is simple columnar epithelium with numerous invaginations known as gastric pits. The gastric pits lead into gastric glands which secrete gastric juice. Mucous cells secrete acidic mucus and function as stem cells for the surface mucosa. Parietal cells secrete hydrochloric acid and intrinsic factor. The chief cells secrete pepsinogen, an inactive form of pepsin. This is activated to pepsin initially by hydrogen ions and by pepsin itself. Neuroendocrine cells secrete multiple hormones into the plasma. The most important of these is gastrin.

The vagus nerve

Both of the vagi enter the abdomen through the oesophageal hiatus. The left vagus nerve passes on to the anterior and the right vagus nerve passes on to the posterior walls of the stomach. The anterior vagus runs along the lesser curve. The nerve of Latarjet supplies the pylorus. The posterior vagus supplies the coeliac ganglion.

Anatomy of the small intestine

The small intestine is the longest part of the alimentary canal. It is divided into three regions

- Duodenum
- Jejunum
- Ileum

Duodenum

The duodenum is approximately 25 cm long and is 'C' shaped. Except for the first part it is retroperitoneal and is divided into four parts:

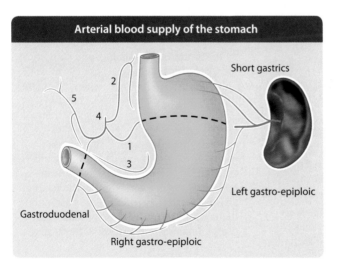

Arterial blood supply of the stomach

Short gastrics

Gastroduodenal

Right gastro-epiploic

Left gastro-epiploic

Figure 12.3 Arterial blood supply of the stomach. 1 = Splenic; 2 = Left gastric; 3 = Right gastric; 4 = Coeliac axis; 5 = Common hepatic.

- First part is continuation of the pylorus and runs transversely
- Second part runs vertically in front of the hilum of the right kidney
- Third part runs horizontally below the pancreas
- Fourth part runs upward to the duodenojejunal junction

The ligament of Treitz connects the duodenojejunal flexure to the right crus of the diaphragm. The duodenal papilla is found on the medial wall of the second part. It is the site of entry of the common bile duct and pancreatic duct. The blood supply of the duodenum is from the superior pancreaticoduodenal artery, a branch of the gastroduodenal artery and the inferior pancreaticoduodenal artery, a branch of the superior mesenteric artery. The venous drainage is into the portal and superior mesenteric vein. The lymphatic drainage is to the coeliac and superior mesenteric nodes.

Jejunum and ileum

The jejunum and ileum are about 6 m long. The proximal 40% is the jejunum. The jejunum begins at the duodenojejunal junction. The ileum ends at the ileocaecal valve. The ileum is connected to the posterior abdominal wall by the small bowel mesentery. The blood supply is from the superior mesenteric artery and branches form arcades within the mesentery. The lower part of the ileum is supplied by the ileocolic artery. The venous drainage is into the superior mesenteric vein. The lymphatic drainage is into the superior mesenteric nodes.

Histology

The small intestine is highly modified for absorption of fluid and nutrients. Structures that maximise the surface area include the:

- Plicae circulares – deep permanent folds of the mucosa and submucosa
- Villi – finger-like extensions of the mucosa
- Microvilli – projections of the plasma membrane of each absorptive epithelial cell

The epithelium of the small intestine is a simple columnar layer with goblet cells. Epithelial invaginations are known as the intestinal glands (crypts of Lieberkuhn). They contain absorptive cells and neuroendocrine cells. The submucosa is unremarkable except in the proximal duodenum and terminal ileum. The proximal duodenal submucosa contains alkaline mucus glands (Brunner's glands) and the terminal ileal submucosa contains aggregates of lymphoid tissue know as Peyer's patches.

Gastric physiology

The motility of the stomach is increased by both distension and parasympathetic activity, via acetylcholine and gastrin. It is decreased by low pH stomach contents which inhibits gastrin release. Fats stimulate the release of cholecystokinin. Acid stimulates the release of secretin. Hyperosmolality of duodenal contents reduces gastric emptying. The rate of emptying also depends on the type of food. Carbohydrate-rich content is faster than protein-rich and fatty food. The stomach produces about 2500 mL of secretion per day. The pH is acidic and can be close to one. Gastric secretions are rich in potassium, hydrogen ions, chloride and bicarbonate. It also contains intrinsic factor and pepsin.

Secretion of gastric acid

A H^+/K^+ ATPase is present in the apical membrane of the parietal cells. It pumps H^+ ions into the gastric gland lumen against their concentration gradient. Potassium is actively pumped into the parietal cell in exchange. Potassium then diffuses back into the lumen of the gastric glands. Chloride diffuses from the parietal cell into the lumen passively down its electrochemical gradient. High concentrations of potassium and chloride are maintained within the parietal cell and chloride and bicarbonate exchanged on the basolateral membrane.

Control of gastric acid

Gastrin acts in two ways. It stimulates gastrin receptors on the parietal cells and stimulates the release of histamine from enterochromaffin-like cells. Gastrin leads to an increase in intracellular Ca^{2+}. Histamine then acts on H_2 on the parietal cells. These are G protein mediated receptors. They lead to an increase in intracellular cAMP and hence in protein kinases which leads to activation of H^+/K^+ ATPase. Acetylcholine activates M3 muscarinic receptors. This increases intracellular Ca^{2+}. Its release is stimulated by vagal action. Prostaglandin E activates an inhibitory G protein. It thus blocks the action of histamine and gastrin by inhibiting protein kinase synthesis. Gastric inhibitory peptide and vasoactive intestinal peptide and secretin act by inhibiting gastrin release.

Oesophageal disease

Gastro-oesophageal reflux disease

Gastro-oesophageal reflux disease (GORD) can be defined as excessive amounts of reflux of gastric secretions associated with significant symptoms or complications. It affects 40% of the adult population. It is due to either acid or bile reflux but delayed oesophageal clearance may also be an important aetiological factor. Gastric acid hypersecretion is rarely implicated. Failure of the function of the lower oesophageal sphincter mechanism is a common finding. Reflux exposes the lower oesophagus to acid or bile, increasing the risk of mucosal injury.

Clinical features

About 20% patients with oesophagitis are symptom free. The commonest symptom is heartburn. This is usually short-lived, intermittent, retrosternal chest pain often associated with an acid taste in the mouth. Symptoms are often worse when supine or at night. Dysphagia may develop if complications occur. There is a poor correlation between symptoms and endoscopic evidence of oesophagitis. A symptom diary may help in the assessment of the patient.

Investigation

Endoscopy may provide histological confirmation of oesophagitis and allow assessment of severity. However, about 30% of patients with symptoms of GORD have no endoscopic evidence of mucosal injury.

The Savary Miller grading of GORD is as follows:

- Grade 1 – Erythaema isolated to one mucosal fold
- Grade 2 – Linear erosions on more than one fold
- Grade 3 – Circumferential erosions
- Grade 4 – Ulceration, shortening or stricture formation
- Grade 5 – Barrett epithelium formation

The Los Angeles classification of GORD is as follows:

- Grade A – Erosions <5 mm on one fold
- Grade B – Erosions >5 mm on one fold
- Grade C – Erosions on two more folds <75% of circumference
- Grade D – Erosions >75% of circumference

In those in whom surgery is being considered, 24-hour pH monitoring and oesophageal manometry are important. During 24-hour pH monitoring a probe is placed 5 cm above lower oesophageal sphincter. A pH of less than 4 for over 1% of the time when erect or 6% of the time when supine is suggestive of GORD.

Management

Most patients gain symptomatic relief with conservative treatment. Lifestyle modifications are important and patients should stop smoking, reduce their alcohol intake and lose weight. Drug treatment involves the use of proton pump inhibitors and prokinetic agents. Proton pump inhibitors will allow 80% of patients to have mucosal healing at 8 weeks. However, about 20% will relapse despite maintenance therapy. Life-long therapy is often required.

Surgical options

The indications for surgery are:

- Failure of conservative management
- Recurrent symptomatic relapse
- Bile reflux
- Documented evidence of deficient lower oesophageal sphincter
- Complications of GORD

Fundoplication is the operation of choice, usually performed as a laparoscopic procedure. Important features are:

- Mobilisation of the gastric fundus
- A tension free wrap possibly around a 50 Fr oesophageal bougie
- A wrap suture line of less than 3 cm

Several types of fundoplication have been described (**Figure 12.4**). Following fundoplication about 3% of patients develop dysphagia and 11% develop gastric bloat. A partial fundoplication, is associated with less dysphagia and fewer gas-related symptoms.

Oesophageal carcinoma

Barrett's oesophagus

Barrett's oesophagus was first described by Norman Barrett in 1950. It consists of a columnar cell-lined distal oesophagus due intestinal metaplasia of the distal oesophageal mucosa. It is a pre-malignant condition and can progress to dysplasia and adenocarcinoma. Barrett's oesophagus increases the risk of malignancy by 30-fold. It is an acquired condition due to gastro-oesophageal reflux. Bile reflux appears to be an important aetiological factor. About 10% of patients with gastro-oesophageal reflux develop Barrett's oesophagus. Approximately 1% of patients with Barrett's oesophagus per year progress to oesophageal carcinoma.

Clinical features

Barrett's oesophagus per se is usually asymptomatic, recognised as an incidental finding at endoscopy. It appears as 'velvety' epithelium extending more than 3 cm above gastro-oesophageal junction. The significance of 'short segment' Barrett's, less than 3 cm long, is unclear.

Management

If recognised at endoscopy, most patients with Barrett's oesophagus are started on life-long acid suppression. There is little evidence that it causes regression of metaplasia. Anti-reflux surgery may reduce progression to dysplasia and cancer. Recent interest has been shown in endoscopic mucosal ablation and this is usually achieved with photosensitisers and laser therapy. The role of endoscopic surveillance of Barrett's oesophagus is controversial. The aim of surveillance is to detect dysplasia before progression to carcinoma. However, about 40% of patients with dysplasia already have a focus of adenocarcinoma. Oesophagectomy for oesophageal dysplasia has an 80% 5-year survival.

Oesophageal carcinoma

Oesophageal cancer is the sixth leading cause of cancer death worldwide. It accounts for about 7000 deaths per year in the UK. Of all oesophageal carcinomas, 90% are squamous cell carcinomas. They usually occur in the upper or middle third of the oesophagus.

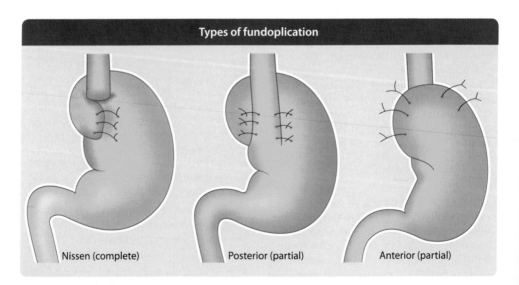

Types of fundoplication

Nissen (complete)　　　Posterior (partial)　　　Anterior (partial)

Figure 12.4 Types of fundoplication

Only 5–10% are adenocarcinomas and these usually occur in the lower third of the oesophagus. Wide variation in incidence has been reported both between countries and in different ethnic groups and populations within a country. There is a clear positive association with social deprivation.

Risk factors for squamous cell carcinoma are:

- Alcohol/tobacco
- Diet high in nitrosamines
- Aflatoxins
- Trace element deficiency – molybdenum
- Vitamin deficiencies – vitamins A and C
- Achalasia
- Coeliac disease
- Genetic – tylosis
- High incidence in Transkei, areas of Northern China and the Caspian littoral region

Clinical features

The classical clinical presentation of oesophageal carcinoma is progressive dysphagia, first with solids and then with liquids. Respiratory symptoms may occur due to overspill of fluid or solids into the respiratory tract or occasionally because of the formation of a trachea-oesophageal fistula. Weight loss is usually a prominent feature.

Investigation

The diagnosis can be confirmed by endoscopy plus biopsy. Most tumours are irresectable and incurable at presentation. The resectability and fitness for surgery can be assessed by:

- CT scanning
- Lung function tests
- Endoscopic ultrasound
- Bronchoscopy
- Laparoscopy

Management

Adenocarcinomas are not radiosensitive and surgery is the mainstay of treatment. Squamous cell carcinomas can be treated with either surgery or radiotherapy.

Surgery

Less than 50% of patients are suitable for potentially curative treatment. Treatment should be in centres that perform the operation regularly. The operative mortality should be less than 5%. Preoperative chemotherapy may improve survival. The operative approach needs to ensure 10 cm proximal clearance to avoid submucosal spread. The approach depends on the site and type of tumour and can involve:

- Total gastrectomy via a thoracoabdominal approach
- Subtotal two-stage oesophagectomy (Ivor-Lewis)
- Subtotal three-stage oesophagectomy (McKeown)
- Transhiatal oesophagectomy

Complications of surgery include:

- Chest infection/pleural effusion
- Anastomotic leak
- Chylothorax
- Recurrent laryngeal nerve damage
- Benign anastomotic stricture

Of those undergoing 'curative' treatment less than 40% survive 1 year. Overall, 5-year survival is very poor and is at best 20%.

Palliative treatment

In those with inoperable disease, the aim of palliative treatment is to relieve obstruction and dysphagia with minimal morbidity. This may be achieved with oesophageal intubation or stenting. Open surgical intubation (Celestin or Mousseau–Barbin tubes) is now obsolete. Endoscopic or radiological placement is now most commonly practiced. An Atkinson tube can be placed endoscopically but requires dilatation with risk of oesophageal perforation. There has been a recent increased use of self-expanding stents that require no pre-dilatation. Complications of stents and tubes include oesophageal perforation, tube displacement or migration and tube blockage due to ingrowth or overgrowth of tumour. Endoscopic laser ablation produces good palliation in over 60% of cases buy may need to be repeated every 4 to 6 weeks. It is associated with the risk of oesophageal perforation in about 5% cases. Squamous carcinomas are radiosensitive and its use may produce some palliation but at the risk of forming a tracheo-oesophageal fistula.

Oesophageal perforation

Oesophageal perforation is a rare condition associated with a high mortality. Management and outcome depends on the time from injury to diagnosis. 'Early' injuries are those identified within 24 hours. 'Late' injuries are those identified later than 24 hours. The causes of oesophageal perforation are multiple and include:

- Endoscopic intubation
- Sclerotherapy of oesophageal varices
- Endoscopic prostheses
- Traumatic intubation
- Perioesophageal surgery
- Trauma
- Caustic ingestion
- Barotrauma
- Tumours
- Infections

Boerhaave's syndrome

Boerhaave's syndrome is post-emetic rupture of the oesophagus. It was first described by Herman Boerhaave in 1723. His patient was Baron Jan von Wassenaer, Grand Admiral of the Dutch Fleet who vomited after a meal and developed left-sided chest pain. He died 18 hours later. At post mortem, he was shown to have a tear of the left posterior wall of the oesophagus, 5 cm above the diaphragm, surgical emphysema and food in the left pleural space.

Clinical features

Oesophageal rupture occurs after 0.1% of standard endoscopies and 2% of endoscopies at which an oesophageal dilatation is performed. The diagnosis requires a high index of suspicion. Typical symptoms include chest pain and dyspnoea. Signs include pyrexia, tachycardia, hypotension and tachypnoea. Subcutaneous emphysema may be present. Undiagnosed, systemic sepsis rapidly develops and death often occurs with 48 hours. A chest x-ray may show a pleural air/fluid level and mediastinal emphysema. The diagnosis can be confirmed by water-soluble contrast swallow or CT scan.

Management

Conservative management may be appropriate for small perforations without systemic upset or those with a small contained thoracic leak. It requires the patient to be 'nil by mouth' and to receive antibiotics and intravenous fluids. Failure of conservative management will need surgery. The surgical management principals for thoracic perforations include:

- To control the oesophageal leak
- Eradicate mediastinal/pleural sepsis
- Re-expand lung
- Prevent gastric reflux
- Nutritional and pulmonary support
- Antibiotics
- Postoperative drainage of residual septic foci

The methods of treatment include:

- Primary closure with a buttress or patch
- Exclusion and diversion
- T-tube fistula
- Thoracic drainage and irrigation
- Resection
- Decompression gastrostomy and feeding jejunostomy

If operated on within 24 hours the mortality is 5 to10%. If the operation is delayed more than 48 hours, the mortality is more than 50%.

Achalasia

Dysphagia can result from either extrinsic or intrinsic mechanical oesophageal compression or primary or secondary neuromuscular problems. The causes include:

- Carcinoma of the bronchus
- Thoracic aortic aneurysm
- Goitre
- Benign stricture
- Oesophageal carcinoma
- Bolus obstruction
- Achalasia
- Diffuse oesophageal spasm
- Nutcracker oesophagus
- Multiple sclerosis
- Systemic sclerosis
- Chagas disease
- Autonomic neuropathy

Achalasia is due to a reduced number of ganglion cells in the oesophageal myenteric plexus. The vagus nerves show axonal degeneration of the dorsal motor nucleus and nucleus ambiguous. The aetiology is unknown but a neurotropic virus may be important. The pathological features are similar to Chagas disease which is due to *Trypanosoma cruzi* infection.

Clinical features

Achalasia is most commonly seen in patients between 40–70 years. The incidence is the same in either sex. Symptoms include dysphagia, weight loss, regurgitation and chest pain. About 5% of patients develop squamous carcinoma of the oesophagus. The differential diagnosis includes:

- Diffuse oesophageal spasm
- Infiltrating carcinoma
- Hypertrophic lower oesophageal sphincter
- Scleroderma
- Chagas disease

Investigation

A chest x-ray may show widening of the mediastinum with an air/fluid level and absence of the gastric fundus gas bubble. A barium swallow may show oesophageal dilatation, with food residue, small tertiary contractions and a 'rat tail' appearance of the distal oesophagus. Oesophageal manometry will show an absent primary peristaltic wave and non-propulsive tertiary contractions. An endoscopy is essential to exclude 'pseudoachalasia' due to a submucosal oesophageal carcinoma. It will also show a tight lower oesophageal sphincter which relaxes with gentle pressure.

Management

Management of achalasia is by either balloon dilatation or cardiomyotomy. In balloon dilatation, a Rider Moeller balloon is placed across the lower oesophageal sphincter and is inflated to 300 mmHg for 3 minutes. With this approach 60% of patients are dysphagia free at 5 years. The procedure may need to be repeated. The risk of oesophageal perforation following balloon dilatation is about 3%.

Cardiomyotomy was described by Heller (1914) and Grenveldt (1918). It may be performed laparoscopically. The muscle fibres of the lower oesophagus are incised along an 8–10 cm length down to the mucosa. Following this procedure 85% of patients are dysphagia free. About 10% develop oesophageal reflux and 3% a peptic stricture. Some centres combine a cardiomyotomy with an antireflux operation.

Gastric disease

Gastric cancer

Gastric cancer is one of the commonest causes of cancer deaths world wide. It accounts for 7000 deaths per year in the UK. The incidence increases with age. The male: female ratio is 2:1. Despite an overall decline in the incidence rates of gastric cancer, several countries, including the UK, have seen an increase in the incidence of adenocarcinomas of the gastric cardia, sometimes referred to as proximal gastric cancer.

Risk factors include:

- Diet low in Vitamin C
- Blood group A
- Pernicious anaemia
- Hypogammaglobulinaemia
- Post gastrectomy

Precursor states include:

- *Helicobacter pylori* infection
- Atrophic gastritis
- Intestinal metaplasia
- Gastric dysplasia
- Gastric polyps

Pathology

Macroscopically, the appearance of tumours vary. Malignant gastric ulcers typically have raised everted edges and sometimes a necrotic base (**Figure 12.5**). Colloid tumours are large gelatinous growths. Linitis plastica is a diffusely infiltrating tumour of the mucosa and submucosa with marked fibrosis leading to a shrunken thickened stomach that fails to distend. Most tumours are adenocarcinomas with varying degrees of differentiation. Anaplastic signet-ring tumours have a poor prognosis. Spread is typically via the lymphatics or portal system. Transcoelomic spread to the ovaries can occur (Krukenberg tumours).

Clinical features

New onset dyspepsia over the age of 50 years is suspicious of a gastric carcinoma as is

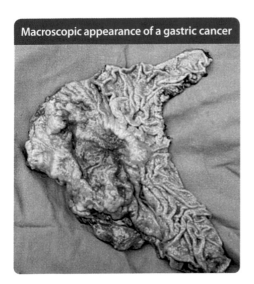

Macroscopic appearance of a gastric cancer

Figure 12.5 Macroscopic appearance of a gastric cancer

constant or worsening dyspepsia that fails to respond to treatment. Weight loss and an epigastric mass are worrying signs. Some patients will develop an iron-deficiency anaemia. Dysphagia and early postprandial vomiting occur with proximal obstructing tumours. Late postprandial vomiting especially of altered food and with no bile suggests gastric outlet obstruction. Most patients present late and are not amenable to radical surgery.

Investigation

Upper gastrointestinal endoscopy should be considered in patients with dyspeptic symptoms over the age of 40 years. It will confirm the diagnosis, site and extent of tumour. Staging requires a combination of preoperative investigations and intraoperative assessment. Endoscopic ultrasound may allow assessment of intramural tumour penetration. Abdominal CT will allow assessment of nodal spread and the extent of metastatic disease. Laparoscopy will show peritoneal seedlings and peritoneal lavage will allow detection of free tumour cells. The Birmingham Staging System is a clinicopathological staging system (**Table 12.1**). It does not require detailed assessment of the lymph node status.

Management

Surgery offers the only prospective of cure. Antral tumours may be suitable for a partial gastrectomy usually with Polya reconstruction. Other tumours will need a total gastrectomy with oesophagojejunal anastomosis and Roux-en-Y biliary diversion. A tumour is considered resectable if it is confined to the stomach or only the N_1 or N_2 nodes involved. Nodes less than 3 cm from tumour are N_1 nodes. Nodes greater than 3 cm from tumour are N_2 nodes.

If the tumour and N_1 nodes are resected it is regarded as a D_1 gastrectomy. If the tumour and N_2 nodes are resected then it is regarded as a D_2 gastrectomy. The evidence to support the use of D_2 gastrectomy is incomplete. A D_2 gastrectomy is associated with increased postoperative mortality but may have improved long-term survival. Even in patients with incurable disease,

Birmingham staging of gastric cancer	
Stage	**Description**
Stage 1	Disease confined to muscularis propria
Stage 2	Muscularis and serosal involvement
Stage 3	Gastric and nodal involvement
Stage 4a	Residual disease
Stage 4b	Metastatic disease

Table 12.1 Birmingham staging of gastric cancer

surgery may palliate symptoms. Results from adjuvant chemotherapy post surgery are disappointing. Chemoradiotherapy may reduce relapse and improve survival. Prognosis is generally very poor and overall, the 5-year survival rate is approximately 5%. Survival is 70%, 32%, 10% and 3% for Stages 1, 2, 3 and 4 respectively.

Other gastric tumours

Gastrointestinal stromal tumours

Gastrointestinal stromal tumours (GIST) is a term that describes all tumours arising from non-epithelial and non-lymphoid tissues of the gastrointestinal tract. They include tumours of benign, malignant and indeterminate potential. Leiomyosarcomas are a form of GIST and account for 2–3% of all gastric tumours. They arise from the smooth muscle of the stomach wall. Lymphatic spread is rare. About 75% present with an upper gastrointestinal bleed and 60% patients have a palpable abdominal mass. The diagnosis can be confirmed by upper GI endoscopy and CT scanning. Partial gastrectomy may allow adequate resection. The 5-year survival is approximately 50%.

Gastric lymphoma

The stomach is the commonest extranodal primary site for non-Hodgkin's lymphoma. Gastric lymphoma accounts for approximately 1% of gastric malignancies. The clinically presentation is similar to gastric carcinoma. About 70% of tumours are resectable and the 5-year survival is approximately 25%. Both adjuvant radiotherapy and chemotherapy may be useful.

Sister Mary Joseph's nodule

Sister Mary Joseph was head nurse to William Mayo in Rochester Minnesota, who was the first to notice that a 'nodule' in the umbilicus was often associated with advanced intra-abdominal malignancy. It usually presents as firm, red, non-tender nodule and results from spread of tumour within the falciform ligament. About 90% of tumours are adenocarcinomas and the commonest primaries are stomach and ovary. The primary tumour is almost invariably inoperable.

Peptic ulcer disease

Peptic ulcer disease is defined as the presence of complete, established defects in the columnar mucosa of the lower oesophagus, stomach or duodenum. Proximal gastric ulcers (type 1) are most commonly found on the lesser curve and antrum of the stomach. Distal gastric and duodenal ulcers (type 2) are found in the pre-pyloric region or duodenum. Type 2 ulcers are four-times more common. Important aetiological factors include:

- *Helicobacter pylori* infection
- Drugs – NSAIDS
- Smoking and alcohol
- Male sex
- High acid production

Helicobacter pylori is a urease-producing Gram-negative spiral flagellated bacterium. It is found in 90%, 70% and 60% of patients with duodenal ulceration, gastric ulceration and gastric cancer respectively.

Clinical features

The number of hospital admissions for uncomplicated peptic ulcer disease is falling. The incidence of complications related to anti-inflammatory use is increasing. Duodenal ulcers usually present with epigastric pain, worse when fasting and relieved by food. Symptoms may be worse at night. The pain often follows a relapsing and remitting course. Gastric ulcers often present with epigastric pain that is worse on eating. Weight loss is a more prominent feature. Patients may also present with iron-deficiency anaemia.

Investigation

The diagnosis can be confirmed by upper gastrointestinal endoscopy. The presence of *Helicobacter pylori* can be detected by:

- Microscopy – silver or Giemsa staining of antral biopsies
- Rapid urease test – colour changes due to change in pH
- ^{13}C or ^{14}C breath test – ingested radioactive urea is broken down to carbon dioxide
- Serology – detected immunologically using an ELISA

Medical management

Proton pump inhibitors produce healing of 90% of peptic ulcers with 2 months of treatment. Recurrence rates are low on long-term maintenance therapy. *Helicobacter pylori* can be eradicated in 80% patients with triple antibiotic therapy. Various drug combinations have been described including amoxycillin, metronidazole and omeprazole. Short-term recurrence rates are low. Long-term recurrence rates are at present unknown.

Drugs have changed the need for ulcer surgery over last 20 years. Admissions for elective surgery have significantly reduced. The number of complications of peptic ulcer disease however remain unchanged due to increased use of anti-inflammatory use in elderly. Bleeding and perforation still have a mortality of more than 10%.

Surgery

A Billroth I gastrectomy was originally described for the resection of distal gastric cancers. It is still used in gastric cancers if radical gastrectomy is inappropriate. It was later applied in the treatment of benign gastric ulcers. It is useful if the ulcer is situated high on the lesser curve. It is less effective than Polya gastrectomy for duodenal ulcers.

A Billroth II or Polya gastrectomy (**Figure 12.6**) was initially described for duodenal ulceration but is rarely performed today. It is useful in recurrent ulceration following previous vagotomy. When constructing the gastrojejunal anastomosis it is necessary to consider whether to form an antecolic or retrocolic anastomosis and whether the anastomosis should be isoperistaltic or antiperistaltic. A Roux-en-Y jejunojejunostomy may also be fashioned (**Figure 12.6b**).

Current surgical options

Current indications for surgical treatment of duodenal ulceration are:

- Intractability
- Haemorrhage
- Perforation
- Obstruction

The aim of surgery is to cure the ulcer diathesis with the lowest risk of recurrence and complications. Operations for duodenal ulceration reduce acid production by the stomach. The cephalic phase of acid production can be reduced by a vagotomy. The antral phase can be reduced by antrectomy. There may be the need for a gastric drainage procedure to overcome the effects of a vagotomy on gastric emptying.

Open surgical procedures include:

- Truncal vagotomy and pyloroplasty
- Truncal vagotomy and gastrojejunostomy
- Highly selective vagotomy
- Anterior seromyotomy and posterior truncal vagotomy

Laparoscopic peptic ulcer operations include:

- Thoracoscopic truncal vagotomy and pyloric stretch
- Highly selective vagotomy
- Posterior truncal vagotomy and selective anterior vagotomy
- Posterior truncal vagotomy and anterior seromyotomy

Post gastrectomy complications include:

- Recurrent ulceration
- Diarrhoea
- Dumping
- Bilious vomiting
- Iron deficient anaemia
- B_{12} deficiency
- Folate deficiency

Post vagotomy complications include:

- Diarrhoea
- Dumping
- Bilious vomiting

Pyloric stenosis

Gastric outflow obstruction due to pyloric stenosis is most commonly secondary to chronic prepyloric or proximal duodenal ulceration. It usually presents with vomiting of undigested food, weight loss, epigastric pain and dehydration. The abdomen is distended and there may be visible peristalsis and a succussion splash. Biochemical assessment may show a hypochloraemic, hypokalaemic metabolic alkalosis. Endoscopy will confirm the diagnosis and may allow balloon dilatation of the stricture. If this fails then surgery is by either gastrojejunostomy or proximal gastric vagotomy with duodenoplasty.

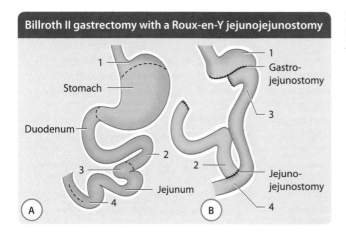

Figure 12.6 (A) Billroth II gastrectomy with a Roux-en-Y jejunojejunostomy (B)

Gastric volvulus

A gastric volvulus is an abnormal rotation of the stomach of more than 180°. It causes closed loop obstruction and can result in incarceration and strangulation of the stomach. Depending on the axis of rotation it is classified as organoaxial or mesentericoaxial (**Figure 12.7**). About 10% cases occur in children and is usually associated with a diaphragmatic hernia. In adults, it is associated with laxity of gastric ligament.

Classification

In organoaxial volvulus, the axis of rotation extends from gastro-oesophageal junction to the pylorus. The gastric antrum rotates in the opposite direction to fundus. This is commonest type of volvulus and is usually associated with diaphragmatic defect. Strangulation occurs in about 10% of cases. In mesentericoaxial volvulus, the axis of rotation bisects the lesser and greater curves. The gastric antrum rotates anteriorly and superiorly and the posterior surface of stomach lies anteriorly. Rotation is usually incomplete. The diaphragm is usually intact and strangulation is rare.

Clinical features

Acute gastric volvulus usually presents with sudden onset of severe epigastric or left upper quadrant pain. If part of the stomach is in the thorax, then chest pain may occur.

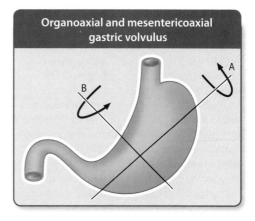

Figure 12.7 Schematic representation of organoaxial (A) and mesentericoaxial (B) gastric volvulus

Progressive distension and non-productive retching may develop. Haematemesis is a late feature. Borchardt triad describes:

- Epigastric pain
- Retching
- Inability to pass a nasogastric tube

Chronic gastric volvulus presents with intermittent epigastric pain and distension. Early satiety, dyspepsia and dysphagia may occur. The symptoms are often minimal and the diagnosis can be difficult.

Investigation

A chest x-ray may shows a retrocardiac gas-filled viscus. A plain abdominal x-ray may show a distended stomach. The diagnosis can be confirmed by a contrast study or abdominal CT scan.

Management

Endoscopic reduction may be attempted in both acute and chronic cases. However, it should not be attempted if there is clinical suspicion of strangulation. A PEG can be inserted after reduction to reduce the risk of recurrence. Surgery is often required and involves reduction of the volvulus, assessment of viability of the stomach and resection if required. An anterior gastropexy may be considered to prevent recurrence. Mortality following surgery for acute gastric volvulus is about 10%.

Coeliac disease

Coeliac disease is an autoimmune disorder of the small bowel. It occurs in genetically predisposed individuals. It affects about 1% of the population and can present in either childhood or adulthood. It is caused by a reaction to gliadin, a gluten protein found in wheat. Long term it leads to an increased risk of both adenocarcinoma and lymphoma. Coeliac disease has been linked with a number of conditions including IgA deficiency, dermatitis hepatiformis, other autoimmune diseases including autoimmune thyroiditis and primary biliary cirrhosis and undefined neurological disorders and epilepsy.

Pathophysiology

The vast majority of coeliac patients have one of two types of HLA DQ, a gene that is part of the MHC class II antigen-presenting receptor. There are seven HLA DQ variants (DQ2 and D4 through 9). Two of these variants – DQ2 and DQ8 – are associated with coeliac disease. The gene is located on the short arm of chromosome 6. The receptors formed by these genes bind to gliadin peptides. Coeliac disease shows incomplete penetrance.

Clinical features

Many patients are asymptomatic. In those with symptoms they include, diarrhoea, weight loss, abdominal pain and fatigue. There may also be features of malabsorption. Anaemia can develop due to iron, folic acid or B_{12} deficiency. Calcium and vitamin D malabsorption may cause osteopenia. A mild coagulopathy may develop due to vitamin K malabsorption.

Investigation

Several investigations can be used to assist in the diagnosis but many tests are only useful if the patient is still on a normal diet containing gluten. Endoscopy with duodenal biopsies is the gold standard.

Multiple biopsies are required. Most patients with coeliac disease have a small bowel that appears normal on endoscopy. Endoscopy may show scalloping of the small bowel folds and a mosaic pattern to the mucosa. Serological tests have a high sensitivity and specificity. Serological tests include the detection of IgA antibodies against reticulin or gliadin. The pathological changes of coeliac disease in the small bowel are categorised by the Marsh classification as follows:

- Stage 0 – Normal mucosa
- Stage 1 – Increased number of intra-epithelial lymphocytes
- Stage 2 – Proliferation of the crypts of Lieberkuhn
- Stage 3 – Partial or complete villous atrophy
- Stage 4 – Hypoplasia of the small bowel architecture

The changes classically improve or reverse after gluten is removed from the diet. Repeat biopsies should be considered after 6 months of gluten exclusion.

Management

The only effective treatment is a life-long gluten-free diet. No medication exists that will prevent damage when gluten is present. Adherence to the diet allows the intestines to heal and leads to the resolution of all symptoms in the vast majority of cases. A tiny minority of patients suffer from refractory disease. Steroids or immunosuppressants may be considered in this situation.

Chapter 13

Hepatobiliary and pancreatic surgery

Applied basic sciences

Anatomy of the liver and pancreas

Liver

The liver is the largest organ in the body (**Figure 13.1**). It occupies the right hypochondrium and extends into the epigastrium. It is protected by the ribs and costal cartilages. Its relations include the abdominal part of the oesophagus, stomach, duodenum, hepatic flexure of the colon and the right kidney and adrenal gland. It is divided into right and left lobes by the falciform ligament. The right lobe is also divided into the quadrate and caudate lobes. The quadrate and caudate lobes are functionally part of the left lobe. It is surrounded by a fibrous capsule. The porta hepatis is found on the posterior–inferior surface. The free edge of less omentum is attached to the margins of the porta hepatis. The porta hepatis contains the:

- Right and left hepatic ducts
- Right and left branches of the hepatic artery
- Portal vein
- Hepatic lymph nodes

The blood supply to the liver is from the hepatic artery and portal vein. Blood is mixed in the central vein of each liver lobule. The venous drainage is via the hepatic veins into the vena cava.

The falciform ligament ascends from umbilicus. Within the falciform ligament runs the ligamentum teres. This is the remains of the umbilical vein. On the surface of the liver the falciform ligament splits in two. The right side forms the upper layer of the coronary ligament. The left side forms the upper layer of left triangular ligament. The extremity of the coronary ligament forms the right triangular ligament. An area devoid of peritoneum is known as the bare area.

Extrahepatic biliary apparatus

The extrahepatic biliary apparatus consists of the:

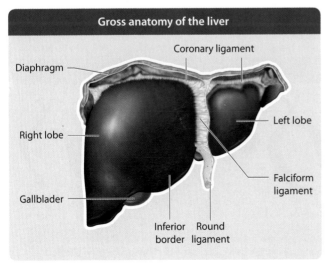

Gross anatomy of the liver

- Diaphragm
- Coronary ligament
- Left lobe
- Right lobe
- Falciform ligament
- Gallbladder
- Inferior border
- Round ligament

Figure 13.1 Gross anatomy of the liver

- Right and left hepatic ducts
- Common hepatic duct
- Common bile duct
- Gallbladder
- Cystic duct

The right and left hepatic ducts emerge from right and left lobes in the porta hepatis. They unite to form the common hepatic duct which is about 4 cm long. The common hepatic duct descends in the free edge of the lesser omentum and is joined by cystic duct to form the common bile duct. The common bile duct is about 8 cm long and also in the free edge of the lesser omentum. It then extends behind the first part of the duodenum, and lies on the posterior aspect of pancreas. It drains into the second part of the duodenum at the ampulla of Vater. The terminal part is surrounded by sphincter of Oddi.

Gallbladder

The gallbladder lies on the viseral surface of liver. It is divided into the fundus, body and neck. The fundus projects from the inferior margin of the liver and comes into contact with abdominal wall at level of tip of 9th costal cartilage. The neck is continuous with cystic duct. Relations of the gallbladder include the anterior abdominal wall, visceral surface of liver, transverse colon and the first and second parts of the duodenum. The blood supply is from the cystic artery, a branch of the right hepatic artery. The cystic vein drains directly into the portal vein. The cystic duct is about 4 cm long but is subject to anatomical variations (**Figure 13.2**).

Pancreas

The pancreas is situated retroperitoneally and is a combined endocrine and exocrine gland. It is divided into the head, neck, body and tail. It develops from the ventral and dorsal pancreatic buds. The ventral bud produces the head and the uncinate process. The dorsal bud gives rise to the body and tail of the pancreas. The head lies within the curve of the duodenum and the uncinate process projects from the head. The superior mesenteric vessels separate the head from the body. The tail extends into the lienorenal ligament along with the splenic artery. The pancreas is closely related to several other organs (**Figure 13.3**). Anterior relations include the transverse mesocolon and stomach. Posterior relations include the inferior vena cava, aorta, portal vein, common bile duct and left kidney. Superior relations include the first part of duodenum and splenic artery.

The pancreas has two ducts – the main and accessory pancreatic ducts (**Figure 13.4**). The main pancreatic duct begins in the tail and drains into the second part of the duodenum together with the common bile duct. The main duct is also known as the duct of Wirsung. The accessory duct begins in the head and is also known as the duct of Santorini. It usually drains into the main duct but can open separately into the duodenum. The blood supply of the pancreas is from the superior and inferior pancreaticoduodenal arteries. The superior pancreaticoduodenal artery is an indirect branch of the hepatic

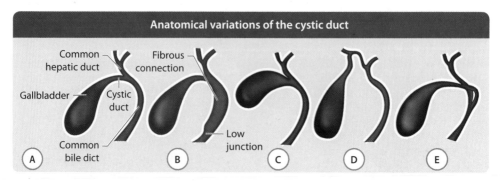

Anatomical variations of the cystic duct

Common hepatic duct
Fibrous connection
Gallbladder
Cystic duct
Common bile dict
Low junction

A   B   C   D   E

Figure 13.2 Anatomical variations of the cystic duct. A = Normal; B = Low insertion of cystic duct; C = No cystic duct; D = Cystic duct joins right hepatic duct; E = Cystic duct passes in front of common bile duct

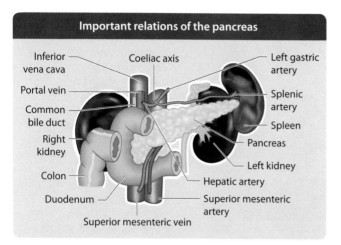

Figure 13.3 Important relations of the pancreas

Important relations of the pancreas

- Inferior vena cava
- Coeliac axis
- Left gastric artery
- Portal vein
- Splenic artery
- Common bile duct
- Spleen
- Right kidney
- Pancreas
- Colon
- Left kidney
- Hepatic artery
- Duodenum
- Superior mesenteric artery
- Superior mesenteric vein

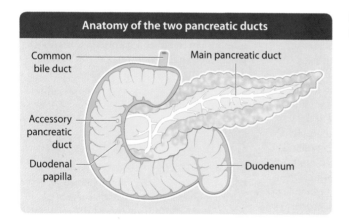

Figure 13.4 Anatomy of the two pancreatic ducts

Anatomy of the two pancreatic ducts

- Common bile duct
- Main pancreatic duct
- Accessory pancreatic duct
- Duodenal papilla
- Duodenum

artery. The inferior pancreaticoduodenal artery is a branch of the superior mesenteric artery. The splenic artery supplies the body and tail. It is a direct branch of the coeliac trunk. The venous drainage corresponds to the arterial supply and drains into the portal system.

About 80% of the mass of pancreas is composed of acinar cells. These form the exocrine portion of the gland. The Islets of Langerhans are dispersed within the gland and are islands of endocrine tissue. The islets consist of Type A (20%), B (70%) and D (10%) cells. Type A, B and D cells produce glucagon, insulin and somatostatin respectively.

Physiology of the liver

Approximately 75% of the blood entering the liver is venous blood from the portal vein.

The remaining 25% is arterial blood from the hepatic artery. Terminal branches of the hepatic portal vein and hepatic artery enter sinusoids in the liver (**Figure 13.5**). Sinusoids are distensible vascular channels lined with highly fenestrated endothelial cells and bounded circumferentially by hepatocytes. As blood flows through the sinusoids, plasma is filtered into the space between the endothelium and hepatocytes. Blood flows through the sinusoids and empties into the central vein of each lobule. Central veins coalesce into the hepatic veins which leave the liver and drain into the vena cava.

The intrahepatic biliary apparatus

The biliary system is a series of channels and ducts that conveys bile from the liver into the lumen of the small intestine. Hepatocytes are

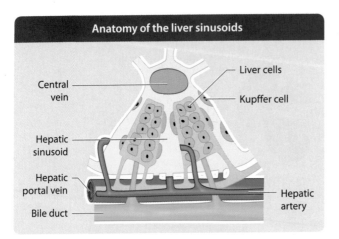

Figure 13.5 Anatomy of the liver sinusoids

arranged in 'plates' with their apical surfaces facing and surrounding the sinusoids. The basal surfaces of adjoining hepatocytes are joined together by junctional complexes to form bile canaliculi. A canaliculus is the dilated intercellular space between adjacent hepatocytes. Hepatocytes secrete bile into the canaliculi which flows parallel to the sinusoids, but in the opposite direction to the blood flow. At the ends of the canaliculi, bile enters into the bile ducts, which are true ducts lined by epithelial cells. Bile ducts are in close proximity to the terminal branches of the portal vein and hepatic artery, and form the portal triad.

Bile is a complex fluid containing water, electrolytes, bile acids, cholesterol, phospholipids and bilirubin. Adults produce approximately 500 mL of bile each day. Bile acids are derivatives of cholesterol synthesised in the hepatocyte. Cholesterol is converted into the bile acids, cholic and chenodeoxycholic acids, which are then conjugated to an amino acid (glycine or taurine) to yield a conjugated form that is actively secreted into canaliculi. Bile acids are important for digestion and absorption of fats and fat-soluble vitamins in the small intestine.

Waste products, including bilirubin, are eliminated from the body by secretion into bile. Bilirubin is a tetrapyrrole and is a normal product of haem catabolism. Unconjugated bilirubin is formed in the reticuloendothelial system of the spleen. It is not water soluble and is transported to the liver bound to albumin. In the liver it is conjugated with glucuronic acid, rendering it water soluble and allowing its excretion in bile.

Hepatobiliary and pancreatic disease
Obstructive jaundice

In healthy individuals, serum bilirubin concentrations are low. When biliary obstruction occurs, the serum levels of conjugated bilirubin are increased, resulting in its accumulation in tissues and its excretion in the urine. The causes of obstructive jaundice are shown in **Table 13.1**. Obstructive jaundice can result in several systemic complications.

Clinical features
Accumulation of bilirubin in tissues produces jaundice, characterised by the deposition of yellow bilirubin pigments in the skin, sclerae, mucous membranes and other tissues. Patients often complain of itch and may notice pale stools and dark urine.

Complications
Vitamin K is required for the γ-carboxylation of the clotting factors II, VII, IX, XI. It is a fat soluble vitamin that is not absorbed in the presence of obstructive jaundice. Deranged production of clotting factors can result in

Causes of obstructive jaundice		
Common	**Infrequent**	**Rare**
Common bile duct stones	Ampullary carcinoma	Benign strictures – iatrogenic, trauma
Carcinoma of the head of pancreas	Pancreatitis	Recurrent cholangitis
Malignant porta hepatis lymph nodes	Liver secondaries	Mirrizi syndrome
		Sclerosing cholangitis
		Cholangiocarcinoma
		Biliary atresia
		Choledochal cysts

Table 13.1 Causes of obstructive jaundice

a bleeding tendency. Active bleeding or the need for urgent surgical intervention requires correction of the clotting disorder with the use of fresh frozen plasma. Parenteral administration of vitamin K should also be considered but its actions are more prolonged.

Hepatorenal syndrome is poorly understood. It is defined as renal failure post intervention in a patient with obstructive jaundice. It is due to Gram-negative endotoxinaemia from the gut. Preoperative lactulose may improve the outcome.

Investigation
Investigation of a jaundiced patient will allow the differentiation of hepatocellular and obstructive jaundice in about 90% cases. In obstructive jaundice, the serum and urine conjugated bilirubin levels are increased. Other liver function tests will also be deranged. The increase in serum ALP and GGT is relatively more than the AST and ALT. The converse is seen in patients with hepatocellular causes of jaundice. The albumin may be reduced and the PTT prolonged.

The normal CBD is less than 8 mm in diameter. The CBD diameter increases with age and after previous biliary surgery. Its diameter is also increased in patients with

bile duct obstruction. Transabdominal ultrasound has a high sensitivity and specificity for the detection of CBD dilatation and it may also allow identification of the underlying cause. CT or MRI scanning is useful in the obese or if there is excessive bowel gas. Both imaging modalities are better at visualising the lower end of the common bile duct and the pancreas. In those with a obstructive jaundice due to a pancreatic tumour, they allow staging and the assessment of operability. ERCP allows biopsies or brush cytology specimens to be taken, stone extraction to occur or the insertion of a biliary stent.

Management
The management of obstructive jaundice involves correction of any complications, decompression the biliary tree and treatment of the underlying cause. Broad spectrum antibiotic prophylaxis should be given. Parenteral vitamin K and fresh frozen plasma may be needed to correct the clotting disorder. Fluid expansion will reduce the risk of the hepatorenal syndrome.

Gallstones

Gallstones are found in about 12% of adult men and 24% of adult women. The prevalence of gallstones increases with advancing age. Only about 10–20% of gallstones ever become symptomatic. Over 10% of those with stones in the gallbladder have stones in the common bile duct.

Pathophysiology

Three types of stones are recognised:

- Cholesterol stones (15%)
- Mixed stones (80%)
- Pigment stones (5%)

Cholesterol stones result from a change in the solubility of bile constituents. Bile acids act as a detergent keeping cholesterol in solution. Bile acids, lecithin and cholesterol result in the formation of micelles. Bile is often supersaturated with cholesterol and this favours the formation of cholesterol microcrystals. Biliary infection, stasis and changes in gallbladder function can precipitate stone formation. Bile is infected in 30% of patients with gallstones. Gram-negative organisms are the most common isolated. Mixed stones are probably a variant of cholesterol stones. Pigment stones are small, dark stones made of bilirubin and calcium salts. They contain less than 20% of cholesterol (**Figure 13.6**). Only about 10% of gallstones are radio-opaque. The clinical presentations of gallstones include:

- Biliary colic
- Acute cholecystitis
- Empyema of the gallbladder
- Mucocele of the gallbladder
- 'Flatulent dyspepsia'
- Mirizzi's syndrome
- Obstructive jaundice
- Pancreatitis
- Acute cholangitis

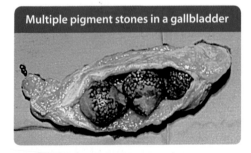

Multiple pigment stones in a gallbladder

Figure 13.6 Multiple pigment stones in a gallbladder

Biliary colic and acute cholecystitis

Biliary colic arises as a result of intermittent obstruction of the cystic duct due to the presence of gallstones within Hartmann's pouch. Acute cholecystitis results from persistent obstruction of the cystic duct. Increased pressure within the gallbladder results in an acute inflammatory response. Secondary bacterial infection may occur in about 20% of cases. The most common organisms implicated are *Escherichia coli*, *Klebsiella* and *Strep. faecalis*.

Clinical features

Biliary colic typically presents with right upper quadrant abdominal pain precipitated by food. The pain may radiate to the back and scapula and usually resolves spontaneously after 30 minutes to a few hours. Systemic upset is mild and abdominal signs may be minimal. In contrast, acute cholecystitis presents with constant pain of longer duration. This is often associated with fever, tachycardia and localised tenderness in right upper quadrant. Murphy's sign, guarding in right upper quadrant on deep inspiration, may be present. Jaundice is uncommon in uncomplicated acute cholecystitis.

Complications of acute cholecystitis include:

- Gangrenous cholecystitis
- Gallbladder perforation
- Cholecystoenteric fistula
- Gallstone ileus

Investigation

Ultrasound is the initial investigation of choice. In patients with biliary colic, stones may be seen within a normal gallbladder. In acute cholecystitis, the diagnostic features include the presence of gallstones, a distended thick-walled gallbladder, pericholecystic fluid and Murphy's sign demonstrated with the ultrasound probe. The common bile duct should also be visualised and its diameter assessed. Liver function tests are often normal but inflammatory markers may be raised. A dilated common bile duct and deranged liver function indicate the need for further assessment for the presence of common bile duct stones.

Management

The initial management of acute cholecystitis is usually conservative. The patient is fasted, given intravenous fluids and opiate analgesia. Intravenous antibiotics should be given to prevent secondary infection. Overall, about 80% patients improve with conservative treatment.

If fit, patients should be considered for a laparoscopic cholecystectomy. The timing of surgery is controversial. Evidence now suggests that early surgery, less than 72 hours after the onset of symptoms, is safe. It has a lower conversion rate and avoids the complications of conservative treatment failure. If patient are unfit for surgery, percutaneous cholecystotomy may be beneficial. It may be particularly useful in patients with acalculus cholecystitis.

Mirizzi's syndrome

The Mirizzi's syndrome refers to common hepatic duct obstruction caused by an extrinsic compression from an impacted stone in the cystic duct or Hartmann pouch of the gallbladder. Obstruction occurs because of either mechanical obstruction or because of inflammation around the common hepatic duct. Patients present with right upper quadrant abdominal pain and jaundice.

Acute cholangitis

Acute cholangitis results from infection in an obstructed biliary tree, usually as a result of gallstones. The classical clinical picture consists of intermittent right upper quadrant abdominal pain, jaundice and fever – the Charcot triad. Patients often have features of severe sepsis and untreated, it can lead to hepatic abscess formation. Management is with parenteral antibiotics and biliary decompression. Operative mortality in the elderly is up to 20% but early endoscopic drainage has been shown to decrease mortality by up to 30%.

Treatment of gallbladder stones

In 1882 the first open cholecystectomy was performed by Langenbuch in Berlin. It was associated with significant complications. Today mortality for open cholecystectomy is still approximately 0.5%. Complications include:

- Bile duct damage
- Retained stones
- Bile leak
- Wound dehiscence
- Pulmonary atelectasis

The morbidity associated with open surgery lead to the development firstly of 'mini' cholecystectomy through a short transverse incision and then laparoscopic cholecystectomy, introduced in 1988. About 40,000 cholecystectomies are performed annually in the UK. More than 4000 common bile ducts are cleared of stones.

Laparoscopic cholecystectomy

Laparoscopic cholecystectomy has been shown to be equally as effective as open cholecystectomy and is associated with reduced morbidity and a faster postoperative recovery. The conversion rate to an open procedure is about 5%.

Preoperative ERCP is indicated if:

- Recent jaundice
- Abnormal liver function tests
- Significantly dilated common bile duct
- Ultrasonic suspicion of bile duct stones

Technique

The routine use of a nasogastric tube and urinary catheter is controversial and both are usually avoided. A CO_2 pneumoperitoneum is induced using either a Veress needle or open technique. The open (Hasson) technique is believed to be safer. Over half of bowel injuries that occur during a laparoscopic cholecystectomy are caused by either the Veress needles or trocars. The abdominal pressure should be set to 12–15 mmHg. Higher intra-abdominal pressure can reduce pulmonary compliance, decrease venous return and result in higher end-tidal CO_2 levels. Surgery is usually performed using four standard ports (2×10 mm and 2×5 mm). The patient is positioned with head up tilt and rolled to the left. Calot triangle is dissected using a retrograde technique. The cystic duct and artery are identified and ligated with clips or endo-loops. About 50% surgeons routinely use intraoperative cholangiography.

Cholangiography allows definition of the biliary anatomy and identification of unsuspected common bile duct stones found in about 10% of patients.

Bile duct injury

Bile duct injury occurs in between 0.1% and 0.5% of patients undergoing laparoscopic cholecystectomy. The risk is related to surgical inexperience and problems identifying the biliary anatomy. The outcome is improved if recognised at time of initial surgery. For most injuries hepaticojejunostomy is the treatment of choice. If the recognition of the injury is delayed, then the complication is associated with higher morbidity and mortality. Management then requires drainage of collections and control of sepsis. Long-term risks include stricture formation and cirrhosis.

Common bile duct stones

Accurate prediction of the presence of common bile duct stones can be difficult. The common bile duct can be imaged by ultrasound, MRCP and ERCP (**Figure 13.7**). The latter is the investigation of choice as it is both diagnostic and therapeutic. A sphincterotomy can be performed and common bile duct stones can be extracted with either balloons or a Dormia basket. If necessary, a biliary stent can be inserted.

Stone extraction is about 90% successful but has a complication rate of approximately 5%. Mortality is less than 1%. If stone extraction fails, patient will require:

- Open cholecystectomy and exploration of the common bile duct
- Laparoscopic exploration of common bile duct
- Mechanical lithotripsy

If stones are retained after exploration of the common bile duct, then consideration needs to be given to:

- Early ERCP
- Exploration via T-tube tract at 6 weeks

Acute pancreatitis

Epidemiology

In the UK, the incidence of acute pancreatitis is about 50 per 100,000 population per year.

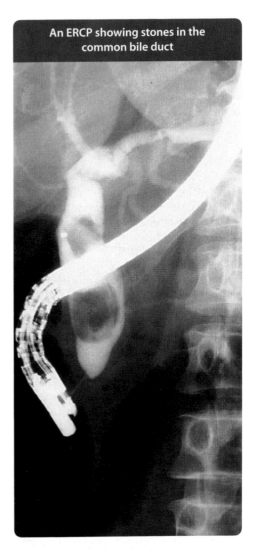

An ERCP showing stones in the common bile duct

Figure 13.7 An ERCP showing stones in the common bile duct

About 80% of patients have mild disease with a low-risk of complications and negligible mortality. However, a small proportion of patients have severe disease. About 40% of these develop life-threatening complications including infected pancreatic necrosis. The mortality associated with infected pancreatic necrosis is about 50%.

Aetiology

Gallstones and alcohol account for 80% of cases of acute pancreatitis. Aetiological factors include:

- Idiopathic
- Obstruction – choledocholithiasis, pancreatic tumours
- Pancreatic structural anomalies
- Toxins – alcohol, drugs (e.g. salicylates, azathioprine, cimetidine)
- Trauma – accidental, iatrogenic
- Metabolic abnormalities
- Infection
- Vascular anomalies

About 20% of cases of acute pancreatitis are idiopathic. Gallstones less than 5 mm in diameter are more likely to cause pancreatitis than larger ones. Less than 5% of patients with gallstones develop pancreatitis.

Clinical features

The classic presentation of acute pancreatitis is with sudden onset severe epigastric pain. The pain is constant in nature and radiates through to the back. Patients are often pyrexial and dehydrated. Tenderness may be localised to epigastrium or generalised. Eponymous signs of retroperitoneal haemorrhage are rare and appear late but include Cullen's and Grey Turner's signs. The differential diagnosis includes perforated peptic ulcer, acute cholecystitis and mesenteric ischaemia. Complications of acute pancreatitis can be local or systemic (**Table 13.2**).

Investigation

Serum amylase has a low sensitivity and low specificity for the diagnosis of acute pancreatitis. A serum amylase of three times the upper limit of normal has a sensitivity and specificity of 60% and 95%, respectively. About 20% of patients with acute pancreatitis have a normal serum amylase, particularly if alcohol is an important aetiological factor. Serum lipase is more sensitive and may remain elevated longer but is not routinely measured. Other causes of hyperamylasaemia include:

- Perforated peptic ulcer
- Cholecystitis
- Generalised peritonitis
- Intestinal obstruction
- Mesenteric infarction
- Ruptured abdominal aortic aneurysm
- Ruptured ectopic pregnancy

CT scanning of the abdomen is the standard imaging modality for evaluating acute pancreatitis and its complications (**Figure 13.8**). Typical CT findings in acute pancreatitis include focal or diffuse enlargement of the pancreas, heterogeneous enhancement of the gland, irregular contour of the pancreatic margins, blurring of the peripancreatic fat planes and the presence of intraperitoneal or retroperitoneal fluid collections. Complications of acute pancreatitis such as pseudocysts, abscess formation, pancreatic necrosis, venous thrombosis, pseudoaneurysm development and haemorrhage can also be recognised. Pancreatic necrosis is recognised by failure of the pancreas to enhance after intravenous contrast administration.

Abdominal ultrasound is the 'gold standard' investigation for the detection of gallstones. Gallstone may not be visible on abdominal CT scanning. Clinical and biochemical that features suggest a gallstone aetiology include:

- Female sex
- Age more than 50 years
- Amylase more than 4000 IU/L
- Bilirubin more than 35 µmol/L
- Increased AST
- Increased ALP

Prognostic factors

Half of all deaths from acute pancreatitis occur within the first week due to multi-organ failure. This usually occurs in the absence of local complications. Late deaths are often

Complications of acute pancreatitis

Local	Systemic
Necrosis possibly with infection	Hypovolaemia and shock
Pancreatic fluid collections	Coagulopathy
	Respiratory failure
Colonic necrosis	Renal failure
Gastrointestinal haemorrhage	Hyperglycaemia
Splenic artery aneurysm	Hypocalcaemia

Table 13.2 Complications of acute pancreatitis

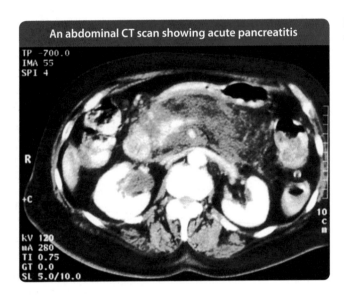

An abdominal CT scan showing acute pancreatitis

Figure 13.8 An abdominal CT scan showing acute pancreatitis

due to local complications. Mortality from pancreatitis is due to:

- Early multiple organ failure
- Late infected pancreatic necrosis
- Haemorrhage
- Associated co-morbidity

Most patients with acute pancreatitis have mild disease which accounts for less than 5% of the mortality from the disease. The aim of prognostic scores is to identify patients with severe disease, allowing them to be more closely monitored in an intensive care environment. The scoring systems need to have a high sensitivity and specificity and ideally should be applicable on admission. Ranson's criteria are measured both on admission and at 48 hours.

Ranson's criteria scored on admission:

- Age more than 55 years
- WCC more than 16,000
- LDH more than 600 U/L
- AST more than 120 U/L
- Glucose more than 10 mmol/L

Ranson's criteria scored within 48 hours:

- Haematocrit fall more than 10%
- Urea rise more than 0.9 mmol/L
- Calcium less than 2 mmol
- pO_2 less than 60 mmHg
- Base deficit more than 4
- Fluid sequestration more than 6 L

Ranson's criteria are not ideal. They can not be applied fully for 48 hours and are also a poor predictor later in the disease. They have been described as a 'single snapshot in a whole feature length of the film'. APACHE II is a multivariate scoring system. It measures objective parameters – vital signs and biochemical analysis. It takes account of the premorbid state and age and can be used throughout the course of the illness.

Management

The aims of treatment of acute pancreatitis are to halt the progression of the local disease and to prevent remote organ failure. In severe disease, this requires full supportive therapy often in ITU or HSU environment.

All patients should be monitored with a urinary catheter. A CVP line and arterial line should be considered in those with significant physiological derangement. There should be regular assessment of serum electrolytes, calcium, blood sugar and liver function tests. Patients require fluid resuscitation with both colloid and crystalloid, correction of hypoxia with an increased F_iO_2 and the administration of adequate analgesia.

Antibiotic prophylaxis is useful in those with severe pancreatitis. ERCP maybe of benefit within the first 48 hours in patients with predicted severe gallstone disease.

Nutritional support is important. Pancreatitis is associated with a catabolic state. The benefit of pancreatic 'rest' by limiting oral intake is unproven and there is evidence that early enteral nutrition is safe. Nasojejunal feeding limits pancreatic secretion and is preferable to oral or nasogastric feeding.

All patients with pancreatitis should undergo an ultrasound within 24 hours of admission. If it confirms gallstones and the patient has severe pancreatitis, then consideration should be given to early ERCP. If the patient fails to settle during the first week of admission, a contrast enhanced CT should be used to assess for the presence of pancreatic necrosis. If there is clinical or radiological suspicion of pancreatic abscess formation, then consideration should be given to CT-guided aspiration. A pancreatic necrosectomy may be required if these is clinical deterioration and bacteriological proof of infection. The operative mortality associated with pancreatic necrosectomy is more than 40%.

Pseudocysts

Peripancreatic fluid collections are common after an episode of pancreatitis. About 35% of patients with acute pancreatitis will develop a peri-pancreatic fluid collection but more than 50% of these will resolve spontaneously over a 3-month period. A pseudocyst is a fibrous walled peri-pancreatic fluid collection. It has no epithelial lining and the fluid has a high amylase content. Acute fluid collections are not pseudocysts and the collection needs to be present for at least a month to be regarded as a pseudocyst. The diagnosis may be suggested by continuing abdominal pain and vomiting and the persistent elevation of the serum amylase. Pseudocysts can be classified as:

- Type 1 – Normal duct anatomy. No fistula between duct and cyst
- Type 2 – Abnormal duct anatomy and no fistula present
- Type 3 – Abnormal duct anatomy and fistula present

Investigation

An abdominal ultrasound will allow assessment of changes in the size of the cyst and an abdominal CT will allow its relationship to adjacent organs to be defined (**Figure 13.9**). An ERCP should be considered to define the pancreatic duct anatomy.

Management

The treatment options for a pancreatic pseudocyst include:

- Percutaneous drainage
- Endoscopic drainage
- Surgical drainage

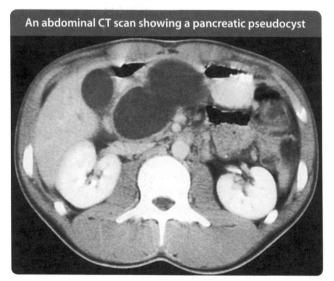

An abdominal CT scan showing a pancreatic pseudocyst

Figure 13.9 An abdominal CT scan showing a pancreatic pseudocyst

Percutaneous drainage can be either by ultrasound or CT guidance. It is about 80% successful in those with Type 1 cysts. The outcome is less certain if there is a fistula to the pancreatic duct or abnormal duct anatomy (Type 2 and 3 cysts). These patients require either endoscopic or surgical drainage. Endoscopic drainage and insertion of pigtail catheter can be performed by a transpapillary or transmural route. Surgical drainage can be by a cystogastrostomy or a Roux-loop cystojejunostomy. Surgery allows adequate internal drainage and a biopsy of the cyst wall can taken to exclude a cystadenocarcinoma. Surgery is associated with a higher risk of complications but a lower cyst recurrence rate.

Pyogenic liver abscess

Pyogenic liver abscesses are usually seen in elderly and infirm patients. They can be multiple or solitary and arise as a result of biliary sepsis. The mortality is high as the diagnosis is often delayed. The commonest organisms involved are:

- *Escherichia coli*
- *Klebsiella*
- *Proteus*
- *Bacteroides* species

Aetiology

The causes of pyogenic liver abscess are:

- Portal pylophlebitis – appendicitis, diverticulitis or pelvic infections
- Biliary disease – cholecystitis, ascending cholangitis or pancreatitis
- Trauma – blunt or penetrating
- Direct extension – empyema of the gall-bladder, subphrenic or perinephric abscess
- Septicaemia
- Infected liver cysts or tumours

Clinical features

Patients are generally systemically unwell. They often have severe abdominal pain usually localised to the right hypochondrium accompanied by a swinging pyrexia, rigors and weight loss. About 25% present with jaundice. Examination may show a hypochondrial or epigastric mass. About 30% of patients have a pleural effusion.

Investigation

Blood tests may show a raised white cell count, increased ESR and deranged liver function tests. Chest x-ray often shows a raised right hemidiaphragm and pleural effusion. An abdominal ultrasound will localise the abscesses and will guide drainage. A CT scan may be useful if the diagnosis is in doubt or if there are multiple abscesses.

Management

Patients should be started on appropriate antibiotics. Percutaneous drainage under ultrasound guidance is the initial treatment of choice. If biliary obstruction is present, consideration should be given to decompression by either ERCP or the use of a percutaneous drain. Surgery may be required if there is failure of resolution with percutaneous drainage or intraperitoneal rupture occurs. Both situations are associated with a high mortality. Laparoscopic drainage may succeed after failure of the percutaneous route.

Amoebic liver abscess

Amoebic liver abscesses are due to infection with the protozoan parasite, *Entamoeba histolytica*. It is found in the stool of carriers in the cystic or trophozoite form. It is transmitted by the faecal–oral route. The liver is the commonest extraintestinal site of infection. About 10% of affected patients develop liver abscesses. The abscesses can be solitary or multiple. About 80% of abscesses develop in the right lobe of the liver. They can present several years after intestinal infection.

Clinical features

Patients present with malaise, pyrexia and weight loss. The right hypochondrial pain is often mild. Less than 20% of patients present with diarrhoea. Jaundice is uncommon. Complications can arise as a result of abscess rupture or extension of infection. Complications occur in 5% of patients and include: ·

- Amoebic empyema
- Hepato-bronchial fistula
- Lung abscess

- Pericarditis
- Peritonitis

Investigation
Blood tests will show a raised white cell count and ESR. A latex agglutination assay is positive in more than 90% patients. Sigmoidoscopy, stool microscopy and rectal biopsy may identify the organism. A chest x-ray may show a raised right hemidiaphragm, atelectasis or abscess. The abscess can often be identified on ultrasound. Aspiration produces a typical 'anchovy sauce' appearing pus. The pus is odourless and sterile on routine culture.

Management
Metronidazole is the antibiotic of choice. If it is ineffective, chloroquine and dehydroemetine may be considered. Ultrasound-guided aspiration may be useful. Surgery is rarely required. The prognosis in uncomplicated cases is good with a mortality of less than 1%. If pulmonary complications occur, mortality can be as high as 20%.

Hydatid disease

Hydatid disease is due to infection with the helminth, *Ecchinococcus granulosa*. The adult worm is normally found in the dog and sheep intestine. Man is an accidental intermediate host. Human infection is most commonly seen in Mediterranean areas, Australia and South America. The liver is the commonest organ involved but the lung, brain and bone can also be infected. Cysts are unilocular, can be up to 20 cm in diameter and may be multiple. Daughter cysts may develop. About 70% of cysts develop in the right lobe of the liver. Pathologically, hydatid liver cysts have three distinct layers:

- Ectocyst – fibrous adventitial layer due to host response
- Middle layer – laminated membrane of proteinaceous material
- Endocyst – inner germinal layer from which the scolices may be detached

Clinical features
The clinical presentation is often non-specific and patients may be asymptomatic. About 60% have right hypochondrial abdominal pain. Only 15% of patients become jaundiced. Other features include skin rashes, pruritus and allergic reactions. Cysts can rupture resulting in a bronchobiliary fistula.

Investigation
About 30% of patients have an eosinophilia. The diagnosis can be confirmed by an indirect haemagglutinin assay. A plain abdominal x-ray may show calcification in the cyst wall. Cysts can be imaged with ultrasound or CT. Aspiration should not be performed if hydatid disease is suspected as this is associated with risk of dissemination of infection or anaphylaxis.

Management
Pharmacological treatment is not curative but is used as an adjunct to surgery to kill spilled scolices. The drugs of choice are albendazole, mebendazole and praziquantel. If surgery is required, a laparotomy is performed to exclude other cysts. The liver is packed off with hypertonic saline-soaked swabs. Cysts are then decompressed with a trocar and cannula Scolicidal agent (e.g. hypertonic saline or 0.5% silver nitrate) can be injected into the cyst cavity. The cavity is filled with saline and a suction drain inserted. Alternatively, liver cysts can be excised. Hepatic resection may be required for recurrent cysts. The recurrence rate is approximately 5% at 5 years.

Hepatocellular carcinoma

Hepatocellular carcinoma (HCC) is a primary malignant tumour of the liver. It is uncommon in northern Europe where hepatic secondaries are 30 times more common than primary liver tumours. The highest incidence is seen in east Africa and south-east Asia. In these areas, it is one of the commonest malignant tumours. The male:female ratio is 4:1. In Europe, the peak age at presentation is 80 years. In Africa and Asia, the peak age at presentation is 40 years.

Aetiology
The incidence of HCC parallels the world-wide prevalence of hepatitis. Aetiological factors include:

- Cirrhosis
- Viral hepatitis – particularly Hepatitis B and C
- Mycotoxins – aflatoxin produced by *Aspergillus flavus*
- Alcohol
- Anabolic steroids
- Primary liver diseases – primary biliary cirrhosis, haemochromatosis

Clinical features

The possibility of a HCC should be suspected in any patient with cirrhosis who shows evidence of clinical deterioration. The commonest clinical features are right hypochondrial pain and an abdominal mass. Malaise, weight loss and low grade pyrexia are often present. Jaundice is a late feature. Haemobilia or haemoperitoneum are often the immediate cause of death. As most tumours present late, screening of high-risk patients has been advocated in countries with a high prevalence.

Investigation

Tumours can be imaged by ultrasound – transabdominal or laparoscopic, CT scanning or CT portography. Assessment of serum α-fetoprotein (αFP) may also be useful. αFP is a normal fetal serum protein produced by the yolk sac and liver. Progressive increases in serum levels are seen in 70–90% of patients with HCC. Slightly increased and often fluctuating serum levels also seen in hepatitis and cirrhosis. In patients with HCC, serum levels correlate with tumour size and the rate of increase in serum levels correlates with growth of the tumour. Tumour resection usually results in a fall in serum concentrations and serial assessment is useful in measuring response to treatment.

Management

Only about 25% patients with HCC are suitable for surgery. The two surgical options are surgical resection or liver transplantation. Surgical resection involves either hemi-hepatectomy or segmental resection. Most tumours are irresectable due to large size, involvement of major vessels, associated advanced cirrhosis or metastatic disease. The presence of cirrhosis increases the operative mortality from about 5% to more than 20%.

After resection, 5-year survival is typically 30–60%. The 5-year recurrence rate is over 80%. Only a small proportion of patients are cured.

Liver transplantation may be considered for irresectable disease confined to the liver. The operative mortality is often 10–20%. Metastases after transplantation occur in 30–40% of patients. After transplantation, 5-year survival is less than 20%.

Most patients are only suitable for palliative treatment. The median survival in those with irresectable disease is 6 months. Possible palliative interventions include:

- Devascularisation procedures
- Chemotherapy
- Cryotherapy
- Chemo-embolisation
- Thermotherapy

Chemo-embolisation improves survival compared to conservative treatment alone.

Cholangiocarcinoma

Cholangiocarcinoma is a rare tumour of the biliary tree. It accounts for about 1000 deaths per year in UK. It arises from the epithelium of the biliary tract. About 25% are intrahepatic. It often presents late with irresectable disease. Cure rates are low and the median survival is less than 12 months. Neoadjuvant and adjuvant therapies have not improved survival. Risk factors for cholangiocarcinoma include:

- Age
- Primary sclerosing cholangitis
- Choledocholithiasis
- Biliary papillomatosis
- Choledochal cysts
- Thorotrast
- Liver flukes (*Clonorchis sinesis*)

Clinical features

Most patients present with obstructive jaundice. Pain and fever are uncommon. Late presentation is associated with fatigue, malaise and weight loss. Some cases are found incidentally when imaging is performed for other reasons.

Investigation

Liver function tests usually show an obstructive picture. Serum CA19.9 and

CA125 may be raised. The diagnosis can be confirmed by CT or MRI. An ERCP can be both diagnostic and therapeutic. Specimens can be obtained for cytology or histology and a biliary stent can be inserted.

Management

Surgery offers the only chance of cure. The tumour is resected and biliary reconstruction is performed. The aim is for resection with tumour-free margins. Determinants of resectability are the extent of the tumour, vascular invasion, hepatic lobar atrophy and the absence of metastatic disease. Liver transplantation in cholangiocarcinoma is controversial due to high recurrence rates.

Pancreatic carcinoma

Pancreatic carcinoma is the second commonest tumour of the digestive system. The incidence is increasing in the Western world. It is uncommon below 45 years of age. More than 80% of cases occur between 60 and 80 years of age. The male:female ratio is 2:1. Most tumours are adenocarcinomas. More than 80% occur in the head of the pancreas. Overall 5-year survival is less than 5%. The prognosis of ampullary tumours is much better.

Clinical features

About 30% of patients present with obstructive jaundice. This is classically described as 'painless jaundice'. However, most patients develop pain at some stage and 50% present with epigastric pain. About 90% of patients develop anorexia and weight loss. Abdominal examination may show the gallbladder to be palpable. Courvoisier's Law states that if in the presence of jaundice the gallbladder is palpable, it is unlikely to be due to gallstones.

Investigation

Abdominal ultrasound has sensitivity of about 80% for the detection of pancreatic cancer. It can detect the level of biliary obstruction, excludes gallstones and may identify the pancreatic mass. Doppler ultrasound allows assessment of the presence of vascular invasion. Spiral CT has improved on the resolution of conventional CT imaging. Contrast-enhanced triple-phase imaging is the imaging modality of choice. It has sensitivity of greater than 95% for detection of pancreatic tumours and until recently was probably the most useful of staging investigations. MRI is increasingly been used for imaging of the pancreas. However, both ultrasound and CT often fail to detect small hepatic metastases. Laparoscopy will identify liver or peritoneal metastases in 25% of patients deemed resectable after conventional imaging. The use of laparoscopic ultrasound may improve the predictability of resection.

Management

Pancreatic resection is the only hope of cure but only 15% of tumours are deemed resectable. Resectability is determined by assessment of tumour size (<4 cm), absence of invasion of the superior mesenteric artery or portal vein and the absence of ascites, nodal, peritoneal or liver metastases. Overall, 75% of patients have metastases at presentation. Preoperative biliary drainage is of unproven benefit and has not been shown to reduce postoperative morbidity or mortality.

Whipple's operation

A Whipple's procedure involves a pancreatico-duodenal resection (**Figure 13.10**). An initial assessment of resectability is performed by dissection and Kocherisation of the duodenum. The head of the pancreas and duodenum are excised followed by an end-to-side pancreaticoduodenostomy, an end-to-side choledochoduodenostomy and gastrojejunostomy. Octreotide can be given for 1 week to reduce pancreatic secretion. Operative mortality in experienced centres is less than 5%. In those suitable for resectional surgery, 5-year survival is still only 30%. Postoperative morbidity is 30–50%. About 10% of patients develop diabetes and 30% of patients require postoperative exocrine supplements. Postoperative adjuvant chemotherapy may improve survival.

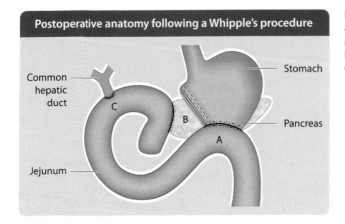

Postoperative anatomy following a Whipple's procedure

Common hepatic duct
C
B
A
Jejunum
Stomach
Pancreas

Figure 13.10 Postoperative anatomy following a Whipple's procedure. A, gastrojejunostomy; B, pancreaticoduodenostomy; C, choledochoduodenostomy.

Complications of a Whipple's procedure include:

- Delayed gastric emptying
- Gastrointestinal haemorrhage
- Operative site haemorrhage
- Intra-abdominal abscess
- Pancreatic fistula

Pylorus-preserving proximal pancreaticoduodenectomy

A pylorus-preserving proximal pancreaticoduodenectomy preserves the gastric antrum and pylorus. Compared with a Whipple's procedure, it is associated with reduced morbidity, fewer post gastrectomy symptoms and less entero-gastric reflux. There is improved postoperative nutrition but no difference in mortality. There are concerns that there may be an associated increased risk of local recurrence.

Palliative treatment

About 85% of patients with pancreatic cancer are not suitable for curative resection. Palliation of symptoms can be achieved either surgically or endoscopically. Surgical palliation has initially a higher complication rate but produces better long-term symptom control. Palliative treatment should achieve relief of jaundice by either endoscopic stenting or surgery, prevention of duodenal obstruction by gastrojejunostomy and relief of pain possibly by a coeliac plexus block. External biliary drainage is rarely required.

Endoscopic stenting of the common bile duct is achievable in over 95% of patients.

Complications include bleeding, perforation, pancreatitis and it has a mortality less than 3%. However, about 20% of patients who undergo palliative stenting will develop duodenal obstruction. The patency of plastic stents is often only 3 to 4 months but this can be improved with the use of self-expanding metal metal wall stents.

Biliary drainage can also be achieved by choledochojejunostomy or cholecystojejunostomy. About 10% of these patients will develop duodenal obstruction. A 'triple bypass' involves a choledochojejunostomy, gastrojejunostomy and entero-enterostomy. This removes the risk of duodenal obstruction and often avoids recurrent jaundice.

Pain occurs in over 80% of patients with advanced malignancy and can be palliated with:

- Slow release morphine
- Coeliac nerve block
- Thoracoscopic section of the splanchnic nerves

Pancreatic neuroendocrine tumours

The pancreas is derived embryologically from the foregut. It has both exocrine and endocrine components. The endocrine components are within the Islets of Langerhans with various cell types:

- α cells secrete glucagon
- β cells secrete insulin
- δ cells secrete somatostatin

Endocrine tumours arise from the Islets of Langerhans and may produce hormones. They may be associated with the multiple endocrine neoplasia (MEN) syndromes.

Insulinomas

Insulinomas are rare. The annual incidence in the UK is 1–2 per million population. They are usually solitary and can occur at any age. They are slightly more common in women. Approximately 90% are less than 2 cm in diameter, 90% are benign and 10% are associated with MEN Type 1 syndrome. The symptoms of an insulinoma are non-specific and variable and may be induced by exercise. The symptoms are those of hypoglycaemia. The diagnosis can be difficult. It is necessary to demonstrate hypoglycaemia in the presence of symptoms. Insulin levels are usually normal or raised. Serum C-peptide levels are often increased. The diagnosis can be confirmed by CT. Resection offers the only chance of cure. The 10-year survival rate is over 90%. Hepatic artery embolisation and chemotherapy maybe required in metastatic disease.

Gastrinomas

Gastrinomas occur in both the duodenum and pancreas. Gastrin over-production results in the Zollinger–Ellison syndrome. Patients presents with severe peptic ulcer disease and diarrhoea. About 20% of patients have MEN type 1 syndrome. Gastric acid hypersecretion can be controlled by either a proton pump inhibitor or surgery. Historically, total gastrectomy was performed and the tumour was left in situ. Today the tumour can be removed by either distal pancreatectomy, enucleation, duodenectomy or a Whipple's procedure. Patients with metastatic disease can be managed with chemotherapy or α-interferon.

Glucagonomas

Glucagonomas are rare and occur as part of the MEN type 1 syndrome. Metastatic disease is often detected at presentation. Symptoms are often non-specific but patients may have a characteristic rash and mucositis. The diagnosis is confirmed by the detection of a raised serum glucagon. Surgery may be beneficial even in

the presence of metastatic disease. Octreotide may help control symptoms.

Chronic pancreatitis

Chronic inflammation of the pancreas results in irreversible destruction of both the endocrine and exocrine pancreatic tissue. The male to female ratio is approximately 4:1. The mean age of onset is 40 years. The incidence is increasing. Chronic pancreatitis increases the risk of pancreatic carcinoma. Early stages of the disease may be characterised by episodes of acute pancreatitis and the pancreas may appear macroscopically normal. The late stages of disease are characterised by pancreatic fibrosis and calcification. Pancreatic duct dilatation and stricture formation may occur. Cysts form within the pancreatic tissue. Aetiological factors include:

- Alcohol
- Tobacco
- Pancreatic duct strictures
- Pancreatic trauma
- Hereditary pancreatitis
- Tropical pancreatitis

Clinical features

Pain is the principal symptom in most patients, usually epigastric and radiating to the back. The pain may be continuous or episodic, often interferes with life and may lead to opiate abuse. Weight lost may occur. Loss of exocrine function produces malabsorption and steatorrhoea. Loss of endocrine function results in diabetes.

Investigation

The serum amylase is often normal. A plain abdominal x-ray may show pancreatic calcification. CT or MRI is the most useful investigation for imaging the pancreas and may confirm pancreatic enlargement, fibrosis and calcification. ERCP has a high sensitivity for detecting chronic pancreatitis. An MRCP will outline the state of the pancreatic ducts. Pancreatic function test rarely provide useful information.

Management

Treatment of the early stages of the disease is with a low fat diet. Alcohol abstention is essential. Opiate analgesia should be avoided if possible. Pancreatic enzyme supplements may reduce both the steatorrhoea and the frequency of painful crises.

Surgery

Surgery is associated with significant morbidity and mortality. It does not arrest the loss of endocrine and exocrine function. The aim of surgery is to remove any mass lesion and relieve pancreatic duct obstruction. A mass lesion can be removed by pancreaticoduodenectomy or a Beger's procedure – resection of the pancreatic head with preservation of the duodenum. Pancreatic duct obstruction can be relieved by pancreaticojejunostomy or a Frey's procedure in which the diseased portion of the pancreatic head is excised and a lateral pancreaticojejunostomy is fashioned. Disease confined to pancreatic tail may require distal pancreatectomy. Surgery relieves symptoms in about 75% of patients.

Portal hypertension

The normal portal venous pressure is 5–10 mmHg. Portal hypertension is defined as a portal pressure more than 12 mmHg.

The aetiology of portal hypertension can be prehepatic, intrahepatic or posthepatic (**Table 13.3**).

Pathophysiology

Increased portal pressure reduces portal venous flow. It encourages the development of porto-systemic anastomoses. Theses develop at sites of connections between the portal and systemic circulation at the:

- Gastro-oesophageal junction
- Lower rectum
- Peri-umbilical veins
- Retroperitoneal veins of Retzius
- Peri-hepatic veins of Sappey

Clinical features

Cirrhosis is the commonest cause of portal hypertension in the UK. Cirrhosis produces features of hepatocellular failure, portal hypertension, variceal bleeding and ascites. About 90% of patients with cirrhosis will develop oesophageal varices. Upper gastrointestinal bleeding will occur in 30% of these patients. The severity of cirrhosis can be assessed using the Child–Pugh classification (**Table 13.4**) and can be divided into three groups:

Aetiology of portal hypertension		
Prehepatic	**Intrahepatic**	**Posthepatic**
Portal vein thrombosis	Presinusoidal	Caval abnormality
Splenic vein thrombosis	Schistosomiasis	Constrictive pericarditis
Tropical splenomegaly	Primary biliary cirrhosis	
Arterio-venous fistula	Chronic active hepatitis	
	Sarcoidosis	
	Sinusoidal	
	Cirrhosis – post hepatitic, alcohol, cryptogenic, metabolic	
	Non-cirrhotic – cytotoxic drugs, Vitamin A intoxication	
	Postsinusoidal	
	Budd–Chiari syndrome	
	Veno-occlusive disease	

Table 13.3 Aetiology of portal hypertension

Child–Pugh classification of the severity of cirrhosis			
Variable	Score		
	1 point	2 points	3 points
Encephalopathy	Absent	Mild/moderate	Severe or coma
Bilirubin (µmol/L)	Less than 34	34–51	More than 51
Albumin (g/L)	More than 35	28–35	Less than 28
Prothrombin time (sec above normal)	1–4	4–6	More than 6
Ascites	None	Mild	Moderate or severe

Table 13.4 Child–Pugh classification of the severity of cirrhosis

- Class A – score 5–6
- Class B – score 7–9
- Class C – score more than 10

Management

In patients with known oesophageal varices, the risk of oesophageal bleeding can be reduced by the use of β blockers. Sclerotherapy of varices does not prevent bleeding. Transjugular intrahepatic portosystemic shunting (TIPPS) involves the creation of an intrahepatic portosystemic shunt. The hepatic vein is cannulated via the internal jugular vein. The intrahepatic portal vein is punctured percutaneously. A guide wire is passed from the portal to hepatic vein. A stent is then passed along guide wire. Complications include encephalopathy and liver failure. The role TIPPS in primary prevention of oesophageal bleeding is at present unknown.

Surgical shunts

The aims of surgical shunts are to reduce portal venous pressure. Portocaval shunts were commonly performed until the mid-1980s. Their use has decreased due to the introduction of TIPPS and liver transplantation in end-stage liver disease. The current roles of surgical shunts are to control variceal bleeding when there is no access to TIPPS, to reduce portal hypertension in those patients awaiting transplantation, to relieve intractable ascites and to reduce bleeding from rectal, colonic or stomal varices. Shunts can be total, partial or selective.

Total shunts have a wide diameter and decompress all of the portal circulation. Following a total shunt, there is no portal venous flow to the liver. Over 90% long-term patency can be achieved but 30–40% of patients will develop encephalopathy. Examples of total shunts are:

- End-to-side portocaval shunt
- Side-to-side portocaval shunt
- Mesocaval C-graft
- Central splenorenal shunt

Partial shunts have a narrow diameter and partially decompress the portal circulation. Some portal vein flow is maintained. About 20% of partial shunts will either stenose or occlude but only 10% of patients will develop encephalopathy. An example of a partial shunt is the small bore portocaval H-graft.

Selective shunts decompress part of the portal circulation and portal vein flow is maintained. Examples of selective shunts are the distal splenorenal and splenocaval shunts.

Ascites

Ascites is free fluid within the abdominal cavity. Over 70% cases are due to liver disease.

Pathophysiology

The normal peritoneal cavity contains approximately 100 mL of fluid. It is a transudate and has a 50% turnover every hour. Peritoneal fluid is produced by the visceral capillaries and is drained via the diaphragmatic lymphatics. In cirrhotic ascites, the pathophysiology is complex.

Portal hypertension results in splanchnic vasodilatation. This results in sodium retention due to alterations in systemic haemodynamics, neurohumeral control and renal function. Impaired free-water excretion results in dilutional hyponatraemia. Renal vasoconstriction can result in the hepatorenal syndrome.

Aetiology

The causes of ascites include:

- Hepatic – cirrhosis, veno-occlusive disease
- Cardiac – right ventricular failure, constrictive pericarditis
- Renal – nephrotic syndrome, renal failure
- Malignancy – ovarian, gastric, colorectal carcinoma
- Infection – tuberculosis
- Pancreatitis
- Lymphatic – congenital anomaly, trauma
- Malnutrition
- Myxoedema

Investigation

A diagnostic peritoneal tap allows peritoneal fluid to be sent for analysis. This includes protein estimation, cytology, bacteriology and biochemistry. A transudate has a total protein less than 30 g/L. Causes of a transudate include cirrhosis and heart failure. An exudate has a total protein more than 30 g/L . Causes of an exudate include carcinomatosis and infection.

Management

Effective treatment of ascites in cirrhosis is difficult. Medical measures include sodium restriction and diuretics. Spironolactone is usually the drug of choice. In those with ascites refractory to medical therapy options include:

- Repeated large-volume paracentesis
- Peritoneovenous shunting
- Portocaval shunting
- Transjugular intrahepatic portosystemic shunting
- Liver transplantation

Applied basic sciences
Anatomy of the large intestine
The caecum and appendix

The caecum is situated in the right iliac fossa and lies below the level of the ileocaecal valve. It is completely covered with peritoneum. Peritoneal folds create the superior, inferior and retrocaecal fossae. Like the remainder of the colon, the caecum has three longitudinal bands of muscle knows as the taeniae coli. These converge on base of the appendix. The anterior relations of the caecum include the greater omentum and anterior abdominal wall. The posterior relations of the caecum include the psoas and iliacus muscle and femoral nerve. The blood supply is from the anterior and posterior caecal arteries. These are terminal branches of the ileocolic artery.

The appendix contains a large amount of lymphoid tissue. It has a complete covering of longitudinal muscle formed from the taeniae coli. The base is attached to the posterior medial surface of the caecum and arises below the level of the ileocaecal valve. It is covered in peritoneum and has a short mesentery known as the mesoappendix. It is related to the anterior abdominal wall one third of the way along a line joining the anterior superior iliac spine and umbilicus (McBurney point). The tip of the appendix can be found in various positions including hanging down into the pelvis related to the right pelvic wall, behind the caecum in the retrocaecal fossa, projecting upward along the lateral side of the caecum or in front or behind the terminal ileum. The blood supply is from the appendicular artery a branch of the posterior caecal artery.

The colon and rectum

The colon is divided into the ascending, transverse, descending and sigmoid colon. The blood supply of the ascending colon is from the ileocolic and right colic arteries, the proximal transverse colon is from the middle colic artery, the distal transverse colon is from the superior left colic artery and the

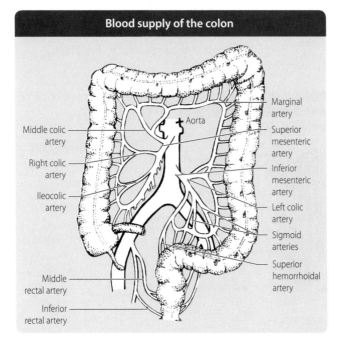

Blood supply of the colon

Middle colic artery
Right colic artery
Ileocolic artery
Middle rectal artery
Inferior rectal artery
Aorta
Marginal artery
Superior mesenteric artery
Inferior mesenteric artery
Left colic artery
Sigmoid arteries
Superior hemorrhoidal artery

Figure 14.1 Blood supply of the colon. (Reproduced from Beck DE. Handbook of Colorectal Surgery, 3rd edn. London: JP Medical Ltd, 2012.)

descending and sigmoid colon is from the inferior left colic artery (**Figure 14.1**). The ileocolic, right and middle colic arteries are branches of the superior mesenteric artery. The superior and inferior left colic arteries are branches of the inferior mesenteric artery. The venous and lymphatic drainage follows the blood supply.

The rectum is about 15 cm long and begins in front of the third sacral vertebra. It passes through pelvic diaphragm and is continuous with anal canal. Peritoneum covers the anterior and lateral surfaces of the upper third and the anterior surface only of the middle third of the rectum. The lower third of the rectum has no peritoneal covering. The rectum has an outer longitudinal and inner circular muscle coat. The mucous membrane forms three transverse folds. The blood supply of the rectum is from the superior, middle and inferior rectal arteries. The superior rectal artery is a branch of the inferior mesenteric artery. The middle rectal artery is a branch of the internal iliac artery. The inferior rectal artery is branch of the internal pudendal artery. The venous drainage corresponds to the arterial supply. The superior rectal vein drains into the inferior mesenteric vein. The middle rectal vein drains into the internal iliac vein. The inferior rectal vein drains into the internal pudendal vein. The lymphatic drainage is into the pararectal nodes. It follows the superior rectal artery to the inferior mesenteric nodes.

The perineum and anal sphincter

The anus has two sphincters – internal and external (**Figure 14.2**). The internal anal sphincter is smooth muscle. The external sphincter is striated muscle. The mucosa of the upper third of anal canal has no somatic sensation. The mucosa of the lower two thirds of the anal canal has somatic innervation from the inferior rectal nerves. Anal glands occur in intersphincteric plane and open at level of the dentate line.

The levator ani muscle is a broad, thin muscle, situated on the side of the pelvis. It is attached to the inner surface of the side of the lesser pelvis and unites with its fellow of the opposite side to form the greater part of the floor of the pelvic cavity. It supports the viscera in the pelvic cavity and surrounds the various structures which pass through it. In combination with the coccygeus muscle, it forms the pelvic diaphragm.

The anal canal above the dentate line is supplied by the terminal branches of the superior rectal artery, which is the terminal branch of the inferior mesenteric artery. The middle rectal artery and inferior rectal artery supply the lower anal canal. Deep to the skin of the anal canal lies the external haemarrhoidal plexus of veins which drain into systemic veins. Above the dentate line lies the internal haemarrhoidal plexus of veins, which drain into the portal venous system. The anorectum is, therefore,

Figure 14.2 Anatomy of the anal canal

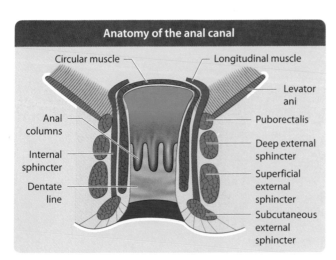

Anatomy of the anal canal

Circular muscle — — Longitudinal muscle

— Levator ani

Anal columns —

— Puborectalis

Internal sphincter —

— Deep external sphincter

Dentate line —

— Superficial external sphincter

— Subcutaneous external sphincter

an important potential portosystemic anastomosis. The lymphatics from the anal canal drain into the superficial inguinal group of lymph nodes.

Colorectal disease
Benign colonic polyps

A polyp is a pedunculated lesion. Not all polyps are tumours. Not all polypoid tumours are benign. Not all benign tumours are polypoid. Large bowel polyps can be classified as epithelial, mesodermal and hamartomas (**Table 14.1**).

Juvenile polyps

Juvenile polyps are the commonest form of polyps in children. They can occur throughout the large bowel but are most common in the rectum. They usually present before 12 years, often with a prolapsing perianal lump or rectal bleeding. They are not pre-malignant and can be treated by local endoscopic resection.

Peutz–Jeghers syndrome

Peutz–Jeghers syndrome is a rare familial condition, inherited as an autosomal dominant disorder characterised by circumoral pigmentation and intestinal polyps. Polyps are found throughout the gut but are more common in the small intestine. The disorder presents in childhood with bleeding, anaemia or intussusception. Polyps can become malignant.

Metaplastic polyps

Metaplastic polyps are small plaques, approximately 2 mm in diameter. The

pathogenesis is unknown and they are not pre-malignant.

Adenomas

Adenomas are benign epithelial neoplasms. They are pre-malignant. The risk of malignancy increases with size. Malignancy is more common in villous rather than tubular lesions. Most adenomas are asymptomatic. Approximately 10% of the population over 45 years have adenomatous polyps. If they do become symptomatic, they usually present with bleeding, mucous discharge or a prolapsing perianal lump. Villous adenomas may produce hypokalaemia but this is rare. Diagnosis is usually by sigmoidoscopy or colonoscopy. A full colonoscopy is essential to exclude other lesions. Treatment is by transanal excision or colonoscopic snaring. Patients require regular colonoscopic surveillance.

Colorectal cancer

Colorectal cancer is the second commonest cancer causing death in the UK. There are 20,000 new cases per year and of these 40% are rectal and 60% are colonic tumours. About 3% patients present with more than one tumour (synchronous tumours). A previous colonic neoplasm increases the risk of a second tumour (metachronous tumour). Some cases are hereditary. Most are related to environmental factors.

Risk factors

Risk factors for sporadic colorectal cancer (75%) include:

- Older age
- Male sex

Classification of large bowel polyps		
Epithelial	**Mesodermal**	**Hamartomatous**
Adenomas – tubular, villous, tubulovillous	Lipoma	Juvenile polyps
	Leiomyoma	Peutz–Jeghers syndrome
Metaplastic polyps	Haemangioma	

Table 14.1 Classification of large bowel polyps

- Cholecystectomy
- Ureterocolic anastomosis
- Diet rich in meat and fat
- Obesity
- Smoking
- Inflammatory bowel disease
- History of colorectal polyps
- History of colorectal cancer
- History of small bowel, endometrial, breast and ovarian cancer

Familial colorectal cancer (20%) is seen in first or second degree relatives with cancer but in whom the criteria for hereditary non-polyposis colorectal cancer (HNPCC) is not fulfilled. The risk increases as follows:

- On first-degree relative increases the risk by 2.3
- Two or more first degree relatives increases the risk by 4.3
- Index case less than 45 years increases the risk by 3.9
- Family history of colorectal adenoma increases the risk by 2.0

Hereditary colorectal cancer (5–10%) is seen in the following syndromes:

- Polyposis syndromes – FAP
- Hereditary non-polyposis colorectal cancer (HNPCC)
- Hamartomatous polyposis syndromes

Of all adenomas, 70% are tubular, 10% are villous and 2% are tubulovillous. Most cancers are believed to arise within pre-existing adenomas. The risk of cancer is greatest in villous adenomas. A series of mutations results in epithelial changes from normality, through dysplasia to invasion.

Inherited syndromes

Familial adenomatous polyposis syndrome

Familial adenomatous polyposis (FAP) is due to a mutation of a tumour suppressor gene on the long arm of chromosome 5. It is inherited as an autosomal dominant condition. The mutation induces proliferation of the mucosa throughout the gastrointestinal tract. FAP syndrome accounts for less than 1% of all colorectal cancers. Patients have widespread colonic polyps that inevitably progress to malignant disease. Polyps usually appear in the second or third decade of life. It is associated with:

- Duodenal adenomatous polyps
- Upper gastrointestinal malignancy
- Congenital hypertrophy of the retinal pigment epithelium
- Desmoid tumours
- Tumours of the central nervous system, thyroid and adrenal cortex

Extra-colonic manifestations include osteomas and epidermoid cysts (Gardener's syndrome).

At risk family member should undergo genetic testing. Screening can be by either rigid or flexible sigmoidoscopy. Sigmoidoscopy is a safe alternative to colonoscopy as rectal sparing is rarely seen. Screening should start in late teens and should continue until 40 years of age and polyp free. Affected individuals should have prophylactic surgery. The surgical options include:

- Panproctocolectomy and ileostomy
- Restorative panproctocolectomy
- Subtotal colectomy and ileorectal anastomosis

The latter option will require surveillance of the rectal stump for polyps.

Hereditary non-polyposis colorectal cancers (Lynch syndrome)

Hereditary non-polyposis colorectal cancers are a heterogeneous group of familial cancers. They account for 3–5% of colorectal cancers and often occur in the right-side of the colon. Tumours arise from polyps although the widespread polyposis seen in FAP is not present. Accelerated progression from polyps to cancer occurs. They occur due to microsatellite instability a result of inheritance of a mutated mismatched repair gene. This increases the risk of the following cancers:

- Colorectal
- Gastric
- Endometrial
- Ovary
- Urothelial

The Amsterdam criteria were developed to standardise the diagnosis of hereditary non-polyposis colorectal cancers and the criteria are as follows:

- At least three relatives with colorectal cancer
- One must be a first-degree relative of the other two
- At least two successive generations should be affected
- One colorectal cancer should be diagnosed before the age of 50 years

It is recommended to start colonoscopic screening 5 years before the youngest affected relative.

Clinical features

Colorectal cancer can present via the outpatient clinic or as an emergency. About 40% of cancers present as a surgical emergency with either obstruction or perforation. Right-sided colonic lesions may present with iron deficiency anaemia due occult blood loss, weight loss or a right iliac fossa mass. Left-sided colonic lesions often present with abdominal pain and alteration in bowel habit or rectal bleeding. Emergency presentation and management is associated with a poorer outcome.

Investigation

In elective cases, the diagnosis can be confirmed by a combination of flexible sigmoidoscopy, colonoscopy or CT scanning. In patients presenting with large bowel obstruction a CT scan is the investigation of choice. CT scanning also allows staging of the disease.

Management

Any surgical resection for a colorectal cancer requires 5 cm proximal and 2 cm distal clearance for colonic lesions (**Figure 14.3**). A 1 cm distal clearance of rectal lesions is adequate if the mesorectum is resected. The mesorectum is fatty tissue directly adjacent to the rectum that contains blood vessels and lymph nodes. The radial margin should be histopathologically free of tumour if possible. Lymph node resection should be performed to the origin of the feeding vessel including an 'en bloc' resection of adherent tumours. The value of a 'no-touch' techniques remains unproven. Depending on site of the tumour the surgical options are:

- Caecum, ascending colon, hepatic flexure – Right hemicolectomy
- Transverse colon – Extended right hemicolectomy
- Splenic flexure, descending colon – Left hemicolectomy
- Sigmoid colon – High anterior resection
- Upper rectum – Anterior resection
- Lower rectum – Abdomino-perineal resection

Transanal microsurgery is an option for small lower rectal cancers. Laparoscopic surgery is increasingly utilised. Early studies raised

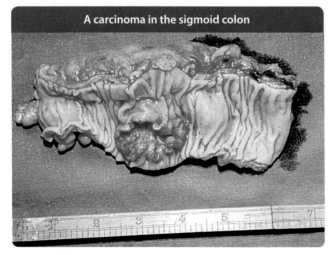

A carcinoma in the sigmoid colon

Figure 14.3 A carcinoma in the sigmoid colon

concerns about port site recurrence. Recent studies suggest equivalence in terms of overall and disease-free survival. Laparoscopic surgery is associated with shorter postoperative recovery and a reduced hospital stay.

The risk of local recurrence following surgery for rectal cancer is reduced by performing a total mesorectal excision. The pelvic peritoneum and lateral ligaments are divided. The plane between the visceral (rectum, mesorectum) and somatic structures is dissected. The middle rectal vessels are divided laterally. The rectal stump should be washed out with cytocidal fluid (water, Betadine) from below. The anastomosis can be either hand-sown or stapled. It can be either a straight anastomosis or a colonic pouch can be fashioned. A colonic pouch is often a J-pouch which provides a better functional outcome. Consideration should be given to a defunctioning loop ileostomy if the anastomosis is less than 12 cm from the anal margin.

Duke's Classification

This was developed by Cuthbert Duke in 1932 for rectal cancers and is as follows:

- Stage A – Tumour confined to the mucosa
- Stage B – Tumour infiltrating through the muscle
- Stage C – Lymph node metastases present

The 5-year survival is 90%, 70% and 30% for Stages A, B and C respectively.

Adjuvant radiotherapy

In patients with rectal cancer, 50% undergoing curative resection develop local recurrence. The median survival with local recurrence is less than 1 year. Risk factors for local recurrence include:

- Local extent of tumour
- Nodal involvement
- Circumferential margin status

The risk of local recurrence can be reduced by radiotherapy. This can be given either pre or postoperatively. Preoperative radiotherapy is given as short course immediately prior to surgery and has been shown to:

- Reduce local recurrence
- Increase time to recurrence
- Increase 5-year survival

A combination chemotherapy and radiotherapy may produce better outcome.

Adjuvant chemotherapy

Adjuvant chemotherapy improves survival in Duke's C tumours. It is of no benefit in Duke's A tumours which already have a good prognosis. Its role in Duke's B tumours remains to be defined.

Colorectal liver metastases

Approximately 20% of patients with colorectal cancer will have liver metastases at the time of their initial presentation. A further 50% of patients with colorectal cancer, will develop liver metastases in the future. Half of these patients will develop liver metastases within 5 years of a potentially 'curative' resection. The median survival with liver metastases is about 1 year.

Detection

The value of intensive radiological follow-up after curative resection of colorectal cancer is controversial. Ultrasound has a limited sensitivity for the detection of liver metastases and will identify lesions more than 0.5 cm in diameter. CT has a higher sensitivity and will also allow assessment of resectability. It is currently recommended that patients undergoing potentially curative colorectal resection should be followed up by CT scanning for at least 2 years. Serial serum tumour marker measurement (CEA) may also be useful in the detection of metastases.

Management

Resectional surgery is the only chance of cure for patients with liver metastases. Only 10% of patients with metastases are suitable for 'curative' hepatic resection. The aim is to resect the tumour with more than a 1 cm margin by segmentectomy, lobectomy or hepatectomy. Following liver resection the 5-year and 10-year survivals are 35% and 20%, respectively. The relative indications for surgical resection are:

- Single lobe involvement
- Less than three lesions without evidence of satellite lesions
- No invasion of the inferior vena cava
- More than 20% of liver can be spared

The relative contraindications for surgical resection are:

- Hilar and coeliac nodal involvement
- Distant metastases
- Poor cardiovascular reserve
- Preoperative portal vein embolisation – atrophy of segments to be excised
- Neoadjuvant chemotherapy

Liver metastases can be palliated by:

- Cryotherapy
- Hepatic artery infusion therapy
- Laser photo-coagulation

Pseudomyxoma peritonei

Pseudomyxoma peritonei is a rare borderline malignant condition. There are approximately 100 cases per year in UK. It is more common in women than men. It is characterised by the production of large volumes of mucinous ascites. It often presents with advanced disease and may be associated with ovarian or appendicular pathology. Depending on the degree of cytological atypia, the pathology has been classified as either disseminated peritoneal adenomucinosis or peritoneal mucinous carcinomatosis.

Clinical features

The clinical features of pseudomyxoma peritonei are those of raised intra-abdominal pressure including bloating, an abdominal wall hernia and a uterovaginal prolapse. There may be features mimicking appendicitis. Patients may have a palpable abdominal mass. There may be features of advanced malignancy including anorexia, weight loss and ascites.

Investigation

Abdominal CT is the first line investigation of choice. An omental cake is often apparent. Scalloping of the diaphragmatic surface of the liver is characteristic. Segmental narrowing of the small bowel is a poor prognostic sign. Patients are often anaemic. Serum inflammatory markers can be raised. Tumours markers (CEA, CA19.9 and CA125) are often elevated.

Management

The management of pseudomyxoma peritonei is controversial. Surgery consists of either complete cytoreduction with curative intent or palliative debulking. Complete cytoreduction is usually combined with intraperitoneal chemotherapy. Careful patient selection is required. Complete cytoreduction is a major undertaking and the postoperative mortality is about 5%. Intra-abdominal sepsis occurs in about 30% patients. Surgery is indicated if complete removal of tumour is achievable or palliative debulking will improve quality of life.

Debulking involves removal of mucin and tumour bulk. Limited resectional procedures may be performed. The aim of cytoreduction is to remove all the macroscopic disease. No tumour deposits more than 3 mm should be left. This will maximise the effect of chemotherapy. Six peritonectomy procedures may be necessary including:

- Greater omentectomy and splenectomy
- Stripping of the left hemidiaphragm
- Stripping of the right hemidiaphragm
- Cholecystectomy and lesser omentectomy
- Distal gastrectomy
- Pelvic peritonectomy and anterior resection

Intraperitoneal chemotherapy

Systemic chemotherapy if of limited value in pseudomyxoma peritonei. Intraperitoneal chemotherapy may be beneficial and should be give after adequate cytoreduction. It is of limited benefit if significant residual disease exists. Intraoperative Mitomycin C is followed by postoperative 5-flurouracil. Chemotherapeutic agents are heated to 41°C as heat seems to have a synergistic effect to the drugs. It does, however, increases the risk of fistula formation and anastomotic leak.

Anal carcinoma

Anal carcinoma is a relatively uncommon tumour. However, the incidence appears to be increasing. There are about 300 cases per year in the UK and they account for 4% of anorectal malignancies.

Aetiology

Anal carcinoma is more common in homosexuals. It is also increasingly seen in those with genital warts. Patients with genital warts often develop intraepithelial neoplasia which appears to be a premalignant condition. The natural history of this premalignant state is, however, unknown. Human papilloma virus (types 16, 18, 31 and 33) is an important aetiological factor. Approximately 50% of anal tumours contain viral DNA.

Pathology

Approximately 80% of anal cancers are squamous cell carcinomas. Other rare tumour types include melanoma, lymphoma and adenocarcinoma. Tumour behaviour depends on its anatomical site. Anal margin tumours are usually well differentiated, keratinising lesions. They are more common in men and have a good prognosis. Anal canal tumours arise above the dentate line. They are usually poorly differentiated and non-keratinising lesions. They are more common in women and have a worse prognosis. Tumours above the dentate line spread to the pelvic lymph nodes. Tumours below the dentate line spread to the inguinal nodes.

Clinical features

The diagnosis can difficult and about 75% of tumours are initially misdiagnosed as benign lesions. About 50% of patients present with perianal pain and bleeding. Only 25% of patients have identified a palpable lesion. In about 70% of patients, the anal sphincter is involved. This can result in faecal incontinence. Neglected tumours can cause a rectovaginal fistula. The inguinal lymph nodes may be enlarged but only 50% of patients with palpable inguinal nodes have metastatic disease.

Investigation

Rectal examination under anaesthetic and biopsy is the most useful 'staging' investigation. Endoanal ultrasound is often impossible due to pain. Abdominal and pelvic CT or MRI can be used to assess pelvic spread.

Management

The management of anal carcinoma has significantly changed over the last 15 years. It was once considered a 'surgical'

disease requiring radical abdominoperineal resection. Now, most patients are managed with radiotherapy. The role of chemotherapy is currently being investigated. Radiotherapy is given to both the primary tumour and the inguinal nodes. About 50% of patients respond to treatment and over 5-year survival is 50%. Surgery should be considered for:

- Tumours that fail to respond to radiotherapy
- Large tumours causing gastrointestinal obstruction
- Small anal margin tumours without sphincter involvement

Diverticular disease

Colonic diverticulae are outpouchings of the colonic wall. They usually result from herniation of the mucosa through the muscular wall and occur at sites where mesenteric vessels penetrate the bowel wall. They are most common in the sigmoid colon. The prevalence increases with age. It affects 10% of the population at 40 years and 60% of the population at 80 years. It is more common in developed countries.

Pathology

Diverticular disease is believed to result form a lack of dietary fibre commonly seen in Western diets. Low dietary fibre results in low stool bulk. This induces increased segmentation of the colonic musculature resulting in hypertrophy. Increased intraluminal pressure results in herniation of the mucosa at sites of weakness of the colonic musculature. Complications of diverticular disease include:

- Diverticulitis
- Pericolic abscess
- Purulent peritonitis – due to rupture of a pericolic abscess
- Faecal peritonitis – due to free perforation of a diverticulum
- Fistula – to vagina, bladder or skin
- Colonic stricture

Inflammation of a segment of diverticular disease results in acute diverticulitis. If the lumen of an inflamed diverticulum becomes obstructed then a pericolic abscess may form. Intraperitoneal rupture of an pericolic abscess can result in purulent peritonitis. Intraperitoneal rupture of an inflamed diverticulum, allowing direct communication between the lumen and peritoneal cavity, can result in faecal peritonitis. A fistula can form if there is rupture into an adjacent organ such as the bladder or vagina.

Clinical features

Uncomplicated diverticular disease is often asymptomatic or at worse causes intermittent left iliac fossa pain. There may be a tendency towards constipation. Acute diverticulitis usually presents with more severe and persistent left iliac fossa pain. The patient may be pyrexial and tachycardic and on examination they may have left iliac fossa tenderness with signs of peritonism. A diverticular abscess often causes prolonged left iliac fossa pain associated with signs of systemic sepsis and swinging pyrexia. Both purulent and faecal peritonitis cause generalised abdominal pain and signs of generalised peritonitis. Patients are more likely to have features of severe sepsis with faecal peritonitis. A colovesical fistula usually presents with recurrent urinary tract infections and pneumaturia – the passage of air *per urethra*. A colovaginal fistula usually presents with the passage of faeces from the vagina. A colonic stricture presents with features of large bowel obstruction, often against the background of repeated episodes of acute diverticulitis.

Investigation

A plain abdominal x-ray with positive diagnostic features (e.g. free intraperitoneal gas or gas in the bladder) is a useful examination but a normal abdominal x-ray can not exclude complications of diverticular disease. An abdominal CT with intravenous and rectal contrast may be useful for imaging abscesses or fistulae and identifying the site of perforation. A flexible sigmoidoscopy may be required to differentiate a benign and malignant colonic stricture.

Management

Minimally symptomatic diverticular disease should be managed by dietary modification, stool bulking agents and the cautious use of laxatives. In patients with acute diverticulitis, the bowel should be 'rested' by restricting oral intake and the use of intravenous fluids. Intravenous antibiotics should be administered and active observation maintained for the development of complications.

If pericolic abscess formation occurs, then percutaneous drainage under radiological guidance is usually possible. Subsequent elective resection and primary anastomosis is often required. Patients who develop generalised peritonitis invariably require emergency surgery. Sigmoid resection and an left iliac fossa end colostomy (Hartmann's procedure) is usually required. The postoperative mortality is high especially (about 40%) in those with faecal peritonitis.

Inflammatory bowel disease

Colonic inflammation is common and the causes include:

- Infection – bacteria, viruses, parasites
- Ulcerative colitis
- Crohn's disease
- Radiation enteritis
- Ischaemic colitis
- Microscopic colitis
- Drug-induced colitis

Epidemiology

Inflammatory bowel disease has a bimodal age distribution with peaks in adolescence and the elderly. Ulcerative colitis is more common than Crohn's disease with a prevalence of 80 and 40 per 100,000 population, respectively. The incidence of both conditions is increasing, possibly due to increased recognition. Ulcerative colitis is slightly more common in men. Crohn's disease is slightly more common in women. Both diseases tend to occur in higher socio-economic groups.

Pathophysiology

Crohn's disease and ulcerative colitis have some pathophysiological features in common. They both result from inappropriate activation of the mucosal immune system. This process seems to be driven by the normal luminal bacteria flora. The pathological processes may result from defective barrier function of the intestinal epithelium. Genetic factors contribute to the susceptibility as demonstrated by a variable prevalence in different populations and increased incidence in first degree relatives, increased concordance in monozygotic twins and concordance in site and type of disease in affected families. Possible environmental factors include smoking, and the use of anti-inflammatory drugs. The pathological features of ulcerative colitis and Crohn's disease are summarised in **Table 14.2**.

Clinical features of ulcerative colitis

In 30% of patients with ulcerative colitis, the disease is confined to the rectum. However, 15% of patients develop more extensive disease over a 10-year period. About 20% patients have total colonic involvement from the outset. Patients generally fall into the following categories:

- Severe acute colitis
- Intermittent relapsing colitis
- Chronic persistent colitis
- Asymptomatic disease

Assessment of disease severity depends on measurement stool frequency and observation of the systemic response.

Systemic features include tachycardia, fever, anaemia, hypoalbuminaemia. Disease can be categorised as:

- Mild – Less than 4 stools per day. Systemically well
- Moderate – More than 4 stools per day. Systemically well
- Severe – More than 6 stools per day. Systemically unwell

Clinical features of Crohn's disease

The clinical features of Crohn's disease depends on the site of disease. About 50% of patients have ileocaecal disease and 25% present with colitis. Extraintestinal manifestations may occur and systemic features are more common than in ulcerative colitis. Extraintestinal manifestations associated with disease activity affect the skin, joints, eyes and liver. They include erythema nodosum, pyoderma gangrenosum, an asymmetrical non-deforming arthropathy, anterior uveitis, episcleritis, conjunctivitis and acute fatty liver. Extraintestinal manifestations unrelated to disease activity include sacroiliitis, ankylosing spondylitis, primary sclerosing cholangitis, cholangiocarcinoma, chronic active hepatitis, amyloid and nephrolithiasis.

Pathological features of inflammatory bowel disease	
Ulcerative colitis	**Crohn's disease**
Lesions continuous – superficial	Lesions patchy – penetrating
Rectum always involved	Rectum normal in 50%
Terminal ileum involved in 10%	Terminal ileum involved in 30%
Granulated ulcerated mucosa	Discretely ulcerated mucosa
No fissuring	Cobblestone appearance with fissuring
Normal serosa	Serositis common
Muscular shortening of colon	Fibrous shortening
Fibrous strictures rare	Strictures common
Fistulae rare	Enterocutaneous or intestinal fistulae in 10%
Anal lesions in <20%	Anal lesions in 75%
	Anal fistulae and chronic fissures
Malignant change well-recognised	Possible malignant change

Table 14.2 Pathological features of inflammatory bowel disease

Investigation

In patients presenting with acute colitis, lower gastrointestinal endoscopy is the investigation of choice. It confirms the presence of colitis, allows assessment of the extent of disease and biopsies can be taken to possibly differentiate ulcerative colitis from Crohn's disease. Ulcerative colitis is usually confluent, extending proximally from the rectum. Crohn's disease may be patchy with 'skip lesions'. Caution should be exercised in performing a colonoscopy in those with severe disease. The endoscopic grading of ulcerative colitis is as follows:

- 0 – Normal
- 1 – Loss of vascular pattern or granularity
- 2 – Granular mucosa with contact bleeding
- 3 – Spontaneous bleeding
- 4 – Ulceration

In those with severe colitis, investigation of the degree of systemic inflammation is important. Useful markers are haemoglobin, white cell count, serum albumin and C-reactive protein. A plain abdominal x-ray is useful is there is suspected toxic megacolon or perforation.

Management

The management of inflammatory bowel disease depends on the type and site of disease and its severity. Different drugs may be used for those with active disease and those in remission.

5-Aminosalicylic acid

5-aminosalicylic acid (5-ASA) is used in mild to moderate ulcerative colitis and Crohn's disease. It blocks the production of prostaglandins and leukotrienes. Sulfasalazine was the first agent described. Now compounds are available that release 5-ASA at the site of disease activity. Mesalazine is 5-ASA conjugated in such a way so as to prevent absorption in the small intestine. Topical preparations may be used in those with left-sided colonic disease. Maintenance therapy is of proven benefit in those with ulcerative colitis but is of unproven benefit in those with Crohn's disease.

Corticosteroids

Corticosteroids are often used in those in whom 5-ASA therapy is inadequate. They are also used in those presenting with acute severe disease. They can be given orally, topically or parenterally. Their use should be limited to acute exacerbations of disease. They are of no proven value as maintenance therapy in either ulcerative colitis or Crohn's disease and their use must be balanced against potential side effects.

Immunosuppressive agents

Immunosuppressive and immunomodulatory agents are often used in those in whom steroids can not be tapered or discontinued. Agents used include:

- Azathioprine
- Methotrexate
- Cyclosporin
- Infliximab

Surgery for ulcerative colitis

Approximately 20% of patients with ulcerative colitis will require surgery at some time and 30% of those with total colitis will require a colectomy within 5 years. Surgery may be required as an emergency. Emergency indications include:

- Toxic megacolon
- Perforation
- Haemorrhage
- Severe colitis failing to respond to medical treatment

Elective indications include:

- Chronic symptoms despite medical therapy
- Carcinoma or high-grade dysplasia

In an emergency, often the only option appropriate is a subtotal colectomy with ileostomy and mucus fistula formation. For elective surgery, the options include:

- Panproctocolectomy and ileostomy
- Subtotal colectomy and ileorectal anastomosis
- Restorative proctocolectomy with ileal pouch formation.

A subtotal colectomy and ileorectal anastomosis maintains continence but proctitis often persists within the rectal stump.

For a restorative proctocolectomy, the patient needs adequate anal musculature. The need for a defunctioning ileostomy following a proctocolectomy is unresolved. The functional results of restorative proctocolectomy are often good but the morbidity can be high. The mean stool frequency is six times per day. Perfect continence is achieved during the day in 90% patients and at night in 60% of patients. Gross incontinence occurs in 5%. About 50% of patients develop significant complications including small bowel obstruction, pouchitis, genitourinary dysfunction, pelvic sepsis, pouch failure and anal stenosis. Larger capacity pouches reduce the stool frequency (**Figure 14.4**).

Surgery for Crohn's disease

Absolute indications for surgery in Crohn's disease include:

- Perforation with generalised peritonitis
- Massive haemorrhage
- Carcinoma
- Fulminant or unresponsive acute severe colitis

Elective indications for surgery in Crohn's disease include:

- Chronic obstructive symptoms
- Chronic ill health or debilitating diarrhoea
- Intra-abdominal abscess or fistula
- Complications of perianal disease

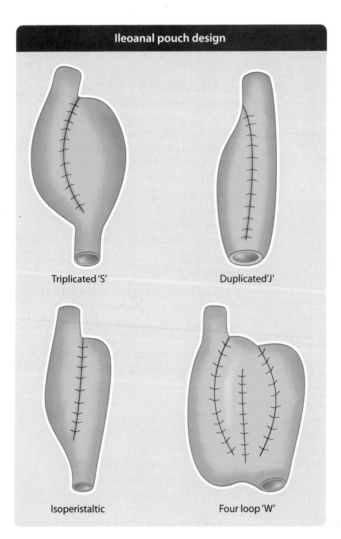

Ileoanal pouch design

Triplicated 'S'

Duplicated 'J'

Isoperistaltic

Four loop 'W'

Figure 14.4 Ileoanal pouch design

Surgery should be as conservative as possible. There is no evidence that increased resection margins reduce the recurrence rate. If possible, the preoperative nutritional state of the patient should be improved prior to surgery. The best surgical option is limited resection. About 30% of patients undergoing ileocaecal resection require further surgery later in life. Strictureplasty is often successful and bypass procedures are rarely required.

Perianal disease
Anorectal sepsis

Aetiology

An abcess is a localised collection of pus. A fistula is an abnormal communication between two epithelial surfaces. Anorectal fistulae occur between the anal or rectal mucosa and the perianal skin (**Figure 14.5**). Most anorectal abscesses and fistulae are believe to arise from infections of the anal glands in the intersphinteric space. The anal glands are found at the level of the dentate line. This theory of origin is known as the cryptoglandular hypothesis. Depending on the route and extent of sepsis, abscesses can classified as:

- Perianal
- Ischiorectal
- Intersphinteric
- Supralevator

Anorectal fistulae can be classified as:

- Intersphinteric
- Transphinteric
- Suprasphinteric
- Extrasphinteric

Clinical features

Anorectal abscesses usually present as painful perianal lumps. Patients may give a history of a previous lump, at the same site, that may have discharged spontaneously. Examination may show a fluctuant lump close to the anal margin. Some patients, particularly those with an intersphinteric abscess, may present with severe anal pain with no visible signs of an abscess. Rectal examination is often impossible due to anal spasm. Patients with ischiorectal fossa abscess often have clinical features of severe sepsis.

An anorectal fistula usually presents with a recurrent perianal purulent discharge. The site of the external opening may give an indication of the site of the internal opening. Goodsall's Rule states than an external opening situated behind the transverse anal line will open into the anal canal in the midline posteriorly. An anterior opening is usually associated with a radial tract. The rule is not absolute and sometimes the path of the fistula can be complex (**Figure 14.6**). Extrasphinteric fistulae are not always

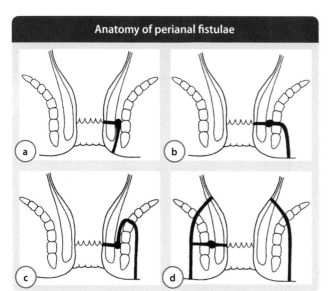

Anatomy of perianal fistulae

a b c d

Figure 14.5 Anatomy of perianal fistulae: (a) intersphincteric fistula; (b) trans-sphincteric fistula; (c) suprasphincteric fistula; (d) extrasphincteric fistula. (Reproduced from Beck DE. Handbook of Colorectal Surgery, 3rd edn. London: JP Medical Ltd, 2012.)

associated with intersphincteric sepsis and consideration should be given to the possibility inflammatory bowel disease or neoplasia as the underlying cause.

Management

The initial surgery for anorectal sepsis should simple and usually requires no more than incision and drainage of an acute abscess. An inexperienced surgeon should avoid looking for a fistula at the time of the initial surgery as, in the presence of acute inflammation, this may result in damage to the anal sphincter. If there is clinical suspicion of an underlying fistula, this can be further assessed by MRI or a subsequent elective admission for an examination under anaesthetic. About 80% of recurrent abscesses are associated with a fistula. Deferred elective surgery has less risk of damage to the sphincter.

In those with an anorectal fistula, the puborectalis muscle is the key to future continence and damage to this and the other sphincter muscles should be avoided.

A low fistula can often simply be laid open with either a fistulotomy or fistulectomy. A high fistula requires staged surgery, often with the placement of a seton. A seton is a non-absorbable suture or surgical-grade cord of material passed along the fistula tract, out through the anus and tied loosely to encourage drainage. The seton may be sequentially tightened to 'cut through' tissue and allow healing of the tract. In some patients, an anorectal advancement flap may be considered to allow early wound healing.

Haemorrhoids

Haemorrhoids are dilated veins in the lower rectum and anal canal. They affect 50% of the population over the age of 50 years. The following factors appear to be important in their aetiology:

- Dilatation of venous plexus
- Distension of arterio-venous anastomoses
- Displacement of the anal cushions

About 80% of patients have high resting anal pressures.

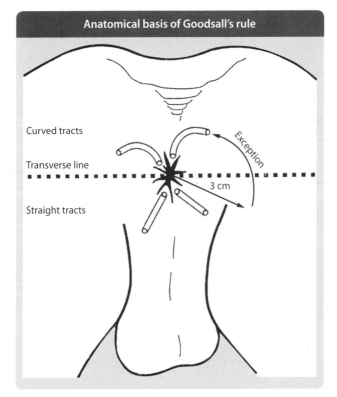

Anatomical basis of Goodsall's rule

Curved tracts

Transverse line

Straight tracts

Exception

3 cm

Figure 14.6 Anatomical basis of Goodsall's Rule. (Reproduced from Beck DE. Handbook of Colorectal Surgery, 3rd edn. London: JP Medical Ltd, 2012.)

Clinical features

Haemorrhoids usually presents with painless, bright red rectal bleeding, a prolapsing perianal lump or acute pain due to thrombosis. Faecal soiling or pruritus ani may occur. Haemorrhoids are often classified as internal or external. Internal haemorrhoids arise above the dentate line and can be sub-classified as:

- First degree – bleeding only
- Second degree – prolapse but reduce spontaneously
- Third degree – prolapse but can be pushed back
- Fourth degree – permanently prolapsed

External haemorrhoids occur below the dentate line and usually present as a perianal lump that my become painful if the tissue becomes thrombosed.

Management

All patients should be advised to have a high residue diet. Local preparations and creams rarely produce long-term clinical benefit. Outpatient treatment options for first and second degree internal haemorrhoids include injection with 5% phenol in arachis or almond oil or rubber band ligation. The latter may have better long-term outcomes. Surgical options include further banding and haemorrhoidectomy. Haemorrhoidectomy is usually performed as an open procedure (Milligan–Morgan).

Haemorrhoidectomy is the treatment of choice for 3rd degree haemorrhoids. The haemorrhoidal tissue is excised with skin-bridges maintained between each wound. The incidence of secondary infection and the severity of postoperative pain may be reduced with oral metronidazole. Botulinum toxin injection may also reduce postoperative pain. Complications of haemorrhoidectomy include:

- Bleeding (3%)
- Urinary retention (10%)
- Anal stenosis may develop if adequate skin bridges are not maintained

Other haemorrhoidectomy techniques include closed or stapled procedures. The recently described stapled technique is associated with:

- Reduced operating time
- Less postoperative pain
- Shortened hospital stay
- More rapid return to normal activity

Thrombosed external haemorrhoids can be managed conservatively. If the pain is intense, the haematoma can be evacuated under local anaesthesia.

Anal fissures

An anal fissure is a break in the skin of the anal canal often occurring as a result of mucosal ischaemia secondary to muscle spasm. They were previously regarded as a 'tear' in the skin due to the passage of a hard stool – pecten band theory. This theory has been largely discounted. About 5% are associated with a chronic intersphinteric abscess. Most acute fissures heal spontaneously. Chronic fissures, with symptoms more than 6 weeks in duration, are associated with increased intra-anal pressure. Treatment is aimed at reducing the anal sphincter pressure.

Clinical features

Anal fissures usually present with pain on defecation, bright red bleeding and pruritus ani. They are seen most commonly between 30 and 50 years of age. About 90% are in the posterior midline. About 10% are in the anterior midline. Anterior fissures are more common in women especially post partum. The fissure is often visible on parting of the buttocks and is seen above a 'sentinel pile' – a small skin tag. Features of chronicity include:

- Symptoms for more than 6 weeks
- Papilla
- Undermined edges
- Visible internal sphincter

If multiple fissures are seen or the fissure is at an unusual site, it is necessary to consider a diagnosis of:

- Crohn's disease
- Syphilis
- Tuberculosis

Management

Stool bulking agents and topical local anaesthesia produces symptomatic improvement. About 50% of acute fissures will heal with this treatment. The use of 0.2%

GTN ointment for treatment of fissures has recently been shown to be beneficial. GTN is a nitric oxide donor that relaxes the internal anal sphincter. It induces a 'reversible chemical sphincterotomy' and reduces the anal resting pressure by 30–40 %. Its use heals more than 70% fissures by 6 weeks with about a 10% risk of early recurrence. The commonest side-effect of GTN is headache. Botulinum toxin can also be used to produce a chemical sphincterotomy.

Surgery should be considered the last resort in the management of anal fissures as it is associated with a high risk of faecal incontinence. Following surgery, 95% achieve prolonged symptomatic improvement but 20% of patients have some degree of incontinence (faecal soiling or incontinence of flatus). Anal dilatation or internal sphincterotomy are the two most common procedures. Sphincterotomy is more effective and has a reduced risk of incontinence. Lateral sphincterotomy is preferred. Posterior sphincterotomy or fissurectomy should be avoided.

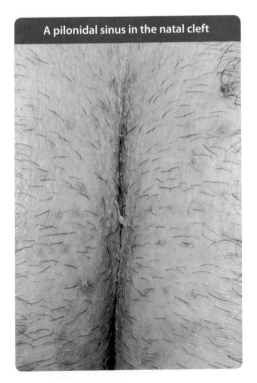

A pilonidal sinus in the natal cleft

Figure 14.7 A pilonidal sinus in the natal cleft

Pilonidal sinus

A pilonidal sinus is a subcutaneous sinus containing hair. It is lined by granulation tissue rather than epithelium and most commonly occurs in the natal cleft (**Figure 14.7**). Pilonidal sinuses are also occasionally seen in the interdigital clefts, in barbers, and in the axilla. A pilonidal sinus is generally believed to be an acquired condition. Inflamed hair follicles in the cleft result in abscess or sinus formation. Hair becomes trapped in the cleft and enters the sinuses. This results in a foreign body reaction which perpetuates sinus formation.

Clinical features

Pilonidal sinuses are usually seen in young adults and are rare after the age of 40 years. The male:female ratio is 4:1. About 80% present with recurrent pain and 80% present with a purulent discharge from the natal cleft.

Management

Surgery is the treatment of choice. Consideration should be given to injection of methylene blue to identify all of the tracts. Antibiotic prophylaxis may be of benefit. The surgical options available include:

- Excision and healing by secondary intention
- Excision and primary closure
- Lord procedures
- Phenol injections
- Skin flap procedures (e.g. Karydakis procedure)

Excision and healing by secondary intention requires regular wound dressing and shaving. This can produces about 70% healing at 70 days but the recurrence rate is about 10%. Excision and primary closure produces 70% healing at 2 weeks but 20% of patients develop a wound infection. Lord procedure involves excision of pits, removal of hair and brushing of tracts. Skin flap procedures aim to excise the sinus, flatten the natal cleft and keep the resulting scar away from the midline (**Figure 14.8**). In expert hands it produces good results and failure rates as low as 5% have been reported.

Rectal prolapse

A complete rectal prolapse is a full thickness prolapse of the rectum through the anus.

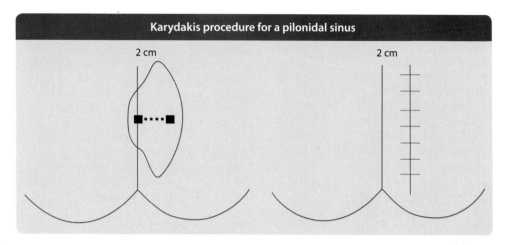

Figure 14.8 Karydakis procedure for a pilonidal sinus.

It contains two layers of the rectal wall and has an intervening peritoneal sac. It usually occurs in elderly adults. The female to male ratio is approximately 6:1. It is invariably associated with weak pelvic and anal musculature. The sigmoid colon and rectum are often floppy and redundant.

An incomplete rectal prolapse is limited to the rectal mucosa. It occurs in both children and adults and is often associated with excessive straining, constipation and haemorrhoids. In children, it is associated with cystic fibrosis. A concealed prolapse is an internal intussusception of the upper into the rectum. The prolapse does not emerge through the anus.

Clinical features

Rectal prolapse occurs in the extremes of life. A rectal prolapse in a child is usually noted by parents and need to be differentiated from colonic intussusception and a juvenile rectal polyp. In adults, it usually presents with a prolapsing anal mass after defaecation. It may be reduce spontaneously or manually. Bleeding, mucus discharge or incontinence may be troublesome. Examination usually shows poor anal tone and the prolapse may be visible on straining. Most prolapses that are longer than 5 cm in length are complete. The differential

diagnosis in an adult is haemorrhoids, a prolapsing rectal tumour or anal polyp and abnormal perineal descent.

Management

Many patients with a complete prolapse are elderly and too frail for surgery. They should be given bulk laxatives and carers taught how to reduce the prolapse. Urgent treatment is however required if the prolapse is irreducible or ischaemic. If the patient is fit for surgery, the operation can be performed via either a perineal or abdominal approach. Abdominal procedures may be performed laparoscopically. Perineal options include:

- Perineal sutures (Thiersch procedure)
- Delorme procedure
- Perineal rectopexy

Abdominal or sacral options include:

- Abdominal rectopexy
- Anterior resection rectopexy

In children, improvement of incomplete rectal prolapse is often seen with dietary advice and the treatment of constipation. Surgery is rarely required. In adults, the management is similar to that of haemorrhoids. This includes injection sclerotherapy, mucosal banding or formal haemorrhoidectomy. Occasionally an anal sphincter repair is required.

Applied basic sciences

Breast anatomy

The breast is made up of both fatty and glandular tissue (**Figure 15.1**) the ratio of varies amongst individuals and the proportions change with age. After the menopause, the relative amount of fatty tissue increases as the glandular tissue diminishes. The base of the breast overlies the pectoralis major muscle between the second and sixth ribs. The gland is fixed to the pectoralis major fascia by the suspensory ligaments, first described by Astley Cooper in 1840. These ligaments run throughout the breast tissue parenchyma from the deep fascia beneath the breast and attach to the dermis of the skin.

The blood supply to the breast skin is based on the subdermal plexus, which communicates with deeper vessels supplying the breast parenchyma. The blood supply is derived from the:

- Internal mammary perforators
- Thoracoacromial artery
- Vessels to serratus anterior
- Lateral thoracic artery
- Intercostal perforators

The sensory innervation of the breast is dermatomal in nature. It is derived from the anterolateral and anteromedial branches of thoracic intercostal nerves. Supraclavicular nerves from the lower fibers of the cervical plexus also provide innervation to the upper and lateral portions of the breast. The sensation to the nipple is from the lateral cutaneous branch of T4.

Breast disease

Assessment of breast disease

The commonest symptoms of female breast disease are:

- A breast lump
- Breast pain
- Nipple discharge
- Nipple retraction
- Axillary lymphadenopathy

Most symptomatic breast cancers present as a painless lump. Breast pain is an uncommon

Figure 15.1 Breast anatomy

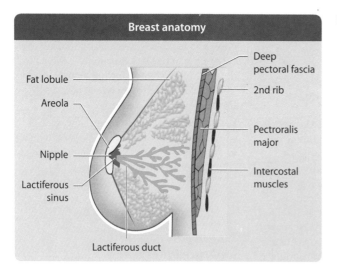

Breast anatomy

Fat lobule

Areola

Nipple

Lactiferous sinus

Lactiferous duct

Deep pectoral fascia

2nd rib

Pectoralis major

Intercostal muscles

presentation of breast cancer. Assessment of most breast problems is by triple assessment comprising of:

- A clinical history and examination
- A radiological assessment – mammography or ultrasound
- A pathological assessment – cytology or biopsy

Each aspect of the triple assessment is reported as:

- 1 = Normal
- 2 = Definitely benign
- 3 = Probably benign
- 4 = Suspicious of malignancy
- 5 = Definitely malignant

Clinical assessment, radiology, cytology and biopsy is given the prefix P, R, C and B respectively. In the pathological assessment, B5a is DCIS and B5b is invasive cancer. Each aspect of the triple assessment needs to be considered in reaching an overall diagnosis.

Breast imaging

The breast can be imaged with mammography, ultrasound or MRI. Mammography is the most sensitive of breast imaging modalities but sensitivity is reduced in young women due to the presence of increased glandular tissue. For symptomatic patients, breast imaging should always be performed as part of a triple assessment.

Mammography

Abnormalities detected on mammography are classified as:

- Spiculate masses
- Stellate lesions
- Circumscribed masses
- Microcalcification

Spiculate masses appear as soft tissue mass with spicules extending into surrounding tissue. About 95% of spiculate masses are due to invasive cancer. Other causes of a spiculated masses include radial scar/ complex sclerosing lesion and fat necrosis. Stellate lesions are localised distortion of the breast parenchyma with no perceptible mass lesion. Other causes of stellate lesions include radial scar and surgical scars. Circumscribed masses should be analysed according to density, outline and size. Causes of well-circumscribed

masses include fibroadenomas, cysts, mucinous or medullary carcinoma and lipomas. Microcalcification is due to debris within the duct wall or lumen and is the sole feature of 33% of screen-detected cancers. Malignant microcalcification is usually linear or branching. Benign microcalcification is usually rounded and punctuate. Causes of microcalcification include DCIS, invasive cancer, papillomas, fibroadenomas and fat necrosis.

Breast ultrasound

Ultrasound is useful in the assessment of breast lumps. It complements mammography and is able to differentiate solid and cystic lesions. It is also able to guide fine needle aspiration and core biopsies. It can be used to assess tumour size and response to therapy. In the diagnosis of malignancy, it has a sensitivity and specificity of 75% and 97%, respectively. Cysts and solid lesions have typical appearances. On ultrasound examination, cysts have smooth walls, sharp anterior and posterior borders and hypoechoic centres without internal echoes. Solid lesions have internal echoes. Malignant tumours have hypoechoic areas, irregular edges and cast hypoechoic shadows. Benign tumours have isoechoic or hypoechoic patterns, smooth walls, well defined borders and cast no shadows.

Breast MRI

Breast MRI is a recently developed technique and has a high sensitivity for multifocal carcinoma. It has low specificity. Lesions detected by MRI need further assessment by ultrasound and biopsy. Uses of breast MRI include:

- Assessing the size of breast cancers
- Determining the focality of lobular cancers
- Imaging the breast for occult disease in presence of axillary metastases
- Differentiating between scar tissue and recurrence
- Assessment of breast implants

Fine needle aspiration and core biopsy

Fine needle aspiration (FNA) is performed without anaesthesia using an 18 Fr needle and 10 mL syringe. Gentle suction is applied whilst the needle is advanced and withdrawn through the lesion. In the management of cysts, FNA will allow the cyst to be drained. In the assessment of a solid lesion, FNA allows tissue to be obtained for cytological assessment. The material is washed from the hub of the needle into an alcohol-containing solution for fixation. The specimen is then centrifuged, applied to a microscope slide and stained.

A core or Tru-cut needle biopsy is obtained under local anaesthesia. A core of tissue is removed from the lesion and fixed in formalin. It is be submitted for histopathological assessment. A core biopsy allows more information to be obtained about the lesion then with FNA but the risks associated with the procedure are higher. The procedure can result in quite extensive bruising. Rare complications include a pneumothorax.

Benign breast disease

Benign breast conditions are practically a universal phenomenon. Previously there was a tendency to include all benign breast disorders under the designation of fibrocystic disease, implying a pathological process. Aberrations of normal development and involution (ANDI) is now the preferred term used to describe most benign breast diseases (**Table 15.1**). It is based on the fact that most benign breast disorders are relatively minor aberrations of the normal processes of development, cyclical hormonal response and involution.

Breast pain

Breast pain or mastalgia is the commonest reason for referral to a breast clinic and accounts for 50% of all referrals. Only 7% of patients with breast cancer report breast pain. Assessment may be helped by the keeping of a breast pain chart. The pain can be divided into cyclical and non-cyclical mastalgia.

Cyclical mastalgia

Cyclical mastalgia is usually bilateral, affects the upper outer quadrant, is mostly minor and accepted by many women as 'part of normal life'. The average age of onset is about 24 years. No consistent hormonal abnormality has been identified. Prolactin levels may be increased. Essential fatty acid profiles may be abnormal. No evidence of psychopathology has been demonstrated. In those with no palpable mass

	Classification of benign breast disease		
	Normal	**Benign disorder**	**Benign disease**
Development	Duct development Lobular development Stromal development	Nipple inversion Fibroadenoma Adolescent hypertrophy	Mammary fistula Giant fibroadenoma
Cyclical change	Hormonal activity	Mastalgia and nodularity	
Epithelial activity			Benign papilloma
Pregnancy and lactation	Epithelial hyperplasia	Bloodstained discharge	Galactocele
Involution	Ductal involution	Duct ectasia nipple retraction	Periductal mastitis
Lobular involution	Cysts Sclerosing adenosis Involutional epithelial hyperplasia	Hyperplasia Micropapillomatosis	Lobular and ductal hyperplasia with atypia

Table 15.1 Classification of benign breast disease

no imaging is required.

Treatment

Most women require no treatment other than simple reassurance. Treatment should be considered if symptoms persist for more than 6 months for more than 7 days per cycle. Evening primrose oil is often used, but there is little scientific evidence to support its use. It requires treatment for at least 4 months and can result in a 50% response rate. Complications are rare with about 1% of patients developing nausea. Danazol has an 80% response rate but 25% patients develop complications including acne, weight gain and hirsutism. Patients taking Danazol require mechanical contraception. Bromocriptine has a 50% response rate with 20% patients developing complications including postural hypotension. Tamoxifen is effective at reducing breast pain but it is not licensed for use in mastalgia. Diuretics or progestogens are not advised.

Non-cyclical mastalgia

Non-cyclical mastalgia usually affects older women. The average age of onset is 45 years and it is usually unilateraland is often localised. True non-cyclical mastalgia often has a musculoskeletal cause. Treatment should involve a supportive bra and anti-inflammatory analgesia.

Fibroadenomas

Fibroadenomas are derived from the breast lobule. They have both epithelial and connective tissue elements. Their pathogenesis is unclear. They are not true neoplasms being polyclonal rather than monoclonal in nature. They should be considered as an ANDI.

Simple fibroadenoma

Most simple fibroadenomas are smooth or slightly lobulated. They usually present between 16 and 24 years of age. The incidence decreases approaching the menopause. They may present as a hard calcified mass in the elderly. Approximately 10% of fibroadenomas are multiple. Recently there has been an improvement in the understanding of natural history. Over a 5-year period, 50% increase in size, 25% remain stable and 25% decrease in size. The risk of malignant transformation is approximately 1 in 1000 and the resulting carcinoma is often a lobular carcinoma. Most fibroadenomas do not require surgical excision but this should be considered with increasing age, particularly if there is any discord between the various aspects of the triple assessment.

Giant fibroadenoma

Giant fibroadenomas have a bimodal age presentation in teens and the premenopausal. They are more common in Afro-Caribbeans and Orientals. They rapidly grow to a large size. They present with pain, breast enlargement, nipple displacement and characteristically have shiny skin changes with dilated veins. Treatment should involve enucleation through a cosmetically appropriately sited scar. Any resulting breast distortion is usually self-correcting. There is no evidence that these tumours recur.

Phyllodes tumour

Phyllodes tumours occur in premenopausal women. They show a wide spectrum of activity, varying from benign to locally aggressive. They have both a cellular and fibrous element and can be classified as benign, borderline and malignant. They should be excised with 1 cm margin of normal tissue and re-excision or mastectomy should be considered for local recurrence. Malignant phyllodes tumours usually do not require adjuvant therapy.

Breast cysts

Approximately 7% of women will develop a clinically palpable cyst at some stage in their lives. They usually occur in peri-menopausal women and the highest prevalence is between 45 and 55 years. Cysts are often multiple, may appear suddenly and are frequently painful. Initial treatment is by simple aspiration. Cytological assessment of cysts fluid is unnecessary but cytology should be considered if there is a blood-stained aspirate. Surgical excision should be considered if a cyst recurs rapidly or repeatedly or there is a residual lump after aspiration.

Breast infections

Lactational breast abscess

Lactational breast sepsis is usually due to *Staphylococcus aureus* infection. Any resulting abscess is usually peripherally situated. Surgery may be pre-empted by early diagnosis. If the diagnosis is suspected then there should be an attempt at aspiration, ideally under ultrasound guidance. Repeated aspiration may be required and formal incision and drainage can often be avoided. Appropriate antibiotics should be given. Patients should be advised to express milk from the affected side and to continue breast feeding from the opposite breast. There is no need to suppress lactation.

Non-lactational breast abscess

Non-lactational breast sepsis often occurs in the periareolar tissue (**Figure 15.2**). Bacterial culture often yields *Bacteroides*, anaerobic streptococci or enterococci. It is usually a manifestation of duct ectasia or periductal mastitis. It most commonly occurs in women between 30 and 60 years. It is more common in smokers who often give a history of recurrent breast sepsis. Repeated aspiration is the treatment of choice. Formal incision and drainage through small incision should be considered if an abscess does not resolve with conservative management. Definitive treatment may be necessary when sepsis is quiescent with appropriate antibiotic prophylaxis. This usually involves a major duct excision. Spontaneous discharge or surgical excision can result in a mammary duct fistula.

Nipple discharge

A nipple discharge is the efflux of fluid from the nipple and accounts for about 5% of referrals to a breast clinic. A discharge can be elicited in approximately 20% of all women by squeezing the nipple and this can often be regarded as 'physiological' especially during the neonatal period, pregnancy, lactation and following mechanical stimulation. It can also represent duct pathology such as:

- Duct ectasia
- Duct papilloma
- Breast cancer

Description of nipple discharge

A nipple discharge can be described as:

- Unilateral or bilateral
- Single or multiple ducts

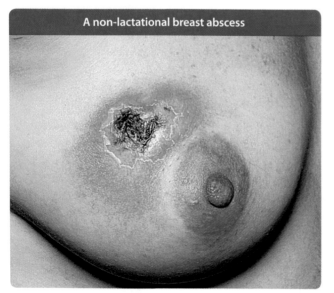

A non-lactational breast abscess

Figure 15.2 A non-lactational breast abscess

- Colour and nature
- Blood-stained
- Spontaneous or expressed

Coloured or opalescent discharge is usually bilateral, multi-duct, creamy or green in colour. It usually occurs in late reproductive life. Symptoms may be intermittent. The commonest cause is duct ectasia. Blood-stained and serosanguinous discharge are more worrying. It is often due to a hyperplastic epithelial lesions and the risk of malignancy increases with age. About 12% of breast cancers present with nipple discharge and 70% of cases of blood-stained discharge have either a duct papilloma or breast cancer.

Investigation

A detailed history will often indicate the underlying cause. Haemostix can be used to test for the presence of blood. Nipple smear cytology is rarely useful. Mammography should be performed in all women over 35 years. Ultrasound may identify a retroareolar lesion. If a lump is present, investigation should be by triple assessment. If there is a suggestion of galactorrhoea the serum prolactin should be measured.

Management

Most women with multi-duct, creamy discharge can be reassured after appropriate investigation. Surgery is only required if the discharge is profuse and embarrassing or malignancy can not be excluded. In women with a single-duct blood-stained discharge consider microdochectomy in younger women or total duct excision in older women.

Galactorrhoea

Galactorrhoea is milk secretion unrelated to breast feeding. It is usually bilateral, multi-duct, milky discharge. Volumes are often copious and can occur spontaneously. The causes of galactorrhoea are shown in **Table 15.2**.

Gynaecomastia

Gynaecomastia is the commonest condition affecting the male breast. It is due to enlargement of both ductal and stromal tissue (**Figure 15.3**). 'True' gynaecomastia is enlargement of the breast glandular tissue. 'Pseudo' gynaecomastia is due to excess adipose tissue. Gynaecomastia is benign and often reversible. The causes of gynaecomastia are shown in **Table 15.3**. Most cases are idiopathic. Physiological causes are due to relative oestrogen excess. Physiological gynaecomastia is seen in the neonatal period, at puberty and in old age.

Clinical features

Gynaecomastia usually presents as unilateral or bilateral non-tender breast enlargement. The history or examination may give an indication of an underlying cause. A detailed drug history should be taken and assessment should include an abdominal and testicular examination. The diagnosis is essentially

Causes of galactorrhoea			
Physiological	**Drugs**	**Pathological**	**Other**
Mechanical stimulation	Dopamine receptor-blocking agents – phenothiazines, haloperidol	Hypothalamic and pituitary stalk lesion	Oestrogens
Extremes of reproductive life		Pituitary tumours	Opiates
	Dopamine-depleting agents – methyldopa	Ectopic prolactin secretion	
Post lactation		Hypothyroidism	
Stress		Chronic renal failure	

Table 15.2 Causes of galactorrhoea

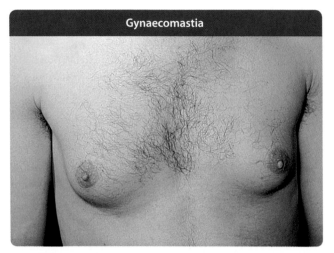

Gynaecomastia

Figure 15.3 Gynaecomastia

Pathological causes of gynaecomastia

Causes	Examples
Primary testicular failure	Anorchia Klinefelter's syndrome Bilateral cryptorchidism
Acquired testicular failure	Mumps Irradiation
Secondary testicular failure	Generalised hypopituitarism Isolated gonadotrophin deficiency
Endocrine tumours	Testicular Adrenal Pituitary
Non-endocrine tumour	Bronchial carcinoma Lymphoma Hypernephroma
Hepatic disease	Cirrhosis Haemochromatosis
Drugs	Oestrogens and oestrogen agonists – digoxin, spironolactone Hyperprolactinaemia - methyldopa, phenothiazines Gonadotrophins Testosterone target cell inhibitors – cimetidine, cyproterone acetate

Table 15.3 Pathological causes of gynaecomastia

clinical and often extensive investigation is not required. Gynaecomastia can be classified according to the degree of breast enlargement and the extent of redundant skin as follows:

- Grade 1 – Minor breast enlargement without skin redundancy
- Grade 2a – Moderate breast enlargement without skin redundancy
- Grade 2b – Moderate breast enlargement with skin redundancy
- Grade 3 – Gross breast enlargement with breast ptosis

Treatment

Most patients simply need reassurance that gynaecomastia is a benign and self-limiting condition without any underlying cause. There are a limited number of studies of the results of medical therapy. Danazol may reduce breast size in 80% of patients. Tamoxifen may reduce both breast size and pain. However, tamoxifen is not licensed for the treatment of gynaecomastia in the UK.

The results of cosmetic surgery can be disappointing. Patients are often unhappy with the cosmetic appearance both before and after surgery. An operation can be considered if gynaecomastia is painful or cosmetically embarrassing. Small areas of gynaecomastia can be excised through periareolar incision. More extensive areas require either liposuction or a breast reduction via a circumareolar incision.

Breast cancer

Breast cancer affects 1 in 9 women worldwide. In UK there are 48,000 new cases and 20,000 deaths each year. It is the commonest cause of cancer death in women. It accounts for 6% of all female deaths. Britain has one of the highest breast cancer mortalities in both Europe and the rest of the world. The WHO classifies breast cancer as either non-invasive or invasive. Non-invasive disease is classified as:

- Ductal carcinoma in situ (DCIS)
- Lobular carcinoma in situ (LCIS)

Invasive disease is classified as:

- Ductal (85%)
- Lobular (10%)
- Mucinous
- Papillary
- Medullary

Ductal carcinoma in situ

Ductal carcinoma in situ (DCIS) is a pre-malignant condition. On histological assessment, malignant cells remain within the basement membrane. Not all cases progress to invasive cancer. True DCIS does not cause lymph node metastases. It is usually asymptomatic and was rarely identified prior to the establishment of breast screening. It usually presents as malignant microcalcification on screening mammography. It is often a multifocal disease process. Management depends on the extent of lesion and the nuclear grade. Surgery alone is often adequate. In those undergoing breast conserving surgery for high-grade DCIS, postoperative radiotherapy should considered. The role of tamoxifen in the management of DCIS is controversial.

Invasive breast cancer

Clinical features

Symptomatic breast cancer usually presents with a painless breast lump. This may be associated with skin dimpling or nipple retraction. Clinical evaluation should assess tethering or fixation to the skin or pectoral muscle. There should also be an examination of the axillary and supraclavicular lymph nodes. Uncommon clinical presentations of breast cancer include inflammatory breast cancer and Paget's disease of the nipple (**Figure 15.4**). Asymptomatic breast cancers may be picked up through the breast screening programme.

Breast cancer surgery

The aims of breast cancer surgery are to achieve cure if excised before metastatic spread has occurred and to prevent the unpleasant sequelae of local recurrence.

Breast surgery

The surgical options for the treatment of breast cancer are:

- Breast conserving surgery
- Simple mastectomy
- Mastectomy +/– breast reconstruction

Tumours considered suitable for breast conservation are usually small single tumours in a large breast, often in a peripheral location with no evidence of local advancement or extensive nodal involvement. Patients undergoing breast conserving surgery should also be considered for adjuvant radiotherapy. There is no difference in survival when breast conserving surgery with radiotherapy is compared to mastectomy. Radical mastectomy is now obsolete.

Axillary surgery

Overall, 30–40% of patients with early breast cancer have nodal involvement. The aims of

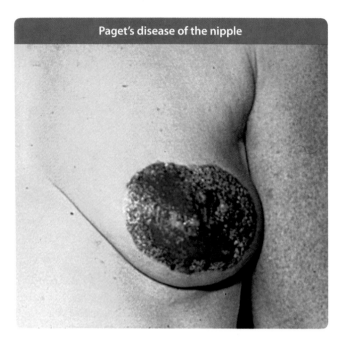

Paget's disease of the nipple

Figure 15.4 Paget's disease of the nipple

axillary surgery in breast cancer is to eradicate local disease and to determine prognosis to guide adjuvant therapy. Clinical evaluation of the axilla is unreliable. Axillary ultrasound and fine needle aspiration or core biopsy may provide preoperative staging information and may allow a tailored approach to the axilla. Surgical evaluation of the axilla is important and should be considered for all patients with invasive cancer.

The axilla can be staged by:

- Axillary node clearance
- Axillary four node sample
- Sentinel lymph node biopsy

The levels of axillary clearance are assessed in relation to the pectoralis minor muscle as follows:

- Level 1 – Below pectoralis minor
- Level 2 – Up to the upper border of pectoralis minor
- Level 3 – To the outer border of the 1st rib

The arguments for axillary clearance include:

- Axillary clearance both stages and treats the axilla
- Axillary sampling potentially misses nodes and under stages the axilla

- Axillary clearance possibly gains better local control
- Avoids complications of axillary radiotherapy
- Avoids morbidity of axillary recurrence

The arguments for axillary sampling include:

- Avoids morbidity of axillary node clearance
- Axillary sampling only stages the axilla
- Must be followed by axillary in those with lymph node involvement
- Avoids unnecessary surgery in 60% of patients with node negative disease
- The combination of axillary clearance and radiotherapy is avoided
- Reduces the risk of lymphoedema

Sentinel lymph node biopsy is now regarded as the optimal method of staging in those with a clinically and radiologically negative axilla. It aims to accurately stage the axilla without the morbidity of axillary clearance. The technique is used to identify the first nodes that tumour drains to by mapping the axilla following the injection of either:

- Radioisotope
- Blue dye
- Combination of isotope and blue dye

The technique allows more detailed examination of nodes removed. The significance of micrometastatic deposits identified in sentinel nodes is unclear. Histological assessment of the nodes removed can now be performed intraoperatively, allowing those with nodal disease to proceed on to an axillary clearance under the same anaesthetic.

Prognostic factors

About 50% of women with operable breast cancer who receive locoregional treatment alone will die from metastatic disease. Prognostic factors have three main uses:

- To select appropriate adjuvant therapy according to prognosis
- To allow comparison of treatment between similar groups of patient at risk of recurrence or death
- To improve the understanding of the disease

Prognostic factors can be chronological, giving an indication of how long the disease has been present and the stage of disease at presentation or biological, relating to the intrinsic behaviour of the tumour. Chronological prognostic factors include:

- Age
- Tumour size
- Lymph node status
- Metastases

Biological prognostic factors include:

- Histological type
- Histological grade
- Lymphatic/vascular invasion
- Hormone and growth factor receptors

Although individual prognostic factors are useful, combining independent prognostic variables in the form of an index allows identification of patients with different prognoses. The Nottingham Prognostic Index (NPI) incorporates the three factors of tumour size, nodal status and histological grade (**Table 15.4**). The Nottingham prognostic index (NPI) = 0.2 × size (cm) + Node stage + Tumour grade.

Chemotherapy

Chemotherapy can be given as either primary systemic therapy prior to locoregional treatment or as adjuvant therapy following locoregional treatment.

Primary (neoadjuvant) chemotherapy

Chemotherapy can be given prior to surgery for large or locally advanced tumours. It may shrink the tumour often allowing breast conserving surgery rather than mastectomy. About 70% tumours show a clinical response. In 30% of patients this response is complete. Surgery should be considered even in those with complete clinical response as 80% of these patients still have histological evidence of tumour. Primary systemic therapy has not to date been shown to improve survival.

Adjuvant chemotherapy

The use of adjuvant chemotherapy depends primarily on risk of recurrence. Important factors to consider include age/menopausal status, nodal status, tumour grade and receptor status. Combination chemotherapy is more effective than a single drug, and is usually given as six or eight cycles at 3-weekly intervals. There is no evidence that more than 6 months treatment is of benefit and the greatest benefit is seen in premenopausal

The Nottingham Prognostic Index		
NPI = L + G + (0.2 × size in cm)		
Number of nodes involved	Lymph node score (L)	Tumour grade (G)
0	1	1
1–3	2	2
>3	3	3

Table 15.4 The Nottingham Prognostic Index

women. High-dose chemotherapy with stem cell rescue produces no overall survival benefit.

Endocrine therapy

Tamoxifen

Tamoxifen is an oral anti-oestrogen. It is an oestrogen receptor antagonist. It is effective in both the adjuvant setting and in advanced disease. It is only effective in those with oestrogen receptor positive disease. Little benefit is seen in oestrogen receptor negative tumours. In the adjuvant setting, it has been shown that 5 years of treatment is better than 2 years. The value of treatment beyond 5 years is unknown. The risk of contralateral breast cancer is reduced by 40%. Benefit is seen in both pre- and post-menopausal women.

Aromatase inhibitors

Several new endocrine therapies are available. The aromatase inhibitors reduce the peripheral conversion of androgens to oestrogens. They are only effective in post-menopausal women and may be superior to tamoxifen in high-risk women. To date, they have not been shown to have survival benefit compared with tamoxifen.

Biological therapy

The human epidermal growth factor receptors are proteins embedded in the cell membrane. They regulate cell growth, adhesion and migration. The HER2 gene is over amplified in 20% of breast cancers. HER2 positivity is an independent poor prognostic factor. Trastuzumab (herceptin) is a monoclonal antibody that binds selectively to the HER2 receptor. It has been shown to improve survival in both the adjuvant and metastatic setting. It only works in patients with HER2 positive cancers. Response to therapy can be predicted by immunocytochemistry and fluorescent in situ hybridisation (FISH) testing. The major side effects are cardiac and its use is associated with cardiac dysfunction in 5% cases.

Locally advanced breast cancer

Locally advanced breast cancers can be regarded as tumours that are not surgically resectable (**Figure 15.5**). Clinical features of locally advanced tumours include:

- Skin ulceration
- Dermal infiltration
- Erythema over the tumour
- Satellite nodules
- Peau d'orange
- Fixation to chest wall, serratus anterior or intercostal muscles
- Fixed axillary nodes

If locally advanced tumours are oestrogen receptor-positive, they can usually treated with primary hormonal therapy. If oestrogen receptor-negative, chemotherapy may be useful. Radiotherapy may be useful in the

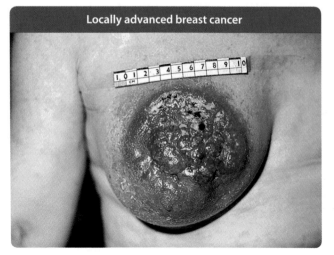

Locally advanced breast cancer

Figure 15.5 Locally advanced breast cancer

local control of disease. If an adequate response to treatment is seen, then a salvage mastectomy can be considered.

Recurrent breast cancer

Most local recurrence of breast cancers are symptomatic (**Figure 15.6**) and are often associated with the development of metastatic disease. Restaging is therefore essential. Local recurrence can be described as single spot, multiple spot of field change recurrence. The commonest sites for metastases from a ductal carcinoma are the liver, bone and lung. Lobular carcinoma is less predictable often spreading to the bowel and retroperitoneum. Consideration should be given to further surgery for isolated 'spot' recurrence after mastectomy or local recurrence in the conserved breast. Radiotherapy should also be considered if not previously given. A change of hormonal agent to an aromatase inhibitor may be appropriate if the tumour is oestrogen receptor positive.

Male breast cancer

About 1% of all breast cancers occur in men. Pathologically, the disease is similar to that which occurs in women. The principles of treatment are the same though obviously the proportion of men undergoing mastectomy is higher. Adjuvant therapy is the same as for women.

Breast reconstruction

Breast reconstruction is increasing in popularity. It can be performed as immediate or delayed procedure. Breast reconstruction is oncologically safe. It does not delay adjuvant therapy or delay the detection of recurrent disease. There are no absolute contraindications. Relative contraindications include old age, diabetes, smoking and collagen diseases. Preoperative counselling about the risks and potential benefits is essential. There are three broad types of breast reconstruction:

- Tissue expanders or implant
- Pedicled myocutaneous flaps
- Free tissue transfer

Each has specific uses and complications. A nipple reconstruction may be considered and the contralateral breast may require surgery to produce symmetry.

Tissue expanders

Tissue expander or an implant-based reconstruction is a simple and reliable technique. However, when used alone it often produces a poor cosmetic result. Capsular contracture can result in firmness and discomfort. Capsulectomy and replacement of the implant may be required. Radiotherapy may increase the risk of capsular contracture. Textured implants reduce the risk of capsule formation.

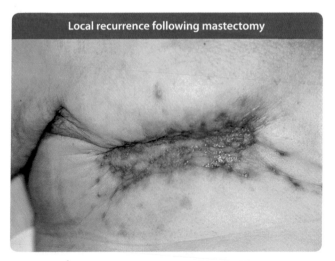

Local recurrence following mastectomy

Figure 15.6 Local recurrence following mastectomy

Pedicled myocutaneous flaps

The two commonest flaps are:

- The latissimus dorsi (LD) flap based on the thoracodorsal vessels
- The pedicle transverse rectus abdominis (TRAM) flap based on the superior epigastric vessels

Either type of flap can be performed as an immediate or delayed procedure. Pedicled flaps produce a better cosmetic result than the use of an implant or tissue expander alone. The use of an LD flap is often combined with tissue expander or prosthesis. TRAM flaps often provide enough autologous tissue to avoid the need for a tissue expander. General complications associated with flaps include necrosis and flap loss. The LD flap leaves a scar on the back and some shoulder weakness. A TRAM flap can result in abdominal donor site hernia and weakness.

Free flaps

Several flaps have been described based on perforator vessels. The most commonly used is the deep inferior epigastric perforator (DIEP) flap. Other flaps have been described based on the superficial inferior epigastric artery or gluteal artery. Free flaps allow tissue transfer with reduced risk of donor site morbidity. The flap failure rates are higher than with pedicled flaps.

Nipple reconstruction

Nipples can be reconstructed using several techniques including:

- Nipple sharing
- Skate flaps
- Labial grafts
- Nipple tattooing
- Prosthetic nipples

Applied basic sciences

Endocrine physiology

Hormones are blood-borne messengers. They are produced by one organ, secreted into the blood and carried to other parts of the body. Only those organs that have specific receptors respond to the hormone. Hormones have a short half-life and are rapidly destroyed. They are involved in homeostasis and adaptation. Some hormones control the activity of other endocrine glands.

Control of salt, water and osmotic pressure

Homeostasis requires close regulation of body salt and water. ADH (antidiuretic hormone) causes water resorption in the collecting ducts of the kidney. Aldosterone increases sodium reabsorption by the kidney. If the blood osmotic pressure is increased ADH secretion is increased. If the blood volume falls aldosterone production in the renal cortex will increase. A number of hormones are also involved in the control of serum calcium.

Reproductive function

Growth of the ovaries and testes and secretion of sex hormones is controlled by follicle stimulating hormone (FSH) and luteinising hormone (LH). Oxytocin produced by the posterior pituitary causes contraction of uterine muscles. Milk production involves many hormones, including prolactin. Milk ejection during lactation is controlled by oxytocin.

Growth and metabolism

Thyroxine increases the metabolic rate of many tissues. Several hormones aid metabolism by raising blood glucose including glucagon, adrenaline, cortisol and growth hormone. Insulin lowers blood glucose. Erythropoietin supports metabolism by regulating the number of red cells in the blood. Important hormones regulating growth include growth hormone and thyroxine.

Thyroid anatomy and physiology

Thyroid embryology

The thyroid gland develops from the floor of embryological pharynx (**Figure 16.1**). This occurs at a point between the tuberculum impar and the copula linguae at the junction of the anterior two-thirds and the posterior one-third of the tongue. This is known as foramen caecum. A diverticulum known as thyroglossal duct invaginates and descends in close relation to the hyoid bone. The gland becomes bilobed to form the thyroid lobes.

Thyroid anatomy

The thyroid gland lies below the thyroid cartilage. The carotid sheath is posterior and lateral. The parathyroids glands lie posterior. The recurrent laryngeal nerve and external laryngeal nerve lie medially. The recurrent laryngeal nerve is closely related to the inferior thyroid artery. The two lobes of the thyroid gland are connected at an isthmus.

The blood supply is from the superior and inferior thyroid arteries. The superior thyroid artery is a branch of the external carotid artery. The inferior thyroid artery is a branch of the thyrocervical trunk. The thyrocervical trunk is a branch the subclavian artery. The venous drainage is into the superior, middle and inferior thyroid veins. The superior thyroid vein drains into the internal jugular vein. The middle thyroid vein drains into the internal jugular vein. The inferior thyroid vein drains into the brachiocephalic vein. The lymphatic drainage is into the deep cervical nodes

Thyroid histology

The thyroid gland is composed of follicles that selectively absorb iodine and concentrate it to produce thyroid hormones. About 25% of all the body iodine is in the thyroid gland. The

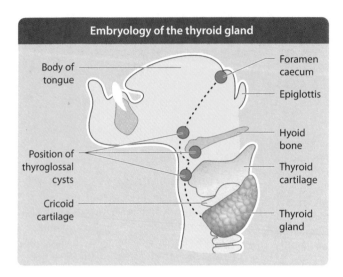

Embryology of the thyroid gland

- Body of tongue
- Foramen caecum
- Epiglottis
- Position of thyroglossal cysts
- Hyoid bone
- Thyroid cartilage
- Cricoid cartilage
- Thyroid gland

Figure 16.1 Embryology of the thyroid gland.

follicles are made of a single layer of thyroid epithelial cells. These secrete thyroxin (both T3 and T4). Inside the follicles is a colloid which is rich in a thyroglobulin. It serves as a reservoir of materials for thyroid hormone production. The spaces between the thyroid follicles contain other type of thyroid cells – parafollicular cells C cells. These secrete calcitonin.

Thyroid physiology

The gland is composed of follicles lined by cuboidal epithelium, which produce T3 and T4. Within the follicles T3 and T4 is stored bound to thyroglobulin. When and as needed, they are secreted. In the circulation T3 and T4 are bound to albumin, thyroxine binding pre-albumin and thyroxine binding globulin. Only about 1% of the hormones remain unbound. Unbound hormones are physiologically active. T3 is quick acting (hours) and T4 is slow acting (days). rT3 (reverse T3) is T3 produced in the peripheries from conversion of T4.

Thyroid hormones promote carbohydrate, protein and lipid metabolism. They act on most cells of the body except the brain. They increase basal metabolic rate and oxygen consumption. They regulate tissue growth and development.

Calcitonin is produced by the parafollicular C cells. Its main action is to lower serum calcium. It acts on skeletal tissue and bone. It inhibits osteoclast activity and bone resorption. It stimulates osteoblast activity. It inhibits release of ionic calcium from bone.

Parathyroid anatomy and physiology

Parathyroid embryology

The parathyroid glands are derived from the pharyngeal pouches (**Figure 16.2**). The 3rd pharyngeal pouch gives rise to the inferior parathyroid glands. The 4th pharyngeal pouch gives rise to the superior parathyroid glands. Abnormalities of position and number of the parathyroid glands are common. About 5% of the population have less than four glands and 25% have supernumerary glands often in aberrant positions.

Parathyroid anatomy

There are four small (20–40 mg) parathyroid glands found near the posterior aspect of the thyroid gland. They have a distinct, encapsulated, smooth surface that differs from the thyroid gland. They are typically light brown in colour, which relates to their fat content and vascularity.

The superior parathyroid glands are located close to the superior pole of the thyroid gland near the cricothyroid cartilage.

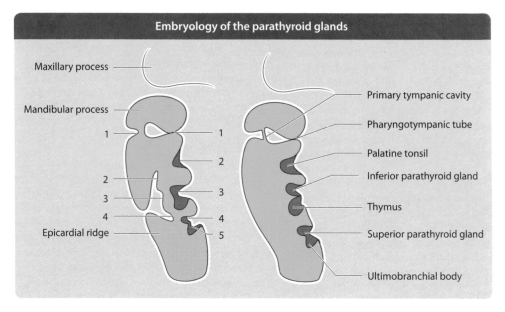

Embryology of the parathyroid glands

Maxillary process

Mandibular process

1

1

2

2

3

3

4

4

5

Epicardial ridge

Primary tympanic cavity

Pharyngotympanic tube

Palatine tonsil

Inferior parathyroid gland

Thymus

Superior parathyroid gland

Ultimobranchial body

Figure 16.2 Embryology of the parathyroid glands. Numbered structures are the pharyngeal pouches and sinuses.

They are most commonly found 1 cm above the intersection of the inferior thyroid artery and the recurrent laryngeal nerve. The inferior parathyroid glands are more variable in location and are most commonly found near the lower pole of the thyroid.

Parathyroid physiology

Parathyroid hormone is an 84 amino acid protein. It has half life measured in minutes. It acts on cell membrane receptors to increase intracellular cAMP. In bone, it increases turnover and calcium release. In the kidney it increases the production of 1,25 dihydroxy-vitamin D3. In the gut it increases calcium absorption.

Pituitary anatomy and physiology

Anatomy of the pituitary gland

The pituitary gland is situated below the 3rd ventricle. It lies in the pituitary fossa of the sella turcica of the sphenoid bone. It is covered by a fold of dura mater known as the diaphragma sellae. It is connected to the brain by the infundibulum and is divided into anterior and posterior lobes.

The anterior lobe of the pituitary is formed in the embryo from Rathke's pouch and consists of the pars anterior and pars intermedia. Its blood supply reaches the lobe via the infundibulum and transports hormones from the hypothalamus. Cells are classified as chromophils or chromophobes. Chromophils are either basophilic or eosinophilic. The posterior lobe is a downgrowth of the floor of the 3rd ventricle. Nerve fibres extend from hypothalamus to the posterior pituitary.

The gland is overhung by the anterior and posterior clinoid processes, dorsum sellae and diaphragma sellae. The infundibulum passes posterior to optic chiasma. Superior to optic chiasma is the anterior communicating artery. A cavernous sinus lies on each side of the gland. In the lateral wall of each cavernous sinus lies the III, IV, ophthalmic branch of V, VI cranial nerves and the internal carotid arteries.

Symptoms of pituitary tumours occur due to endocrine effects and pressure on adjacent structures. Visual changes include:

- Bitemporal hemianopia
- III nerve palsy
- Palsies of IV and VI nerves are rare
- Proptosis

The hypothalamus

The hypothalamus is a major control centre for homeostasis. It constantly measures the condition of the body and regulates functions using both nerves and hormones. It is responsible for control of emotional response, temperature regulation, appetite and water balance. Hormonal control is exerted through the anterior and posterior pituitary. It controls both lobes of the pituitary gland.

Anterior pituitary physiology

The hypothalamus controls the anterior pituitary through a series of releasing hormones. Releasing hormones travel in a portal system to the pituitary gland. They either stimulate or inhibit the release of anterior pituitary hormones. The anterior pituitary is in turn controlled by negative feedback loops. The anterior pituitary produces six major hormones.

- ACTH – acts on the adrenal cortex
- TSH – acts on the thyroid
- LH/FSH act on the ovaries and testes
- Prolactin – acts on the breast
- Growth hormones – has diverse actions

Adrenocorticotrophic hormones

Corticotrophin-releasing hormone (CRH) is produced in hypothalamus. It stimulates the release of adrenocorticotrophic hormone (ACTH) from the anterior pituitary. ACTH stimulates the adrenal cortex to release several hormones including glucocorticoids, androgens and mineralocorticoids. Increased levels of glucocorticoids reduce ACTH release. ACTH levels are increased in fever, stress and hypoglycaemia.

Thyroid stimulating hormone

Thyrotropin-releasing hormone (TRH) is produced in the hypothalamus. It stimulates the release of thyroid-stimulating hormone (TSH) from the anterior pituitary. TSH stimulates thyroid hormone production. Raised levels of thyroid hormones inhibit release of TRH and TSH. TRH levels are increased during exercise and as part of the stress response.

Gonadotrophins

Gonadotrophin-releasing hormone (GnRH) is produced by the hypothalamus. It stimulates the release of LH and FSH from anterior pituitary. FSH stimulates sperm and egg production. LH causes ovarian follicle maturation and ovulation. LH also causes release of the gonadal hormones – testosterone and oestrogen. Rising levels of gonadal hormones inhibits GnRH, LH and FSH.

Growth hormone

Growth hormone-releasing hormone (GHRH) is produced by the hypothalamus. It stimulates release of growth hormone (GH) by the anterior pituitary. Growth hormone is non-trophic and has direct action on non-endocrine cells. It is an important anabolic hormone. It stimulates many cells to grow and divide. It also promotes bone and skeletal muscle growth. It increases protein production by liver and muscle and stimulates gluconeogenesis. It converts glucose to glycogen stores.

Posterior pituitary physiology

Nerves pass directly from two nuclei in the hypothalamus (supraoptic and paraventricular) to the posterior pituitary. Posterior pituitary hormones are made in the cell bodies of the nerves. Hormones travel down the nerve axons by axoplasmic transport to the posterior pituitary. Hormones are released from the pituitary as needed by neurosecretion. The posterior pituitary releases two hormones. Antidiuretic hormone (ADH) acts on collecting duct of the kidney to increase water retention. Oxytocin stimulates the uterus to contract during childbirth. It also causes vasoconstriction and raises blood pressure.

Thyroid and parathyroid disease

Thyroglossal cysts

Thyroglossal cysts arise from the thyroglossal duct. They are present in about 7% of the population. The male to female ratio is approximately equal. About 40% of cases present less than 10 years of age. Thyroglossal cysts are usually found in the subhyoid portion of the tract and 75% present as a midline swelling (**Figure 16.3**). The remainder

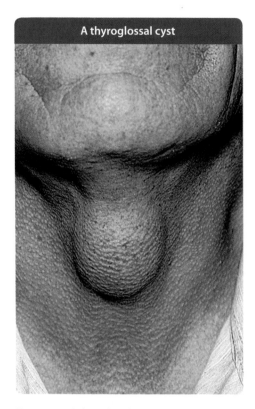

A thyroglossal cyst

Figure 16.3 A thyroglossal cyst

can be found as far lateral as the lateral tip of hyoid bone. As they are attached to the foramen caecum, they move up on protruding the tongue. They often present as an infected cyst due lymphoid tissue in the cyst wall. A fistula may occur following rupture or drainage of an infected thyroglossal cyst.

Treatment

A Sistrunk operation is the surgery of choice. A transverse skin crease incision is made. Platysma flaps are raised and the cyst dissected. The middle third of the hyoid bone and any suprahyoid tract extending into the tongue is dissected and excised.

Thyrotoxicosis

Thyrotoxicosis is due to over production of thyroxine. It affects 2% women and 0.2% of men. The commonest causes of thyrotoxicosis are:

- Grave's disease
- Toxic nodular goitre
- Toxic solitary nodule
- Thyroiditis

Clinical features

The clinical features of thyrotoxicosis are numerous and include:

- Palpitations, tachycardia, cardiac arrhythmias, cardiac failure
- Sweating and tremor
- Hyperkinetic movements
- Nervousness
- Myopathy
- Tiredness and lethargy
- Weight loss
- Heat intolerance
- Diarrhoea and vomiting
- Irritability
- Emotional disturbance
- Behavioural abnormalities
- Ophthalmic signs
- Irregular menstruation and amenorrhoea
- Pretibial myxoedema
- Thyroid acropachy
- Vitiligo
- Alopecia

Pretibial myxoedema occurs in 1–2% of patients with Grave's disease. It presents with painless thickening of the skin in nodules or plaques. They usually occurs on the shins or dorsum of foot. The presence of pretibial myxoedema is strongly associated with ophthalmopathy. Thyroid acropachy occurs in less than 1% of patients with thyrotoxicosis. It closely resembles finger clubbing. Almost all patients also have ophthalmopathy or pretibial myxoedema.

Grave's disease

Grave's disease usually occurs in women between 20 and 40 years. It is an immunological disorder due to production of thyroid stimulating IgG antibodies. These bind to TSH receptors stimulating thyroid hormone production. It produces a diffuse goitre. Clinically, patients have features of thyrotoxicosis often with eye signs including:

- Exophthalmos and proptosis – usually bilateral

- Diplopia due to weakness of the external ocular muscles
- Chemosis and corneal ulceration

Investigation

The diagnosis of thyrotoxicosis can be confirmed by measurement of TSH level. A normal TSH excludes the diagnosis of thyrotoxicosis (except in rare case of TSH secreting pituitary tumours). The serum free T_4 is normally increased. The serum total T_4 can be variable due to changes in thyroid binding globulin. Occasionally free T_3 is increased in isolation in T_3-toxicosis.

Management

In patients with severe thyrotoxicosis, rapid symptomatic relief can be achieved with β-blockers. Thyroid function can be reduced by anti-thyroid drugs, radioactive iodine or surgery.

Anti-thyroid drugs

Anti-thyroid drugs inhibit the synthesis of thyroxine by reducing the incorporation of iodine into tyrosine residues. The most commonly used drug is carbimazole. It can be used short-term (3–4 months) prior to definitive treatment (radioiodine or surgery) or long-term (12–24 months) to induce remission in Grave's disease. Overall, 40% of patients with Grave's disease respond to carbimazole. The side effects include agranulocytosis, aplastic anaemia and hepatitis. Patients need to be warned to seek medical attention if they develop a sore throat or other signs of infection. The advantage of anti-thyroid drugs is that surgery or the use of radioactive materials may be avoided. The disadvantages are that treatment is prolonged; the failure rate after 2 years' treatment is approximately 50%. It is impossible to predict which patients will remain in remission.

Radioactive iodine

^{131}I is the commonest isotope used for the treatment of thyrotoxicosis. A dose of 400 MBq renders 50% patients hypothyroid, but about 20% remain hyperthyroid. Its use is contraindicated in children, pregnancy and breast feeding. Pregnancy should be avoided for 4 months after treatment. The advantage of radio-iodine treatment is that surgery or prolonged drug therapy are avoided. The disadvantages are that 80% of patients will be hypothyroid at 10 years and long-term follow-up is required.

Surgery

Surgery is indicated in patients with Grave's disease if there is relapse after an adequate course of anti-thyroid drugs, a large goitre or high T_4 levels at diagnosis. Subtotal thyroidectomy is the treatment of choice. It preserves about 4 g (10%) of thyroid tissue. Patients must be euthyroid prior to operation. The advantages of surgery are that the goitre is removed and the cure rate is high. The disadvantages are that 5% develop recurrent thyrotoxicosis, 20% develop postoperative hypothyroidism and 0.5% develop parathyroid insufficiency.

Thyroid storm

A thyroid storm is an uncommon life-threatening exacerbation of thyrotoxicosis. It has a mortality of up to 50%. Precipitating factors include thyroid surgery, radioiodine and withdrawal of antithyroid drugs. Clinical features include severe thyrotoxicosis, fever, delirium, seizures and jaundice. Treatment is with propylthiouracil, Lugol's iodine, a β-blocker and supportive measures.

Goitre

Goitre is a non-specific term describing enlargement of the thyroid gland. It does not imply the presence of any specific pathology. Goitres can be either diffuse or multi-nodular (**Table 16.1**). Causes of diffuse goitres include a simple goitre, Grave's disease, thyroiditis, lymphoma and amyloidosis.

Solitary thyroid nodules

About 5% of the population have a clinically palpable solitary thyroid nodule and 50% of the population have a solitary nodule identifiable at autopsy. Over 80% of solitary thyroid nodules occur in women. The risk of malignancy is increased three-fold in men. Malignancy is more common in children and those more than 60 years of age. Approximately 50% solitary thyroid nodules in children are cancers and 70% will have cervical and 15% pulmonary metastases on presentation. However, childhood tumours have good prognosis with greater than 80% 10-year survival.

Overall, If all nodules were removed less than 10% would prove to be malignant. Thyroid surgery is not without complications. There is a need for a selective surgical excision policy for thyroid nodules. Conservative management is appropriate if malignancy can be reasonably excluded.

Clinical features

Rapid painless growth suggests malignancy. Sudden painful growth suggests haemorrhage into a degenerating colloid nodule. Family history is important. About 20% medullary carcinomas are familial and associated with multiple endocrine neoplasia (MEN) 2 syndrome. A history of radiation exposure should also be sought. In 1940s to 1960s large numbers of children were exposed in the USA to low dose irradiation. It was used in the treatment of many benign conditions including tonsillar hypertrophy, acne, thymic enlargement. Radiation exposure increases the incidence of thyroid malignancy – usually papillary tumours.

Examination needs to assess whether the lesion is a true solitary nodule or a dominant nodule within goitre. True solitary nodules have 10% risk of malignancy. Dominant nodules in a multinodular goitre have a 2–5%

risk of malignancy. Evidence of fixation or nodal involvement suggests malignancy. Most patients will be clinically and biochemically euthyroid. Obstructive signs include stridor, tracheal deviation, neck vein engorgement. Hoarseness and vocal cord paralysis suggests a recurrent laryngeal nerve palsy.

Investigation

Investigation of a solitary thyroid nodule should include:

- Biochemical assessment of thyroid functional status
- Ultrasound
- Isotope scanning
- Fine needle aspiration cytology

Biochemical assessment

The thyroid functional status should be assessed by measurement of free T_4 and TSH. Anti-thyroglobulin and anti-microsomal antibodies should also be measured. If there is a family history suggestive of medullary carcinoma then serum calcitonin should also be measured. If there is suspicion of MEN2 syndrome, the patient will need 24-hour urinary catecholamine estimation to exclude a phaeochromocytoma prior to surgery.

Ultrasound

An ultrasound scan will define whether a lesion is a solitary or dominant nodule. It will also distinguish between solid and cystic lesions. Most sonographically solid lesions are benign and cancers can occur in the

Thyroid examination and functional assessment		
Thyroid examination	**Thyroid function**	**Causes**
Diffuse goitre	Euthyroid	Physiological goitre Autoimmune thyroiditis
Diffuse goitre	Hyperthyroid	Primary hyperthyroidism
Multinodular goitre	Euthyroid	Multinodular goitre
Multinodular goitre	Hyperthyroid	Toxic nodular goitre
Solitary nodule	Euthyroid	Thyroid cyst Thyroid adenoma Thyroid carcinoma
Solitary nodule	Hyperthyroid	Functioning adenoma

Table 16.1 Thyroid examination and functional assessment

wall of a cystic lesion. There are no reliable sonographic criteria to distinguish benign and malignant lesions. Features that might suggest malignancy include:

- Hypoechogenicity
- Microcalcification
- Irregular margins
- Increased blood flow on Doppler
- Regional lymphadenopathy

Isotope scanning

^{131}I , ^{123}I or ^{99}Tch scanning provides a functional assessment of the thyroid. Nodules can be classified as cold, warm or hot. Isotope scanning is unable to differentiate benign and malignant nodules. Most solitary thyroid nodules are cold. Most cancers arise in cold nodules. The risk of cancer in a cold nodule is about 10%. The risk of tumour in a hot nodule is negligible. As a result, scintigraphy is of minimal use in the evaluation of solitary thyroid nodules. It is of increased use in the assessment of recurrent thyroid swellings and retrosternal goitres.

Fine needle aspiration cytology

Fine needle aspiration cytology (FNAC) should be one of the first-line investigations of a solitary thyroid nodule. With an experienced cytologist, the diagnostic accuracy can be more than 95%. The accuracy is improved if the sample is performed under ultrasound guidance. Possible cytopathological diagnoses are:

- Benign
- Malignant
- Indeterminate
- Inadequate

FNAC can distinguish benign and malignant tumours, except for follicular neoplasms. The diagnosis of follicular carcinoma depends on visualisation of capsular involvement. If a follicular neoplasm is found on FNAC, the lesion will require surgical excision. Indications for surgery after FNA cytology are:

- All proven malignant nodules
- All cytologically diagnosed follicular neoplasms
- All lesions exhibiting an atypical but non-diagnostic cellular pattern
- Cystic nodules which recur after aspiration

- When on clinical grounds the index of suspicion of malignancy is high even if the cytology report suggests it is benign

A definitive FNAC allows:

- Non-operative treatment of benign disease
- Appropriate surgical treatment of thyroid cancers at the initial operation
- Surgery to be avoided in anaplastic tumours and lymphomas
- A reduction in the total number of thyroid lobectomies
- Increased yield of thyroid cancers

Thyroid neoplasms

Thyroid tumours can be classified as either benign of malignant (**Table 16.2**). The commonest malignant tumours are papillary and follicular carcinomas.

Benign thyroid tumours

Most benign thyroid tumours are follicular adenomas. Papillary adenomas are rare. All papillary tumours should be considered malignant.

Follicular adenoma

Of all follicular lesions, 80% are benign and 20% are malignant. They are encapsulated, smooth and discrete lesions with a glandular or acinar pattern. Follicular adenomas can not be differentiated from carcinoma on FNAC alone. The diagnosis requires histological assessment to exclude capsular invasion.

Toxic adenoma

Toxic adenomas account for 5% of all cases of thyrotoxicosis. The female to male ratio is approximately 9:1. Clinical presentation is with a thyroid nodule (50%) or thyrotoxicosis (40%). Thyrotoxicosis is not usually associated with the eye signs seen in Grave's disease. Scintigraphy shows a hot nodule with suppression of normal thyroid uptake. Treatment is by thyroid lobectomy. Postoperative management requires thyroxine until the suppressed gland returns to normal.

Malignant thyroid tumours

Differentiated thyroid cancer accounts for 80% of thyroid neoplasms. The female to male ratio is approximately 4:1. Malignant thyroid tumours usually present with a solitary thyroid nodule in a young or middle age adult. Papillary and follicular tumours are biologically very different (**Table 16.3**).

Papillary tumours

Most papillary tumours are less than 2 cm diameter at presentation. Tumours less than 1 cm diameter should regarded as minimal or micropapillary lesions. Approximately 50% of papillary tumours are multicentric with a simultaneous tumour in the contralateral lobe. Psammoma bodies and 'orphan Annie' nuclei are characteristic histological features. Early spread occurs to the regional lymph nodes. A 'lateral aberrant thyroid' almost always represents metastatic papillary carcinoma. Thyroid lobectomy is adequate for minimal lesions. Total thyroidectomy is otherwise the surgery of choice. Many tumours are TSH dependent and TSH suppression with postoperative thyroxine is appropriate. The role of prophylactic lymph node dissection at time of initial surgery is unclear. Lymph node dissection does not improve survival. If nodal metastases are present, then a modified neck dissection is required.

Follicular tumours

Follicular adenoma and carcinoma can not be differentiated on FNAC alone. Treatment of all follicular neoplasms is by thyroid lobectomy with frozen section. If the frozen section confirms a carcinoma then total thyroidectomy should be performed. If frozen section confirms an adenoma, no further surgery is required. All patients require suppressive thyroxine therapy. Total thyroidectomy allows detection of metastases using ^{123}I scanning during follow-up.

Anaplastic carcinoma

Anaplastic carcinoma accounts for less than 5% of all thyroid malignancies. They occur in the elderly and are usually an aggressive tumour. Local infiltration causes dyspnoea, hoarseness and dysphagia. Incision biopsy should be avoided as it often causes uncontrollable local spread. Thyroidectomy is seldom feasible. Radiotherapy and chemotherapy are important modes of treatment. Death often occurs within 6 months.

Thyroid lymphoma

Thyroid lymphoma accounts for 2% of all thyroid malignancies. It often arises in a thyroid gland with Hashimoto's thyroiditis. It presents as a goitre in association with generalised lymphoma. Diagnosis can often be made by FNAC. Radiotherapy is the treatment of choice. Prognosis is good, often with more than 85% 5-year survival.

Medullary carcinoma

Medullary carcinoma accounts for 8% of all thyroid malignancies. They arises from the

Classification of thyroid tumours	
Benign	**Malignant**
Follicular adenoma	Papillary carcinoma
Teratoma	Follicular carcinoma
	Mixed papillary–follicular carcinoma
	Medullary carcinoma
	Lymphoma
	Miscellaneous – e.g. squamous, sarcoma
	Metastatic

Table 16.2 Classification of thyroid tumours

Comparison of papillary and follicular tumours	
Papillary	**Follicular**
Multifocal	Solitary
Unencapsulated	Encapsulated
Lymphatic spread	Haematogenous spread
Metastasises to regional nodes	Metastasises to lung, bone and brain

Table 16.3 Comparison of papillary and follicular tumours

para-follicular C-cells. About 20% of cases are familial with autosomal dominant inheritance with almost complete penetrance. It can also occur as part of the MEN IIa and MEN IIb syndromes. Genetically determined cases are often bilateral and multifocal. At risk patients can be identified by looking for a missense mutation in the RET proto-oncogene and can be offered prophylactic thyroidectomy. About 80% of cases are sporadic. Sporadic cases are usually unilateral. Tumours metastasise to the regional nodes and also via blood to bone, liver and lung. About 50% of cases have lymph node metastases at presentation. Tumours produce calcitonin, calcitonin gene-related peptide and carcinoembryonic antigen. Serum calcitonin estimation can be used in follow-up to look for the presence of metastatic disease. Total thyroidectomy is the treatment of choice.

Management

The role of either total thyroidectomy or lobectomy in the management of differentiated thyroid is controversial.

Arguments for total thyroidectomy include:

- Multifocal disease occurs in the opposite lobe in 50% cases
- Total thyroidectomy reduces the risk of local recurrence
- Ablation with radioiodine is facilitated
- Serum thyroglobulin can be used as a tumour marker for progression or recurrence
- In experienced hands, the morbidity of total thyroidectomy is low

Arguments for thyroid lobectomy alone include:

- Many patients do not require radioiodine
- Progression to undifferentiated carcinoma is rare
- The significance of micro-foci in the contralateral lobe is uncertain
- No evidence that more extensive surgery is associated with a better prognosis
- The higher incidence of hypoparathyroidism after total thyroidectomy

Complications of thyroidectomy include:

- Haemorrhage
- Respiratory obstruction
- Recurrent laryngeal nerve palsy
- Hypocalcaemia
- Pneumothorax
- Air embolism
- Recurrent hyperthyroidism
- Hypothyroidism

Recurrent laryngeal nerve palsy

The recurrent laryngeal nerve is a branch of the vagus nerve that supplies motor function and sensation to the larynx. The left recurrent laryngeal nerve loops under the arch of the aorta, posterior to the ligamentum arteriosum before ascending. The right recurrent laryngeal loops around the right subclavian artery. The nerves supply all the laryngeal muscles except for the cricothyroid, which is innervated by the external branch of the superior laryngeal nerve. The recurrent laryngeal nerve can easily be damaged during thyroid surgery. If the damage is unilateral, the patient may present with voice changes including hoarseness. Bilateral nerve damage can result in stridor and aphonia. It is essential to document the movement of the vocal cords by indirect or fibreoptic laryngoscopy prior to thyroid surgery as some patients have asymptomatic recurrent laryngeal nerve palsies.

Follow-up of thyroid carcinoma

Annual ^{123}I scanning should be considered in order to detect asymptomatic recurrence. Treatment of such recurrence can still be curative. The patient needs to be off T_4 for at least 1 month with conversion to T_3. Serum thyroglobulin is also important in follow-up. Increasing levels are often the first sign of recurrence and may allow detection of recurrence without the inconvenience of scintigraphy.

Thyroiditis

de Quervain's thyroiditis

de Quervain's thyroiditis is also known as granulomatous or subacute thyroiditis. It is believed to be due to a viral infection. It often follows an upper respiratory tract infection. It presents with a painful swelling of one or both thyroid lobes, usually associated with malaise and fever. Patients often have clinical features of mild hyperthyroidism and the free T_4 and

ESR is usually raised. It is usually a self-limiting illness with spontaneous recovery. Long-term, a few patients develop mild hypothyroidism. Symptomatic improvement can occur with the use of anti-inflammatory drugs. Steroids may speed resolution in those with severe symptoms.

Hashimoto's thyroiditis

Hashimoto's thyroiditis is also known as lymphomatous thyroiditis and is due to an autoimmune disease. It produces diffuse swelling of the thyroid gland. Histologically, the thyroid is infiltrated with lymphocytes and plasma cells. It may progress to secondary lymphoid nodule formation and stromal fibrosis. Serum anti-thyroglobulin and anti-microsomal antibodies are raised. Patients eventually become hypothyroid. Thyroxine replacement therapy suppresses TSH and reduces the size of the gland. Surgery is rarely required. Long-term the risk of thyroid lymphoma is increased.

Riedel's thyroiditis

Riedel's thyroiditis is also known as acute fibrous thyroiditis. It is a rare but important disease as it often clinically mimics malignancy. Histologically there is a diffuse inflammatory infiltrate throughout the thyroid gland which may extend beyond the capsule into adjacent structures. Clinically it is associated with sclerosing cholangitis, retroperitoneal and mediastinal fibrosis. Surgery is rarely required but division of the isthmus may be necessary to decompress the trachea.

Acute suppurative thyroiditis

Acute suppurative thyroiditis is due to a bacterial or fungal infection. It produces an acutely inflamed thyroid gland. The diagnosis is confirmed by fine-needle aspiration cytology. Treatment is by parenteral antibiotics.

Parathyroid disease

Hyperparathyroidism

Hyperparathyroidism is a common disorder affecting approximately 1 in 1000 of the population. It affects 1 in 500 women over 45 years of age. Most patients are asymptomatic and most cases are identified when hypercalcaemia is detected on testing for other conditions. Causes of hypercalcaemia include:

- Primary hyperparathyroidism
- Malignancy
- Granulomatous disease – sarcoidosis, tuberculosis
- Drugs – thiazide diuretics, vitamin D toxicity, lithium, milk alkali syndrome
- Familial hypercalciuric hypercalcaemia
- Endocrine – thyrotoxicosis, adrenal crisis
- Immobilisation
- Renal failure
- Aluminium intoxication

Hyperparathyroidism can be primary, secondary or tertiary. Primary hyperparathyroidism is due to overproduction of parathyroid hormone by the parathyroid glands. Primary hyperparathyroidism can be due to:

- Parathyroid adenoma (85%)
- Parathyroid hyperplasia (15%)
- Parathyroid carcinoma (<1%)

Secondary hyperparathyroidism is a reactive increase in parathyroid hormone production to compensate for a disturbance in calcium homeostasis. Tertiary hyperparathyroidism is a condition in which reactive parathyroid hyperplasia results in parathyroid hormone hypersecretion despite correction of the underlying aberration of calcium homeostasis.

Clinical features

The clinical features of hyperparathyroidism include:

- General – polydipsia, weight loss
- Renal – colic, haematuria, back pain, polyuria
- Cardiovascular – hypertension, heart block
- Musculoskeletal – non-specific aches and pains, bone pain, pathological fractures
- Gastrointestinal – anorexia, nausea, dyspepsia, constipation
- Neurological – depression, lethargy, apathy, weakness, psychosis

Investigation

In primary hyperparathyroidism, the serum corrected calcium and PTH are both increased. About 75% patients have hypercalciuria and 50% have hypophosphataemia. There may also be a mild hyperchloraemic acidosis. In secondary hyperparathyroidism, the serum PTH is increased but the calcium will be either normal or low.

Preoperative parathyroid localisation

Opinion remains divided on the optimum method for the preoperative localisation for primary parathyroid surgery. Some surgeons may consider primary surgery without investigation.

Radiology

Ultrasound is operator dependent with variable accuracy. It may not detect a normal parathyroid gland and the sensitivity for the detection of abnormal glands is about 80%. It is able to identify intra-thyroid parathyroid glands but may miss deep or intra-thoracic glands. CT is equally as accurate as ultrasound and may be more useful for identifying ectopic glands. MRI is a potentially useful investigation with improved resolution with the use of neck surface coils. About 85% lesions less than 0.5 cm in diameter can be detected by MRI.

Scintigraphy

Scintigraphy utilises a combined ^{99}Tch (pertechnate) and ^{201}Th (thallium chloride) subtraction technique. The thyroid gland takes up both ^{99}Tch and ^{201}Th. The parathyroid glands take up only ^{201}Th. Image subtraction leaves only the parathyroid image. It is the best preoperative localisation technique able to localises about 85% of abnormal glands. The specificity of the investigation is reduced by ^{201}Th uptake in thyroid abnormalities (e.g. multinodular goitres, thyroid adenomas).

Selective venous catheterisation

Selective venous catheterisation is an invasive procedure during which multiple venous blood samples are taken from the neck and mediastinal sites. PTH levels double that measured in a peripheral venous sample are considered significant. It is a lateralising rather than localising procedure. With a parathyroid adenoma, there is unilateral elevation. In hyperplasia, there is bilateral elevation. It is of greatest use prior to re-exploration of the neck for recurrent disease.

Management

The indications for surgery in hyperparathyroidism are:

- Significant symptoms
- Corrected calcium more than 2.8 mmol/L
- Complications of hypercalcaemia

The management of mild hypercalcaemia or asymptomatic patients is controversial. Preoperatively, methylene blue is infused intravenously over about 1 hour. It selectively stains the parathyroid glands. Normal glands stain pale green. Pathological glands stain dark blue or black. An experienced parathyroid surgeon can recognise a normal gland, hyperplasia or adenoma. Frozen section may be useful in differentiating an adenoma and hyperplasia. If a parathyroid adenoma and one normal gland are identified then the adenoma can be removed and no further surgery is required. If hyperplasia is found then all four glands should be removed and one gland transplanted into a marked forearm site.

Persistent or recurrent hyperparathyroidism

Persistent hyperparathyroidism

Persistent hyperparathyroidism is hypercalcaemia identified within 6 months of the initial surgery. It is usually due to a missed adenoma.

Recurrent hyperparathyroidism

Recurrent hyperparathyroidism is hypercalcaemia more than 6 months after the initial surgery with an intervening period of normocalcaemia. It is usually due to inadequate surgery for hyperplasia, but there is a need to consider MEN syndromes. Further surgery should be offered if the corrected serum calcium is more 3 mmol/L. Preoperative localisation is essential as recurrent parathyroid surgery has a higher morbidity and greater chance of failure.

Familial hypocalciuric hypercalcaemia

Familial hypocalciuric hypercalcaemia is an autosomal dominant condition with high penetrance. It accounts for less than 1% cases of hypercalcaemia. It is due to increased renal tubule absorption of calcium. PTH levels are normal. It is a benign condition and parathyroid surgery is not required. It should be suspected if hypercalcaemia has been seen in several generations of a family, especially if members have had unsuccessful parathyroid surgery.

Normocalcaemic hypercalciuria

Normocalcaemic hypercalciuria is due to increased absorption of calcium from the gut or a primary renal tubular leak. There is no benefit from parathyroid surgery.

Pituitary and adrenal disease

Adrenal incidentalomas

Adrenal incidentalomas are adrenal masses discovered during imaging for non-adrenal related causes. They are the commonest adrenal 'disorder'. They are found during 1–5% of abdominal CT scans. About 5–10% patients have non-functioning adrenal masses found at postmortem examination. The male to female ratio is equal. Most incidentalomas are benign and hormonally inactive (**Table 16.4**). Very few patients require adrenalectomy. Diagnostic assessment needs to evaluate whether the lesion is hormonally active or malignant.

Assessment

Assessment of function requires:

- Plasma dihydroepiandosterone
- 24-hour urinary catecholamines and metanephrines
- Low dose dexamethasone suppression test
- Serum ACTH

Assessment of the risk of malignancy requires CT or MRI scanning. On CT scan, malignant lesions are irregular non-homogeneous and have high attenuation. On MRI, malignant lesions have bright intensity on T2 weighed images. CT guided cytology may be useful but it is necessary to exclude a phaeochromocytoma prior to this procedure.

Management

If an adrenal incidentaloma is functioning, then the patient should be considered for an adrenalectomy. This can be performed as either an open or laparoscopic procedure. Malignant lesions are best managed by open surgery. If the lesion is non-functioning, treatment depends on the size of the lesion and the risk of malignancy.

Adrenal metastases

The adrenal gland is a common site for metastases. The most common primary sites are breast, lung, renal, melanoma and lymphomas. Adrenal metastases are often bilateral. If the patient has a prior history of carcinoma, then 10–40% of adrenal masses will be metastases. The risk of malignancy increases with size of the lesion. Most malignant adrenal lesions are greater than 5 cm in diameter.

Cushing's syndrome

Cushing's syndrome results from cortisol excess. The commonest cause is iatrogenic from the use of exogenous steroid medication. Cushing's disease, due to an ACTH-secreting pituitary microadenoma, has an incidence of 1 per 100,000 per year. The female : male ratio is 5:1 and the peak incidence 30 to 50 years.

Aetiology

Cushing's syndrome can result from primary (20%) or secondary (80%) adrenal disease.

Primary adrenal causes include:

- Adrenal adenoma
- Adrenal carcinoma
- Adrenal cortical hyperplasia

Secondary adrenal causes include:

- Cushing's disease
- Ectopic ACTH production from a malignancy

The commonest malignancies associated with ectopic ACTH production are:

- Small cell carcinoma of the lung
- Carcinoid tumours
- Medullary carcinoma of the thyroid

Differential diagnosis of adrenal incidentalomas in the absence of prior malignancy	
Diagnosis	Percentage
Non-functioning cortical adenoma	55
Cortisol producing adenoma	8
Aldosteronoma	2
Adrenal carcinoma	5
Phaeochromocytoma	5
Metastases	20
Other (e.g. cyst, myelolipoma)	5

Table 16.4 Differential diagnosis of adrenal incidentalomas in the absence of prior malignancy

Clinical features

The clinical onset of Cushing's syndrome is often insidious (**Table 16.5**). Patients often notice weight gain, in the face, supraclavicular region and upper back. If not noticed by themselves, it may be highlighted by those they live with. There may also be changes in their skin, including purple stretch marks and easy bruising. As a result of progressive proximal muscle weakness, patients may have difficulty climbing stairs, getting out of a low chair, and raising their arms. Menstrual irregularities, amenorrhea, infertility, and decreased libido may occur in women. Men may develop decreased libido and impotence. Psychological problems such as depression, cognitive dysfunction, and emotional lability may occur. New-onset of hypertension and diabetes mellitus, difficulty with wound healing, increased infections, osteopenia and osteoporotic fractures may occur.

Investigation

The clinical presentation often does not identify the cause of Cushing's syndrome. Investigations are aimed at:

- Providing a biochemical confirmation of the diagnosis
- Identifying the site of the pathological lesion
- Identifying the nature of the pathology

The diagnosis can be confirmed by finding an increased 24-hour urinary free cortisol, loss of diurnal rhythm of serum cortisol and failure of suppression of serum cortisol with low dose (0.5 mg) dexamethasone. The anatomical site of lesion can be identified by measuring serum ACTH. This will be low in adrenal disease and high in pituitary and ectopic production. A CRH test will show an increased ACTH following the administration of CRH in pituitary disease. There will be no increase in ACTH following the administration of CRH in ectopic production. A high-dose dexamethasone suppression test will show reduced serum cortisol levels in pituitary disease.

Imaging is vital in identifying that site of the pathological lesion. A pituitary MRI has a high sensitivity for identifying microadenomas but is not 100% predictive. If diagnostic doubt exists, then bilateral inferior petrosal sinus sampling for ACTH may prove diagnostic. Abdominal CT will allow identification of adrenal pathology and somatostatin scintigraphy may identify sites of ectopic hormone production.

Management

Cushing's disease is best managed by transphenoidal microadenectomy. The success rate is approximately 90%. Large tumours occasional require open surgery via the anterior fossa. Postoperative radiotherapy may be required. If pituitary surgery fails, consideration needs to be given to bilateral adrenalectomy. These patients will require postoperative mineralocorticoid and glucocorticoid replacement. Approximately 25% patients undergoing bilateral adrenalectomy develop Nelson's syndrome. Removal of both adrenals eliminates the production of cortisol and the lack of negative feedback allows any pre-existing pituitary adenoma to grow unchecked. Continued growth can cause mass effects due to physical compression of brain tissue, along with increased production of ACTH and melanocyte stimulating hormone (MSH). The signs and symptoms of Nelson's syndrome include muscle weakness and skin hyperpigmentation due to MSH excess.

Clinical features of Cushing's syndrome	
Symptoms	**Signs**
Weight gain	Truncal obesity
Menstrual irregularity	Plethora
Hirsutism in women	'Moon' face
Headache	Hypertension
Thirst	Bruising
Back pain	Striae
Muscle weakness	Buffalo hump
Abdominal pain	Acne
Lethargy/depression	Osteoporosis

Table 16.5 Clinical features of Cushing's syndrome

Adrenal adenomas require adrenalectomy. This can be performed either laparoscopically or via open surgery. Open surgery can be performed via a transabdominal or retroperitoneal approach.

Conn's syndrome

Aldosteronism, excess secretion of aldosterone, can be primary, due to pathology of the adrenal gland or secondary, due to reduced plasma volume and increased angiotensin production. The commonest causes of secondary hyperaldosteronism are cirrhosis, nephrotic syndrome and cardiac failure. Conn's syndrome is primary hyperaldosteronism due to:

- Aldosterone producing adenoma (50%)
- Bilateral idiopathic hyperplasia – idiopathic hyperaldosteronism (40%)
- Aldosterone secreting carcinoma

Pathophysiology

Aldosterone is produced by the zona glomerulosa of the adrenal cortex. It acts on the distal convoluted tubule to increase sodium reabsorption. Sodium reabsorption occurs at the expense of potassium and hydrogen ion loss.

Clinical features

Conn's syndrome usually occurs between 30 and 60 years and accounts for 1% of cases of hypertension. The hypertension often responds poorly to treatment. Biochemically there is usually a hypokalaemic alkalosis. It should be noted that serum potassium may be normal.

Investigation

Investigation is needed to confirm primary hyperaldosteronism and to localise the pathology. The diagnosis depends on demonstration of:

- Reduced serum potassium
- Increased urinary potassium excretion
- Increased plasma aldosterone

An abdominal CT is able to demonstrate 80% of adrenal adenomas. MRI has a similar sensitivity. Assessment of function may require isotope (NP59) scanning or renal vein sampling for aldosterone.

Management

If an adrenal adenoma is demonstrated, then adrenalectomy is the treatment of choice. Patients may require preoperative spironolactone to increase serum potassium. Following surgery, the blood pressure returns to normal in 70% of patients. Hypertension associated with bilateral idiopathic hyperplasia is difficult to control. Spironolactone alone or with an ACE inhibitor is often useful.

Phaeochromocytomas

Phaeochromocytomas are neuroendocrine tumours usually of the adrenal medulla. Overall, 10% are multiple, 10% are extra-adrenal and 10% are malignant. Extra-adrenal tumours are called paraganglionomas. Most secrete adrenaline and some secrete noradrenaline and dopamine. The clinical features and effects are due catecholamine excess.

Clinical features

Phaeochromocytomas account for 0.1% cases of hypertension. Symptoms are often sporadic and paroxysmal. Attacks may last minutes or hours and occur at variable intervals. The clinical features include hypertension, palpitations, tachycardia and sweating. About 50% of patients develop chest pain.

Chronic effects include hypovolaemia and cardiomyopathy. Phaeochromocytomas can be associated with:

- Multiple endocrine neoplasia syndrome (Type 2)
- Neurofibromatosis
- Von Hippel Lindau syndrome

Investigation

To confirm the diagnosis of a phaeochromocytoma, it is necessary to demonstrate catecholamine excess by:

- 24-hour urinary vanniyl mandelic acid (VMA)
- 24-hour urinary total catecholamines
- Serum adrenaline or noradrenaline

Tumour can be localised with either abdominal CT, MRI or meta-iodobenzylguanidine (MIBG) scanning.

Management

Usually, the clinical features of a phaeochromocytoma can not be controlled pharmacologically. Adrenalectomy is invariably necessary after appropriate preoperative preparation. Surgery for a phaeochromocytoma requires close cooperation between the surgeon and anaesthetist. Preoperative preparation requires α-blockade with phenoxybenzamine for at least 2 weeks. β-blockade after α-blockade may be required. β-blockade without α-blockade can cause a hypertensive crisis. Preoperative hypovolaemia should be corrected. Potential intraoperative problems include hypertension associated with handling of the tumour and hypotension following devascularisation of the tumour. Tight intraoperative blood pressure control is necessary and can be achieved with fluids, nitroprusside and dopamine infusions.

Multiple endocrine neoplasia syndromes

The term multiple endocrine neoplasia (MEN) encompasses several distinct syndromes. Each syndrome features tumours of endocrine glands, each with its own characteristic pattern. In some cases, the tumours are malignant, in others they are benign. Benign or malignant tumours of non-endocrine tissues also occur as components of some of these syndromes.

MEN 1 syndrome (Wermer's syndrome)

- Hyperparathyroidism (90%)
- Pancreatic islet cell tumours (60%)
  - Gastrinoma (60%)
  - Insulinoma (10%)
  - Vipoma
  - Glucagonoma
- Pituitary tumours (5%)
  - Prolactinoma
  - GH, ACTH, TSH secreting tumours
- Thyroid adenoma
- Adrenal adenoma
- Carcinoid tumours

MEN 2a syndrome (Sipple's syndrome)

- Medullary thyroid carcinoma (100%)
- Phaeochromocytoma (50%)
- Hyperparathyroidism (10%)

MEN 2b syndrome

- Medullary thyroid carcinoma (100%)
- Phaeochromocytoma (50%)
- Multiple mucosal neuromas (100%)
- Ganglioneuromatosis of the gut (100%)
- Marfanoid appearance (100%)

The MEN 1 gene

MEN1 syndrome follows Knudson's 'two-hit' model for tumour suppressor gene carcinogenesis. The first hit is a heterozygous MEN1 germ line mutation, inherited from one parent. The second hit is a MEN1 somatic mutation that occurs in predisposed endocrine cells. MEN1 gene mutations can be identified in 70–95% of MEN1 patients. The same mutations are also seen in about 20% of familial isolated hyperparathyroidism cases. Almost all patients are heterozygous for mutations. About 50% of patients develop signs and symptoms by 20 years of age. More than 95% or patients have symptoms by 40 years of age. About one-third of patients affected with MEN1 will die early from an MEN1-

related cancer or associated malignancy. Pancreatic gastrinomas and thymic and bronchial carcinoids are the leading causes of morbidity and mortality.

Carcinoid tumours

Carcinoid tumours are rare neuroendocrine lesions. They arise from amine precursor uptake and decarboxylation (APUD) cells. Approximately 1000 carcinoid tumours are identified in the UK each year. Most primary tumours arise from the gastrointestinal tract. The commonest sites of primary tumours are the appendix (30%) and small bowel (20%). When they metastasise to the liver these tumours produce the carcinoid syndrome. Foregut tumours produce little 5-hydroxy indol acetic acid (5HIAA) but often produce other hormones (e.g. gastrin). Midgut and hindgut tumours more often produce increased amounts of 5HIAA.

Clinical features

Carcinoid tumours often produce vague right-sided abdominal discomfort. The symptoms may have been present for a number of years prior to diagnosis and previous investigations have often been normal. The diagnosis is often only made after urgent surgery – usually due to intestinal obstruction. In those with carcinoid syndrome, symptoms include diarrhoea and flushing. The flushing affects the face and neck lasting only several minutes. It is often precipitated by alcohol or chocolate and may be associated with palpitations or hypotension. Abdominal examination is often normal. A right-sided abdominal mass or hepatomegaly may be present. Other clinical features include telangiectasia, pellagra and tricuspid regurgitation.

Investigation

The diagnosis of a carcinoid tumour may be confirmed by finding increased 24-hour urinary 5HIAA excretion. Plasma chromogranin A levels may be increased. Radiological investigations are rarely helpful. An ultrasound may demonstrate an abdominal mass or liver secondaries. ^{111}In-octreotide scintigraphy may identify primary or secondary tumours. Sclerotic bone secondaries occasionally occur.

Management

The diagnosis is often made after resection of the primary tumour. Symptomatic carcinoid syndrome can often be palliated by use of a somatostatin analogue (e.g. octreotide) and embolisation of the hepatic metastases. The prognosis of carcinoid tumours is better than for adenocarcinomas at similar sites. For surgically resectable tumours, ten-year survival rates of more than 60% have been reported.

Appendiceal carcinoid tumours

Carcinoids are the most common tumour of the appendix. They are an incidental finding in 0.5% of appendicectomy specimens and account for 85% of all appendiceal tumours. About 75% occur at the tip, 15% in the middle and 10% at the base of the appendix. 80% are less than 1 cm in diameter and only 5% are greater than 2 cm in diameter. Locoregional spread or metastases are rare, especially if the tumour is less than 2 cm in diameter. Appendicectomy alone is adequate if the tumour is less than 1 cm in diameter. Right hemicolectomy should be considered for tumours greater than 1 cm in diameter. Prognosis is good with 5-year survival rates of more than 90%.

Secondary hypertension

Hypertension affects 10–20% of adult population and is defined as a diastolic blood pressure greater than 95 mmHg and a systolic blood pressure greater than 160 mmHg. It is associated with increased risk of ischaemic heart disease, stroke, peripheral vascular disease and renal dysfunction. In 90% cases no cause is found (essential hypertension). In 10% cases an underlying abnormality is identified (secondary hypertension). The causes of secondary hypertension area shown in **Table 16.6.**

Renal artery stenosis

Renal artery stenosis accounts for about 2% of all cases of hypertension. About 70% of cases are due to atherosclerosis and 20% of

Causes of secondary hypertension			
Renal	**Adrenal**	**Drug-induced**	**Other**
Renal artery stenosis	Primary aldosteronism	Oral contraceptives	Coarctation of the aorta
Glomerulonephritis	Cushing's syndrome	Corticosteroids	Pre-eclampsia
Pyelonephritis	Phaeochromocytoma	Sympathomimetics	Raised intracranial pressure
Interstitial nephritis			
Obstructive nephropathy			
Polycystic disease			

Table 16.6 Causes of secondary hypertension

cases are due to fibromuscular dysplasia. A renovascular cause of hypertension should be suspected if there is:

- Severe hypertension (diastolic pressure greater than 125 mmHg)
- A patient with pulmonary oedema
- A patient with generalised atherosclerosis
- A very young patient

The diagnosis can be confirmed by a duplex ultrasound scan, digital subtraction angiography, increased serum renin levels and renal isotope scan.

Management

The initial management of renal artery stenosis should be pharmacological. If blood pressure is well controlled with drugs then no further intervention is required. In young patients or those with poorly controlled blood pressure, consideration should be give to percutaneous transluminal angioplasty, renal stenting, renal artery endarterectomy or aortorenal bypass graft. The best results from intervention are seen in those with fibromuscular dysplasia.

Applied basic sciences

Arteries of the upper limb

Axillary artery

The axillary artery is a continuation of the subclavian artery. It runs from the lateral border of the first rib to the lower border of teres major. Pectoralis minor crosses anterior to it and divides it into three parts. Branches arise from the three parts of the axillary artery as follows:

- First part – highest thoracic artery
- Second part – lateral and thoracoacromial arteries
- Third part – subscapular, anterior and posterior circumflex humeral arteries

There is a good collateral circulation around the scapula. Branches of the first part of the subclavian artery anastomose with branches of the third part of the axillary artery.

Brachial artery

The brachial artery is a continuation of the axillary artery. It runs from the lower border of teres major to the neck of the radius. It ends by dividing into the radial and ulnar arteries. The branches of the brachial artery are:

- Profunda brachi which travels in the radial groove of humerus
- Superior ulnar collateral artery
- Inferior ulnar collateral artery
- Nutrient artery to humerus
- Radial and ulnar arteries

The median nerve crosses anterior to it from lateral to medial side at the level of the mid arm.

Arteries of the lower limb

Femoral artery

The femoral artery is the continuation of the external iliac artery. It enters the thigh below the inguinal ligament. It lies midway between the anterior superior iliac spine and symphysis pubis. It passes through the lateral compartment of the femoral sheath.

It ends as the popliteal artery at the opening of the adductor magnus. The branches of the femoral artery are the:

- Superficial external iliac artery
- Superficial epigastric artery
- Superficial external pudendal artery
- Deep external pudendal artery
- Profunda femoris artery

The profunda femoris artery arises from the lateral aspect of femoral artery. It then passes behind the femoral artery and gives the medial and lateral circumflex femoral arteries and four perforating branches. It supplies the medial and posterior compartments of the thigh.

Popliteal artery

The popliteal artery is the continuation of femoral artery. It divides into the anterior and posterior tibial arteries. The anterior tibial artery continues as the dorsalis pedis artery.

Arteries of the head and neck

Common carotid artery

The right common carotid artery arises from the brachiocephalic artery. The left common carotid artery arises from the arch of the aorta. Both are embedded in their respective carotid sheath and are related to the internal jugular vein and vagus nerve. They divide at the upper border of thyroid cartilage into the internal and external carotid arteries. Just proximal to the division is the carotid sinus. This contains nerve endings from the glossopharyngeal nerve. The carotid sinus functions as a baroreceptor. Posterior to the bifurcation is the carotid body. This is innervated by glossopharyngeal nerve. The carotid body functions as a chemoreceptor.

External carotid artery

The external carotid artery is a terminal branch of the common carotid artery. It begins at level the level of the upper border of the thyroid cartilage and terminates in the substance of the parotid gland. The terminal branches of the external carotid artery are the:

- Superficial temporal artery
- Maxillary artery

Branches of the external carotid artery in the neck are the:

- Superior thyroid artery
- Ascending pharyngeal artery
- Lingual artery
- Facial artery
- Occipital artery
- Posterior auricular artery

Internal carotid artery

The internal carotid artery is a terminal branch of the common carotid artery. It begins at the level of upper border of the thyroid cartilage and enters the cranial cavity through carotid canal in petrous part of the temporal bone. It is embedded in carotid sheath. It is related to the internal jugular vein and vagus nerve. The internal carotid artery has no branches in the neck.

Veins of the lower limb

Long saphenous vein

The long saphenous vein is a superficial vein – superficial to the deep fascia. It is a continuation of the dorsal venous arch. It passes anterior to the medial malleolus and drains into the femoral vein by passing through the saphenous opening of the fascia lata. It is accompanied by the saphenous nerve and has numerous valves which prevent retrograde blood flow. Tributaries include the:

- Superficial epigastric vein
- Superficial external pudendal vein
- Superficial circumflex iliac vein
- Communicating branches to small saphenous and deep veins

Short saphenous vein

The short saphenous vein is also a superficial vein. It arises from the lateral aspect of the dorsal venous arch. It passes posterior to the lateral malleolus. It ascends in the back of the leg and is accompanied by the sural nerve. It drains into the popliteal vein.

Perforating veins

Perforating veins connect the superficial great and small saphenous veins to deep veins. They have valves which allow blood to flow only from the superficial to deep veins.

Venous physiology

The main purpose of the venous system is to return oxygen-depleted blood back to the heart.

Specific characteristics of the venous system of the leg are important to move blood against gravity in the standing position. The presence of anti-reflux valves and the resistance of the vein walls allows blood to move from the superficial to the deep venous system and from the feet to the heart. The pump mechanism of the lower limb maintains blood flow through the veins.

Vascular pathology

Both arteries and veins have three layers to the vessel wall:

- Tunica intima
- Tunica media
- Tunica adventia

The tunica intima is a thin layer that includes the vascular endothelium. The tunica media is made up of circularly-arranged smooth muscle cells and sheets of elastin. The tunica adventia is mainly made up of fibrous connective tissue.

Arteriosclerosis

Arteriosclerosis describes several conditions which result in narrowing of the arteries including atheroma, Mönckeberg arteriosclerosis and arteriosclerosis. Atheroma is due to lipid deposition within the intima of the arterial wall. Mönckeberg arteriosclerosis (medial calcific sclerosis) is due to calcification of the media of medium-sized arteries. Arteriolosclerosis is characterised by hyaline thickening of small sized arteries and is commonly seen in the kidneys secondary to hypertension or diabetes mellitus.

Atheroma

Atheroma is the single most important cause of morbidity and mortality in Western countries. The outcomes of atheroma formation include ischaemic heart disease, peripheral vascular disease and cerebrovascular disease. The cause of atheroma is unknown, but many risk factors and also factors which accelerate disease progression have been identified. The major risk factors for atherosclerosis are:

- Hyperlipidaemia
- Hypertension
- Smoking
- Diabetes
- Age
- Sex
- Family history
- Alcohol
- Low socioeconomic status

Aetiology

High plasma levels of serum low density lipoprotein (LDL) cholesterol promotes accumulation of cholesterol in the arterial intima and ultimately plaque formation. Endothelial injury is probably an important initiating factor. Lipid rich plaque contents are derived from thrombus formation at sites of endothelial injuries. Growth factors, such as platelet derived growth factor, involved in thrombosis formation, may also promote proliferation of cells in plaques, including cells of smooth muscle origin derived from the arterial media. Inflammation is also a feature of atheromatous plaques and may be involved in disease progression. Macrophages produce various factors which promote inflammation. This results in lymphocyte accumulation, fibroblast proliferation and collagen production.

Pathology

Lipid deposition in the intima is the key feature of atheroma formation. These deposits are known as atheromas or atheromatous plaques and develop from fatty streaks. All arteries down to 1 mm in diameter can be affected. Atheroma formation occurs at sites of haemodynamic stress.

Fatty streaks and fibrous plaques

Fatty streaks are seen as early as infancy. They comprise a slightly elevated zone on the arterial wall caused by accumulation of a small number of lipid laden histiocytes, with some free lipid (**Figure 17.1**). Fibrous plaques

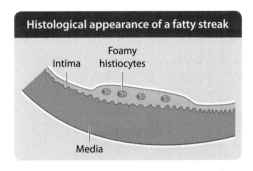

Histological appearance of a fatty streak

Intima · Foamy histiocytes · Media

Figure 17.1 Histological appearance of a fatty streak

are the second stage of atheroma formation. Lipid accumulates both free and in foamy histiocytes. Smooth muscle cells migrate from the media and proliferate. Fibrosis develops around the lipid, and forms a cap over the lesion. The plaques have a classic structure (**Figure 17.2**). There is a central core consisting of cholesterol crystals, foam cells, debris and thrombus. Foam cells are lipid filled macrophages. There is a superficial cap made up of mainly smooth muscle cells and connective tissue. Advanced disease is associated with calcification. Fibrous plaques are usually found in large to medium sized arteries.

Complicated plaques

Ulceration or fissuring of the fibrous cap of an atheromatous plaque reveal plaque contents, resulting in thrombus formation. The plaque may also undergo calcification. There may be inflammation associated with the plaque. This destroys the media which undergoes fibrosis, weakening and aneurysm formation. The vascular consequences of atheroma are:

- Arterial narrowing causing ischaemia
- Arterial occlusion resulting in infarction
- Arterial wall weakening resulting in aneurysm formation
- Arterial embolism

Thrombosis

Thrombus is a solid mass of blood constituents formed within the vascular system. It can occur in both the arterial and venous systems. Thrombosis is different from clot formation. Clotting is coagulation which

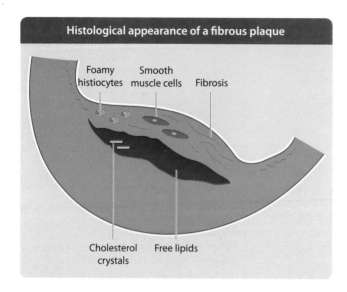

Figure 17.2 Histological appearance of a fibrous plaque

can occur within or outside the vascular system in life or post mortem. Thrombus consists of fibrin, platelets and entrapped red blood cells. Contact with damaged endothelium or atheromatous plaque contents triggers the coagulation cascade. It converts fibrinogen monomer to the fibrin polymer. On contact with fibrin or collagen, platelets release granules which promote aggregation of adjacent platelets. It forms a mass which covers an endothelial defect. Factors which promote thrombosis include:

- Vessel wall changes
- Changes in blood constituents
- Changes in blood flow

These are known as the Virchow Triad. Thrombi can occlude a vessel which may result in infarction. Released fragments of thrombus can travel in the bloodstream to occlude distal vessels. Thrombosis can be cleared by the fibrinolytic system. Plasminogen activator released from endothelial cells converts plasminogen to plasmin which dissolves fibrin. Thrombus can also undergo recanalisation. Endothelial cells grow out from the vessel wall and create new channels through the thrombus.

Embolism

An embolus is a mass of material in the blood which can lodge in a vessel and block its lumen.

Embolism to the lungs (pulmonary arteries) originates in the deep veins. Embolism to organs and the limbs originates in the heart or large arteries. An embolus can be made up of:

- Thrombus
- Atheromatous plaque
- Infected thrombus
- Endocardial or valve vegetations
- Fat
- Gas
- Amniotic fluid
- Tumour
- Foreign material

Ischaemia and infarction

Ischaemia occurs when an organ or tissue has perfusion lower than its metabolic needs. Infarction occurs when tissue necrosis results from ischaemia. Both can occur as a result of arterial, venous or capillary disease. Arterial ischaemia can occur as a result of:

- Atheromatous narrowing
- Thrombosis
- Embolism
- Low flow states
- Vasculitis
- Hypertensive vascular disease
- Spasm

The outcome of ischaemia depends on the:

- Adequacy of cardiac function

- Anatomy of arterial supply
- Speed of onset
- Susceptibility of tissue

Most infarcts are pale. Where there is a dual blood supply (e.g. lung), the infarct can be red. It occurs when some blood continues to get in to the infarcted area. Following infarction polymorphs and macrophages remove dead tissue. Capillaries grow into the area and granulation tissue forms. Fibroblasts grow into the area creating a scar.

Capillary ischaemia

Blocked or damaged capillaries can cause tissue ischaemia. It occurs in:

- Frostbite
- Cryoglobulinaemia
- Disseminated intravascular coagulation
- Diabetic microangiopathy

Aneurysms

An aneurysm is a localised dilatation of a vessel wall anywhere in the circulatory system. It can be classified as true or false aneurysm. A true aneurysm consists of one or more of the vessel wall layers. A false aneurysm is made up of connective tissue. Common sites of true aneurysms are the abdominal aorta and the iliac, popliteal and femoral arteries. Causes of aneurysms include:

- Atherosclerosis
- Vasculitis (e.g. Kawasaki disease)
- Syphilis
- Infective (mycotic)
- Trauma
- Congenital (e.g. Berry aneurysm)

Abdominal aortic aneurysm

An abdominal aortic aneurysm is dilatation of the aortic wall of more than one and a half times the normal aortic diameter. A diameter of more than 3 cm is usually regarded as aneurysmal. They are more common in men. The incidence increases with age. Most arise below the renal arteries.

Raynaud's disease

Raynaud's phenomenon is paroxysmal cyanosis of the digits of hand or feet caused by local spasm of small blood vessels. It most commonly affects the hands and is usually precipitated by cold. It is usually seen in young women. Raynaud's phenomenon can be secondary to conditions such as:

- Scleroderma
- Mixed connective tissue disease
- Atherosclerosis
- Systemic lupus erythematosus
- Buerger's disease

If no cause is found, it is known as Raynaud disease.

Buerger's disease

Buerger's disease results from inflammation of the small and medium sized arteries. It may also involve adjacent nerves. It is also known as thromboangiitis obliterans. It is more common in men and may begins at a young age. It is strongly associated with heavy cigarette smoking. The arterial involvement is often segmental. Occlusive inflammatory thrombi are seen within the lumen. Microscopically, all the layers of the vessel wall are involved. There is polymorphonuclear infiltration of the vessel wall. Clinical features include claudication, rest pain, ulceration and gangrene. Angiography typically shows occlusive thrombi and cork screw collaterals.

Arterial disease
Assessment of arterial disease

Peripheral vascular disease often remains clinically silent until late in life. The clinical condition may progress as the degree of stenosis increases. Arterial investigations are used to:

- Confirm the clinical impression of arterial disease
- Assess the disease severity
- Allow the preoperative planning of surgical or radiological interventions

Non-invasive testing of arterial patency

Hand-held Doppler

Reflection of an ultrasound wave off a stationary object does not change its frequency. Reflection off a moving fluid results in a change of frequency proportional to the velocity of flow. A hand-held 8 MHz

Doppler probe can be used to assess the arterial system. It can be used to measure arterial pressures. Measurements can be made at both rest and after exercise.

In a normal individual, the lower limb arterial pressures are greater than upper limb pressures. The Ankle–Brachial Pressure Index (ABPI) is the ratio of best foot systolic pressure to the brachial systolic pressure and can be used to assess the severity of peripheral vascular disease (**Figure 17.3**). The ratio falls with increasing disease severity. In a normal individual, the ABPI is great than one. In patients with claudication, the ratio is usually 0.4 to 0.7. In patients with critical limb ischaemia it is usually 0.1 to 0.4. In normal individuals, pressures do not fall flowing exercise. In claudicants, the ABPI falls following exercise and recovery is delayed. In the diabetic lower limb, pressures can be falsely elevated due to calcification in the vessel wall.

Toe pressure can provide an accurate assessment of the distal arterial circulation. They are not influenced by calcification in pedal vessels, particularly seen in diabetics. Normal toe pressures are 90–100 mmHg. Toe pressures less than 30 mmHg suggests critical limb ischaemia.

Duplex ultrasound

Duplex ultrasound is a combination of pulsed Doppler and real time B-mode ultrasound. It allows imaging of vessels and any associated stenotic lesion. Both arterial blood flow and pressure wave form can be simultaneously assessed. In normal individuals, a 'triphasic' wave is obtained with rapid antegrade flow during systole, transient reverse flow in early diastole and slow antegrade flow in late diastole. An arterial stenosis results in a reduced rate of rise of the antegrade flow, a decreased amplitude of the forward velocity and loss of reverse flow. This is known as

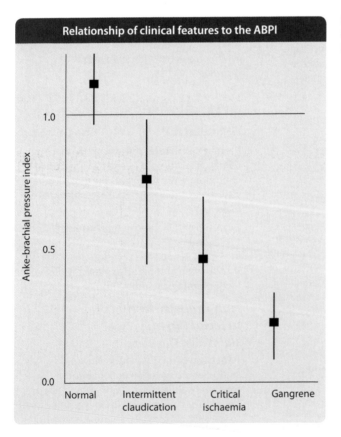

Figure 17.3 Relationship of clinical features to the ankle–brachial pressure index (ABPI)

a 'biphasic' wave form. At the site of the stenosis, velocity is increased. Severe stenosis results in a 'monophasic' wave form (**Figure 17.4**). Duplex ultrasound has sensitivity and specificity of 80% and 90%, respectively for the detection of stenotic lesions in the femoral and popliteal arteries.

Pulse-generated run-off

Proximal occlusion of an artery often causes poor filling of crural vessels. One of the most important prerequisites prior to femoro-distal bypass is the identification of patent distal vessels. Rapid cycling of a proximal cuff, termed pulse generated run-off, artificially generates arterial pulse waves allowing functional testing of distal arterial patency.

Magnetic resonance angiography

Magnetic resonance angiography (MRA) is the use of MR to image blood vessels. A variety of techniques have been described based on flow effects or contrast enhancement. These images, unlike conventional or CT angiography do not display the lumen of the vessel, rather the blood flowing through the vessel. Injection of an MRI contrast agent is currently the most commonly used method of acquiring MRA. The contrast medium is injected into a vein, and images are acquired during the first pass of the agent through the arteries. Time-of-flight methods use a short echo time and flow compensation to make flowing blood much brighter than stationary tissue. This technique avoids the use of contrast.

Invasive vascular assessment

Angiography

Angiography is usually performed using digital subtraction techniques. A catheter is inserted in an accessible artery using a Seldinger technique. The femoral artery is commonest site of vascular access. It is generally a safe procedure performed under local anaesthetic. Potential complications are either technique or contrast related and include:

- Haematoma
- Arterial spasm
- Sub-intimal dissection
- False aneurysm
- Arteriovenous fistula
- Embolisation
- Infection
- Anaphylactic reaction
- Toxic reactions
- Deterioration in renal function

CT angiography

CT angiography requires intravenous contrast and a significant dose of ionising radiation.

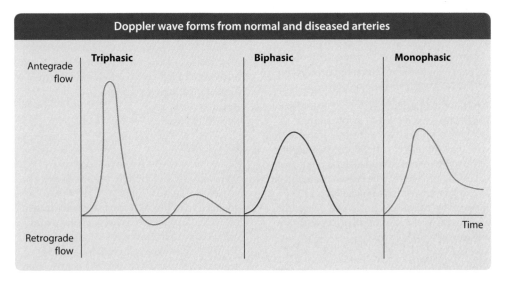

Figure 17.4 Doppler wave forms from normal and diseased arteries

However spiral CT and reconstruction can provide detailed images and is particularly useful for the assessment of aneurysmal disease.

Peripheral vascular disease

Intermittent claudication

About 5% of males over the age of 50 years have intermittent claudication. About 5% of claudicants progress to critical ischaemia each year. However, with appropriate management, more than 75% of patients with intermittent claudication remain stable or even show clinical improvement. Peripheral vascular disease is an independent risk factor for other cardiovascular disease. At 5 years of follow-up, 10% of claudicants and 50% of those with critical ischaemia have had an amputation. Also, 20% of claudicants and 50% of those with critical ischaemia have died, usually from ischaemic heart disease.

Clinical features

Intermittent claudication is calf or thigh pain precipitated by exercise and relieved by rest. It usually occurs after a predictable distance and is often described by patients as 'cramp' or 'tightness'. The location of pain, varies with the vessels that are involved. The usual relationship between the site of the pain and the site of arterial disease can be summarised as follows:

- Buttock and hip – aortoiliac disease
- Thigh – common femoral artery or aortoiliac disease
- Calf – superficial or popliteal femoral artery
- Foot claudication – tibial or peroneal artery

Assessment of progression of symptoms is important – worsening or improvement. Peripheral pulses can be present in patients with intermittent claudication. The impact on social function should also be identified. Claudication needs to be differentiated from spinal stenosis which also causes exercise-induced leg pain. Spinal stenosis is usually associated with neurological symptoms and relieved by spinal flexion.

Investigation

Intermittent claudication is essentially a clinical diagnosis. Measurement of the ABPI will allow assessment of the severity of peripheral vascular disease. Investigation should also be aimed at identifying risk factors such as diabetes and hypercholesterolaemia.

Management

The management of claudication is usually conservative, at least initially. Risk factor reduction is important and should involve stopping smoking, controlling hypertension, the use of lipid-lowering drugs, anti-platelet medication and good diabetic control, if appropriate. Patients should lose weight and undertake regular exercise, as part of a supervised exercise program. Indications for operative intervention in peripheral vascular disease are disabling claudication or critical limb ischaemia. Angiography is essentially a preoperative investigation and is not required in the routine assessment of claudication. The two options for intervention are percutaneous angioplasty or bypass surgery.

Critical limb ischaemia

Critical limb ischaemia (CLI) can be defined as persistently recurring ischaemic rest pain requiring regular analgesia for more than 2 weeks, associated with ulceration or gangrene of the foot or toes, with an ankle pressure of less than 50 mmHg or toe pressures of less than 30 mmHg.

Clinical features

CLI is characterised by rest pain. It occurs or is worsened when foot is elevated (e.g. in bed) and is improved with the foot dependent. It is almost invariably associated with ulceration or gangrene (**Figure 17.5**). Foot pulses are usually absent.

Investigation

CLI requires investigation to confirm the diagnosis and identify the site of any underlying stenosis or occlusion. The diagnosis can be confirmed by measuring the ABPI. The site of the stenosis can be identified using duplex ultrasound. MRA allows more accurate non-invasive assessment of the arterial system and is especially useful when planning interventional radiological or surgical interventions.

Management

Revascularisation of a critically ischaemic limb can be by either balloon angioplasty with stenting or bypass surgery. In recent years, the potential and scope of interventional radiological procedures has improved, widening their indications and use. Also, the outcomes are similar for angioplasty and bypass surgery for both aortoiliac and femoropopliteal disease. As a result, the number of bypass operations performed for critical limb ischaemia has reduced.

Percutaneous transluminal angioplasty is a technique of mechanically widening a narrowed or obstructed blood vessel. An empty and collapsed balloon on a guide wire, is passed into the narrowed segment and inflated to a fixed size using water pressures some 75 to 500 times normal blood pressure. The balloon crushes the fatty deposits, opening up the blood vessel. The balloon is then deflated and withdrawn. Angioplasty of the aorto-iliac segment has a 90% 5-year patency rate. Angioplasty of the infra-inguinal vessels has a 70% 5-year patency rate. The best results are seen in those patients with short segment stenoses, less than 2 cm long. Complications occur in less than 2% of patients and include:

- Wound haematoma
- Acute thrombosis
- Distal embolisation
- Arterial wall rupture

Lesions which display unfavorable anatomy and which might be better treated surgically have either long segment or multifocal stenoses or occlusions. For superficial femoral disease, the surgical option is a femoropopliteal bypass. For popliteal or tibial vessel disease, the surgical option is usually a femorodistal bypass. Arterial bypass grafts can be either biological or synthetic.

Biological grafts include:

- Long saphenous vein in situ or reversed
- Internal mammary artery
- Dacron-coated umbilical vein

Synthetic grafts include:

- Dacron
- Woven or knitted grafts
- Velour
- Polyfluorotetraethylene (PTFE)

The choice of graft material is determined by the long-term patency rates. Autologous vein is the best graft material but not always available. Interposition of vein between a PTFE graft and the artery at a distal anastomosis can improve long-term patency. The vein is often fashioned as either Miller cuff of Taylor patch. Reasons for graft failure depend on the time since surgery and include:

- Less than 30 days – technical failure
- 30 days to 1 years – neointimal hyperplasia at the distal anastomosis
- More than 1 years – progression of distal disease

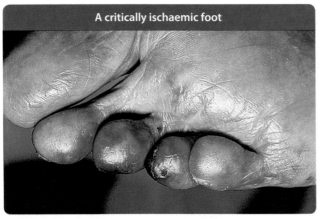

A critically ischaemic foot

Figure 17.5 A critically ischaemic foot

Acute limb ischaemia

The effects of sudden arterial occlusion depend on the state of the collateral supply. In the lower limb, the collateral supply in the leg is usually inadequate unless there is pre-existing occlusive disease.

Aetiology

Acute limb ischaemia (ALI) can result from:

- Embolism
- Thrombosis
- Trauma
- Arterial dissection

An embolus can arise from the left atrium in patients in atrial fibrillation, a mural thrombus after a myocardial infarct, prosthetic and diseased heart valves, an aneurysm or atheromatous stenosis. Rare causes include tumours, a foreign body or a paradoxical embolus from the venous system entering the arterial system via an atrial or ventricular septal defect.

Clinical features

The clinical diagnosis of ALI depends on recognition of the six 'Ps':

- Pain
- Paraesthesia
- Pallor
- Pulselessness
- Paralysis
- Perishing with cold

Fixed staining of the limb is a late sign. Objective sensory loss requires urgent treatment. There is a need to try differentiate embolism from thrombosis. This can be difficult. Important clinical features that may help include:

- Rapidity of onset of symptoms
- Features of pre-existing chronic arterial disease
- Potential source of embolus
- State of the pedal pulses in the contralateral leg

Management

When ALI is recognised, the patient should be heparinised and analgesia given. Associated cardiac disease should be actively managed. The definitive treatment options are different for embolic and thrombotic disease. Patients shown to have embolic disease should be considered for embolectomy or intra-arterial thrombolysis. Those with thrombotic disease should be given intra-arterial thrombolysis with the need for angioplasty and bypass surgery considered.

Emergency embolectomy

Emergency embolectomy can be performed under either general or local anaesthesia. The femoral vessels are displayed and both the inflow and outflow are controlled with slings. A transverse arteriotomy is performed and a Fogarty balloon embolectomy catheter is used to retrieve the embolus. If the embolectomy fails, an on-table angiogram should be performed and consideration given to a bypass graft or intraoperative thrombolysis.

Intra-arterial thrombolysis

During intra-arterial thrombolysis an angiogram is performed and a catheter advanced into the thrombus. Streptokinase and heparin can then be infused. Alternative thrombolytic agents include urokinase or tissue plasminogen activator. A repeat arteriogram should be obtained at 6–12 hours. The catheter can be advanced and thrombolysis continued for 48 hours or until clot lysis occurs. Angioplasty of a chronic arterial stenosis may be necessary. Success rates of 60–70% have been reported after intra-arterial thrombolysis but careful case selection is necessary. Thrombolysis can be accelerated by pulse spray through multiple side hole catheter, aspiration thrombectomy – debulking thrombus by aspiration or by giving a higher dose of thrombolytic agent over a shorter time. Intra-arterial thrombolysis is not suitable if there is severe neuro-sensory deficit.

Diabetic foot

Foot problems are common in both Type-1 and Type-2 diabetics. About 30% of diabetics have a peripheral neuropathy. Many of these patients also have features of peripheral vascular disease (**Figure 17.6**). Approximately, 15% of diabetics will develop foot ulceration. In the UK, diabetes is the

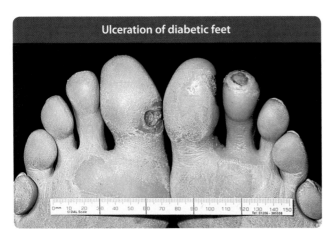
Ulceration of diabetic feet

Figure 17.6 Ulceration of diabetic feet

leading cause of non-traumatic lower limb amputation.

Pathophysiology

The diabetic foot results from a combination of a peripheral neuropathy and ischaemia. The neuropathy has sensory, motor and autonomic components. Sensory loss results in loss of protective sensation and unnoticed foot injuries. Loss of motor control to the small muscles of the feet results in a claw foot deformity. Autonomic neuropathy leads to vasomotor denervation and arteriovenous shunting. This compromises the ability to direct blood flow to the capillary beds. As a result, ischaemia can affect both the large and small vessels. Large vessels disease results in atheroma of the femoral, popliteal and tibial vessels. Small vessel disease affects the microcirculation. Other contributing factors include poor vision, limited joint mobility, cerebrovascular disease and peripheral oedema. In patients with foot ulceration, healing is impaired. This results from impaired fibroblast function, deficiency in growth factors and abnormalities of the extracellular matrix.

Management

Prevention of complications is far preferable to the need for active management. Patients should be monitored and self-care encouraged. They should be educated about washing, care of corns and calluses, toenail cutting and suitable footwear. In those with ulceration, assessment should be made of potential infection and vascular insufficiency.

In diabetic feet, wound swabs often show both Gram-negative, Gram-positive and anaerobic bacteria. If osteomyelitis occurs, it is usually due to *Staphylococcus aureus* infection. Plain radiography or MRI may demonstrate the extent of the infection. The threshold for antibiotic use should be low. The antibiotics selected should be based on culture and sensitivities.

Surgery may be required if there is progression of infection despite antibiotic treatment. All patients with diabetic ulceration should undergo non-invasive vascular assessment. The ABPI should be calculated. This may be falsely elevated due to arterial calcification and normal values may still be recorded in diabetics with significant major vascular disease.

Revascularisation should be considered if arterial insufficiency is present. Diabetics have a predisposition for disease in the medium-sized vessels especially at the popliteal trifurcation. The distal pedal vessels are often spared. Femorodistal bypass grafting may be required.

Abdominal aortic aneurysms

An abdominal aortic aneurysm (AAA) is an increase in the aortic diameter by greater than 50% of normal and is usually regarded as an aortic diameter of greater than 3 cm diameter. It is more prevalent in elderly men. The male:female ratio is 4:1. Risk factors for an AAA include:

- Hypertension
- Peripheral vascular disease
- Family history.

AAAs accounts for 2% of male deaths above the age of 55 years. Approximately 3000 elective and 1500 emergency AAA operations are performed in the UK each year. The mortality following emergency surgery is greater than 50%. The mortality following elective surgery should be less than 5%. The selection of patients for elective surgery depends on assessing the risk of operation against risk of rupture.

In patients with an AAA, the diameter expands exponentially at approximately 10% per year. The risk of rupture increases as the aneurysm expands. Overall, only 15% of aneurysms ever rupture and about 85% of patients with a AAA die from an unrelated cause. For those with an aortic diameter of 5.0 to 5.9 cm, 6.0 to 6.9 cm and more than 7 cm the lifetime risk of rupture is 25%, 35% and 75% respectively.

AAA Screening

AAAs are suitable for a screening programme as elective surgery on asymptomatic aneurysms can reduce the mortality associated with rupture. Who should be screened is controversial. The consensus is that males over 65 years, especially hypertensives, should be screened. Patients with small aneurysms should undergo regular surveillance with repeated ultrasound every 6 months and intervention planned if the aortic diameter increases.

Clinical features

About 75% of AAAs are asymptomatic. Possible symptoms prior to rupture include epigastric pain, back pain, malaise and weight loss (with inflammatory aneurysms). Abdominal examination may show an expansile epigastric mass. A ruptured AAA presents with sudden onset abdominal pain, hypovolaemic shock and a pulsatile epigastric mass. Rare presentations include distal embolic features, an aorto-caval fistula and a primary aorto-intestinal fistula.

Investigation

In patients being considered for elective surgery, preoperative investigation needs to determine the extent of the aneurysm and the fitness for operation. An ultrasound will confirm the presence of an aneurysm. Spiral CT, possibly with 3D reconstruction, allows assessment of the aneurysm size, its relation to renal arteries and involvement of the iliac vessels (**Figure 17.7**). The most significant postoperative morbidity and mortality is related to cardiac disease. If there are preoperative symptoms of cardiac disease, a cardiological opinion will be required. A thallium scan may be useful. Cardiac catheterisation with a view to revascularisation is required in up to 10% patients.

Management

Indications for surgery for a AAA include:

- Rupture
- Symptomatic aneurysm
- Rapid expansion
- Asymptomatic more than 6 cm in diameter

Endovascular aneurysm repair

Over the past few years, endovascular repair of AAA has been introduced into clinical practice. Its exact role remains unclear and medium and late complications have only recently been recognised. The morbidity of conventional open aneurysm surgery is related to exposure and cross clamping of the infra-renal aorta. Endovascular repair may be associated with reduced physiological stress, morbidity and mortality.

Endovascular repair is achieved by either a transfemoral or transiliac placement of a prosthetic graft. Proximal and distal cuffs or stents anchor the graft and exclude the aneurysm from the circulation. The three main types of graft are:

- Aorto-aortic
- Bifurcated aorto-iliac
- Aorto-uni-iliac graft with femoro-femoral crossover and contralateral iliac occlusion

Choice of technique depends on aneurysm morphology (**Figure 17.8**). Only about 40% of aneurysms are suitable for this type of repair. Aorto-aortic grafts are less frequently used due to high complication rate. Successful stenting is associated with reduced aneurysm

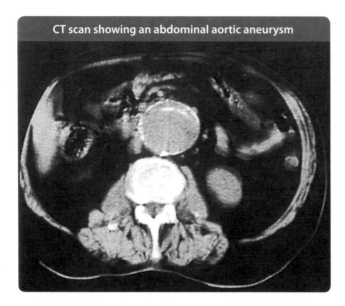

CT scan showing an abdominal aortic aneurysm

Figure 17.7 An abdominal CT scan showing an abdominal aortic aneurysm

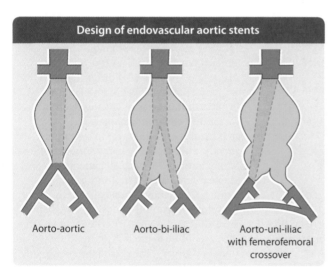

Design of endovascular aortic stents

Aorto-aortic   Aorto-bi-iliac   Aorto-uni-iliac
                                             with femerofemoral
                                                  crossover

Figure 17.8 Design of endovascular aortic stents

expansion but they still have a 1% per year risk of aneurysm rupture. Complications of endovascular repair include:

- Graft migration
- Endovascular leak
- Graft kinking
- Graft occlusion

Popliteal artery aneurysms

A popliteal aortic aneurysm is defined as a popliteal artery diameter greater than 2 cm. It accounts for 80% of all peripheral aneurysms. About 50% of popliteal aneurysms are bilateral and 50% are associated with an abdominal aortic aneurysm. About 50% are asymptomatic. Symptomatic aneurysms present with features of compression of adjacent structures (veins or nerves), rupture or limb ischaemia due to emboli or acute thrombosis. Treatment is by proximal and distal ligation with revascularisation of the leg by a femoropopliteal bypass. About 20% patients with a symptomatic popliteal aneurysm will undergo an amputation.

Carotid artery disease

In the carotid arteries, atherosclerosis is most common at the bifurcation of the common carotid artery. Stenosis of the internal carotid artery is a potentially treatable cause of ischaemic stroke, transient ischaemic attack and retinal infarction. A patient with an asymptomatic 50% carotid stenosis has 1–2% per year risk of a stroke. The risk of stroke increases with the degree of stenosis. Once a stenosis has become symptomatic the risk of a stroke is further increased. Once an ischaemic stroke has occurred the risk of further stroke is about 10% in the first year and 5% in subsequent years.

Clinical features

Carotid artery disease may be asymptomatic or symptomatic. Symptomatic carotid artery disease may result in either a transient ischaemic attack (TIA) or a stroke. A TIA results from a sudden and temporary loss of blood flow to an area of the brain usually lasting only a few minutes to 1 hour. Symptoms usually resolve within 24 hours, with complete recovery. Symptoms of a TIA may include:

- Sudden weakness or clumsiness affecting one side of the body
- Loss of coordination or movement
- Confusion, dizziness or fainting
- Loss of sensation in the face
- Loss of sensation affecting one side of the body
- Temporary loss of vision or blurred vision
- Inability to speak clearly or slurred speech

Investigation

The presence of a carotid bruit is an unreliable guide to the severity of stenosis. A bruit may be absent in patients with severe stenosis. Duplex ultrasound is the best method for initial assessment of carotid artery disease. Doppler recordings allow assessment of flow at any stenosis and ultrasound allows imaging of arterial anatomy. Until recently, carotid angiography was the gold standard method of assessing the degree of stenosis but it has a 4% risk of inducing further neurological event and a 1% risk of permanent stroke. Magnetic resonance angiography is an increasingly used non-invasive technique. Today most surgeons will operate on the basis of non-invasive assessments alone.

Management

The initial management of carotid artery disease is medical. Patients should stop smoking and hypertension and diabetes should be controlled. Prophylactic aspirin prevents 40 'vascular events' per 1000 patients treated for 3 years. It should be given to those with asymptomatic stenoses and those in whom an ischaemic stroke has been confirmed by CT. The combination of aspirin and dipyridamole is no more effective than aspirin alone.

Carotid endarterectomy

All patients with stable neurological symptoms from acute non-disabling stroke or TIA who have a symptomatic carotid stenosis of 50–99% according to the NASCET (North American Symptomatic Carotid Endarterectomy Trial) criteria or 70–99% according to the ECST (European Carotid Surgery Trialists' Collaborative Group) criteria should be assessed and referred for carotid endarterectomy within 1 week of the onset of a stroke or TIA symptoms. Ideally, they should undergo surgery within a maximum of 2 weeks. All patients with stable neurological symptoms from an acute non-disabling stroke or TIA who have symptomatic carotid stenosis of less than 50% according to the NASCET criteria, or less than 70% according to the ECST criteria should not undergo surgery. The reason for the variable criteria is that even though the two trials used angiography to assess the stenosis, the degree of stenosis was assessed differently. Comparison of the two measurements and re-analysis of the ECST trial data using the measurement method used in NASCET has shown that a 50% NASCET stenosis was broadly equivalent to a 70% ECST stenosis and a 70% NASCET stenosis broadly equated to an 85% ECST stenosis.

Patients with an asymptomatic stenosis are at higher risk of stroke than the general population, but not as high a risk as patients with symptomatic stenosis. The incidence of stroke in these patients is 1 to 2% per year. The surgical mortality of endarterectomy ranges from 1% to as much as 10%. Surgeons are divided over whether asymptomatic patients should be treated with medication alone or should be considered for surgery. Surgery is currently not routinely indicated in this group of patients.

Carotid endarterectomy is a surgical procedure used to prevent stroke, by correcting a stenosis in the common carotid artery. The internal, common and external carotid arteries are clamped, the lumen of the internal carotid artery is opened and the atheromatous plaque is removed. Some surgeons use a temporary shunt to ensure the blood supply to the brain during the procedure. The procedure may be performed under general or local anaesthesia. The latter allows for direct monitoring of neurological status by intraoperative verbal contact and testing of grip strength. With general anaesthesia indirect methods of assessing cerebral perfusion must be used such as transcranial Doppler analysis and carotid artery stump pressure monitoring.

Carotid stenting

Angioplasty and stenting is being increasingly used to dilate stenoses. It involves selective catheterisation of common carotid artery. A wire is advanced into the external carotid artery and a sheath is placed in the normal segment of the common carotid artery. The stenotic lesion is negotiated with a distal protection device. This is placed in the internal carotid artery and involves either a balloon occlusion system or polyurethane sac. Its use requires a patent contralateral internal carotid artery. Angioplasty is then performed, a stent deployed and the distal protection device is retrieved.

Vascular trauma

Vascular trauma can result from either blunt or penetrating injury. The pattern of injury differs according to the mechanism of injury. Penetrating injury is more common in the USA than Europe. Blunt vascular trauma is often associated with significant fractures, tissue loss and an increased amputation rate.

The diagnosis of blunt vascular trauma is often delayed. The types of vascular injury are described as:

- Contusion
- Puncture
- Laceration
- Transection

Clinical features

The clinical features depends on site, mechanism and extent of injury. Signs of vascular injury are classically divided into 'hard' and 'soft' sign

Hard signs of vascular injury are:

- Absent pulses
- Bruit or palpable thrill
- Active haemorrhage
- Expanding haematoma
- Distal ischaemia

Soft signs of vascular injury are:

- Haematoma
- History of haemorrhage at scene of accident
- Unexplained hypotension
- Peripheral nerve deficit

Investigation

Hard signs of vascular injury often require urgent surgical exploration without prior investigation. If time permits, angiography should be considered to confirm the extent of the injury in a stable patient with equivocal signs or to exclude vascular injury in a patient without hard signs but a strong suspicion. The role of Doppler ultrasound in vascular trauma remains to be defined.

Management

The management of vascular trauma often requires a multidisciplinary approach with orthopaedic and plastic surgeons. The aims of surgery are to control life-threatening haemorrhage and to prevent limb ischaemia. If surgery is delayed more than 6 hours revascularisation is unlikely to be successful. The use of arterial shunts is controversial but they may reduce ischaemic time and allow early fixation of fractures.

Vascular repair is usually performed after gaining proximal control and wound debridement. The options include:

- Simple suture of a puncture hole or laceration
- Vein patch
- Resection and end-to-end anastomosis
- Interpositional graft

Contralateral saphenous vein is the ideal interpositional graft. A prosthetic graft material may be used if the vein is poor or there is bilateral limb trauma. Primary amputation should be considered if there is severe injury with significant risk of reperfusion injury or if the limb after surgery is likely to be painful and useless.

Complications

A false aneurysm most commonly occurs following catheterisation of the femoral artery. It often presents with pain, bruising and a pulsatile swelling. The diagnosis can be confirmed by Doppler ultrasound. It may be possible to obliterate the aneurysm by ultrasound-guided compression therapy. Suturing of the puncture site or a vein patch may be required.

An arteriovenous fistula often presents several weeks after the injury. The patient complains of a swollen limb with dilated superficial veins. A 'machinery-type' bruit is often present throughout the cardiac cycle. The diagnosis can be confirmed by angiography. The fistula can often be divided and both the vein and artery sutured. A flap of fascia should be interposed between vessels to reduce the risk of recurrence.

Amputations

Approximately 5500 limb amputations are performed each year in the UK. Overall, 75% patients are older than 65 years, 65% patients are men and 70% of amputees having surgery for ischaemia are dead within 3 years. The commonest indications for amputation in the UK are:

- Peripheral vascular disease (85%)
- Trauma (10%)
- Tumours (3%)
- Infection (<1%)

The level of amputation is influenced by the cosmetic appearance, the functional requirement and the viability of soft tissues.

Where possible, amputations should be performed at 'Sites of election.'

For lower limb amputations these are:

- Toe
- Transmetatarsal
- Syme
- Below knee
- Through knee/Gritti–Stokes
- Above knee
- Hindquarter

For upper limb amputations these are:

- Digital
- Forearm
- Through elbow
- Above elbow
- Forequarter

The level of lower limb amputation will influence postoperative mobility. Approximately 80% of below-knee amputees will walk but this is reduced to 40% for above-knee amputees.

Venous disease

Varicose veins

Varicose veins affect 20% of adult females and 10% of adult males. Until recently, 75,000 operations for varicose veins were performed annually in UK. About 20% of operations were for recurrent disease. Surgery is now restricted to those with features of venous hypertension or ulceration.

Clinical features

Varicose veins present as dilated veins in the distribution of either the long saphenous vein (LSV) or short saphenous vein (SSV). A poor correlation exists between the symptoms and signs. It is important to identify from the history, those patients with a history suggestive of a deep venous thrombosis or previous lower limb fracture. Examination should identify the distribution of the varicose veins using a tourniquet testing and a hand-held 5 MHz Doppler probe. Cough, tap and thrill tests are inaccurate means of assessing varicose veins. The presence of complications such as lipodermatosclerosis or venous ulceration should also be documented. Previous treatment should be recorded.

Investigation

Duplex scanning should be considered if there is:

- Suspected short saphenous incompetence
- Recurrent varicose veins
- Complicated varicose veins (e.g. ulceration, lipodermatosclerosis)
- History of deep venous thrombosis

Management

The management of varicose veins can be:

- Conservative
- Radiofrequency ablation
- Endovascular obliteration
- Sclerotherapy
- Surgery

Absolute indications for intervention are:

- Lipodermatosclerosis leading to venous ulceration
- Recurrent superficial thrombophlebitis
- Bleeding from a ruptured varix

Radiofrequency ablation

Radiofrequency ablation uses high frequency alternating current delivered via a bipolar catheter. The catheter is placed intraluminally under duplex guidance. Local heating results in venous spasm and a collagen seal. It is usually performed under general anaesthesia. The long saphenous vein is accessed at the knee using a Seldinger technique and 90% vein occlusion can be achieved in the first week after treatment. It is associated with less pain than open surgery, improved quality of life and an earlier return to work. Complications include paraesthesia and skin burns. Recurrence rates are similar to open surgery.

Endovascular laser treatment

Endovascular laser treatment uses laser energy delivered via a narrow laser fibre used to obliterate the vein. It causes heat injury to the vessel wall. It is usually performed under local anaesthesia. Clinical and symptomatic improvement is seen in 95% of patients. Patient satisfaction is high and early return to work is possible. Complications include

paraesthesia and skin burns. Recanalisation is seen in less than 10% of patients.

Sclerotherapy

Sclerotherapy is only suitable for below knee varicose veins. Before considering sclerotherapy it is necessary to exclude saphenofemoral junction (SFJ) or saphenopopliteal junction (SPJ) incompetence. The main role of sclerotherapy is in persistent or recurrent varicose veins after previously adequate saphenous surgery. The principal sclerosants available are:

- 5% Ethanolamine oleate
- 0.5% Sodium tetradecyl sulphate

Recently foam (a mixture of air and sclerosant) has been shown to be more effective than sclerotherapy alone. The needle is placed in the vein when full with the patient standing. The vein is then empted prior to injection. Immediately after injection, compression is applied and maintained for 6 weeks. The main complications of sclerotherapy are extravasation of sclerosants causing pigmentation or ulceration and deep venous thrombosis.

Surgery

For LSV surgery, the patient should be placed in the Trendelenburg position with 20–30° head down. The legs should be abducted 10–15°. The SFJ is found 2 cm below and lateral to pubic tubercle. It is essential to identify the SFJ before performing flush ligation of the LSV. It is then necessary to individually divide and ligate all tributaries of the LSV which are the:

- Superficial circumflex iliac vein
- Superficial inferior epigastric vein
- Superficial and deep external pudendal vein

The femoral vein should be checked clear of direct branches for 1 cm above and below the SFJ. Stripping of LSV reduces the risk of recurrence. However, the LSV should only be stripped to upper calf. Stripping to the ankle is associated with an increased risk of saphenous neuralgia. Postoperative care should involve elevation of the foot of the bed for 12 hours and Class 2 compression stockings should be worn for at least 2 weeks.

For SSV surgery, the patient should be placed prone with 20–30° head down. The SPJ has a very variable position and preoperative localisation with duplex ultrasound is recommended. It is important to identify and preserve the sural nerve. Stripping of the SSV is associated with a risk of sural nerve damage. Subfascial ligation of the SSV alone is inadequate. The significance of perforator disease is unclear. Perforator disease may be improved by superficial vein surgery alone. Surgery to the perforator veins (e.g. Cockett and Todd procedure) is associated with high morbidity. Subfascial endoscopic perforator surgery (SEPS) has been described but is not indicated for uncomplicated primary varicose veins. It may have a role in addition to saphenous surgery in those with venous ulceration.

Recurrent varicose veins

About 15–25% of varicose vein surgery is for recurrence. The outcome of recurrent varicose veins surgery is less successful. The need for recurrent surgery can be avoided with adequate primary surgery. The reasons for recurrence are often:

- Inaccurate clinical assessment
- Inadequate primary surgery
- Failure to strip the LSV
- Injudicious use of sclerotherapy
- Neovascularisation

Venous hypertension and leg ulceration

Leg ulceration has a high prevalence and presents a considerable economic burden. Most cases of leg ulceration are due to venous hypertension and 40% of venous ulcers are due to superficial venous disease. Management of ulceration due to deep venous disease can prove difficult. However, surgical correction of superficial venous disease often results in healing. Rare causes of ulceration include:

- Rheumatoid arthritis
- Malignancy
- Syphilis

Venous hypertension

Venous hypertension affects 1–2% of the population. It is due to chronic venous insufficiency and distal vein hypertension. It is usually the result of the post thrombotic syndrome but can be due to primary valvular incompetence. Venous insufficiency can be classified as primary or secondary. Primary insufficiency has no obvious cause of valvular dysfunction. Insufficiency results in early refilling of the venous pool after muscle contraction. It causes a progressive and sustained increase in calf vein pressure. This is known as ambulatory venous hypertension and results in capillary dilatation and leakage of plasma proteins. Incompetent perforating veins expose the superficial veins to high pressures during muscle contraction. This is known as the hydraulic ram effect. It produces localised venous hypertension, filtration oedema and continues until tissue pressures rise to restore equilibrium. Accumulation of leukocytes occurs in dependent limbs of those with venous hypertension. Trapping of white cells is associated with activation. Hypoxic endothelial cells stimulate adherence of white cells. Following activation they release O_2 radicals, collagenases and elastases which injure the surrounding tissue.

Clinical features

Patients often have a history of leg swelling and skin changes consistent with chronic venous insufficiency. The history and examination should exclude other causes of leg ulceration. Signs of venous hypertension include:

- Perimalleolar oedema
- Pigmentation
- Lipodermatosclerosis
- Eczema
- Ulceration

Clinical assessment should identify any previous deep vein thrombosis and assess the presence of arterial disease. It should identify varicose veins and underlying valvular incompetencies.

Investigation

A hand-held Doppler can be used to assess the presence of venous reflux. The LSV, SSV and perforators should be assessed. The patency of the femoral and popliteal veins should be checked. Flow can be augmented by compression of the calf, deep inspiration or a Valsalva manoeuvre. Duplex ultrasonography allows anatomical and functional assessment and the flow rate and anatomy can be documented.

Management

The initial management of venous hypertension is usually conservative. Surgery is rarely required and the outcomes can be disappointing. Elastic compression stockings provide graduated compression and produce local alteration of the microvascular haemodynamics. They have minimal effect on deep vein dynamics. They do not cure hypertension, but do protect the skin from the effects.

The aims of surgery are to cure venous hypertension and heal the ulceration. A combination of superficial venous surgery and compression may be beneficial. Possible surgical strategies include:

- Skin grafting
- Free flap grafting
- Superficial vein stripping
- Perforating vein interruption
- Valve plasty
- Thrombolysis, dilation, stenting

Marjolin ulceration

Marjolin ulceration was first described by Jean Nicholas Marjolin in 1828. It is a squamous cell carcinoma arising at sites of chronic inflammation. Recognised underlying causes include chronic venous ulceration, burns and osteomyelitis. There is usually a long period between the injury and malignant transformation. This period may be 10–25 years. About 40% of Marjolin ulcers occur on the lower limb. The malignant change is usually painless and nodal involvement is uncommon. Diagnosis is confirmed by biopsy of the edge of the ulcer. Management involves adequate excision and skin-grafting. Amputations are sometimes required.

Venous thrombosis and thromboprophylaxis

Venous thrombosis is a significant cause of morbidity and mortality. Pulmonary embolus accounts for about 10% of all hospital deaths. At least 20% of patients who develop a deep venous thrombosis (DVT) will progress to a post-thrombotic limb. Most calf DVTs are clinically silent. About 80% of calf DVTs lyse spontaneously without treatment but 20% of calf DVTs will propagate to the thigh and have increased risk of pulmonary embolus.

Pathophysiology

Thrombus formation and propagation depends on the presence of Virchow's triad:

- Venous stasis
- Hypercoagulable state
- Endothelial damage

Risk factors for venous thrombosis are shown in **Table 17.1**. Immobility contributes to venous stasis. A hypercoagulable state can be caused by drugs or malignancy. Endothelial damage can result from external compression. It is estimated that about 1:250 of the population have a congenital thrombophilia. The potential for venous thrombosis can be investigated by a thrombophilia screen:

- FBC and blood film
- Clotting studies – APPT/PT/TT
- Reptilase test
- Protein C and S and antithrombin III assay
- Lupus anticoagulant

Risk assessment

The risk of venous thrombosis depends on the age of the patient, their co-morbidity and the nature of the procedure. Surgical procedure can be divided into low, moderate or high-risk.

Low-risk is defined as:

- Minor surgery (less than 30 min) + no risk factors other than age
- Major surgery (more than 30 min), age less than 40 years + no other risk factors
- Minor trauma or medical illness

Moderate risk is defined as:

- Major general, urological, gynaecological, cardiothoracic, vascular or neurological surgery + age more than 40 years or other risk factor
- Major medical illness or malignancy
- Major trauma or burn

Risk factors for venous thrombosis	
Patient factors	**Disease or surgical procedure**
Age	Trauma or surgery to pelvis, hip, lower limb
Obesity	Malignancy
Varicose veins	Heart failure
Immobility	Recent myocardial infarction
Pregnancy	Lower limb paralysis
Puerperium	Infection
High-dose oestrogen therapy	Inflammatory bowel disease
Previous deep vein thrombosis or pulmonary embolism	Nephrotic syndrome
Thrombophilia	Polycythaemia
Deficiency of antithrombin III	Paraproteinaemia
Antiphospholipid antibody	Paroxysmal nocturnal haemoglobinuria
Lupus anticoagulant	Behçet's disease
	Homocystinuria

Table 17.1 Risk factors for venous thrombosis

- Minor surgery, trauma or illness in a patient with previous DVT, PE or thrombophilia

High-risk is defined as:

- Fracture or major orthopaedic surgery of the pelvis, hip or lower limb
- Major pelvic or abdominal surgery for cancer
- Major surgery, trauma or illness in a patient with previous DVT, PE or thrombophilia

Prevention of thromboembolism

The risk of venous thromboembolic disease can reduced by both patient education, physical and pharmacological mechanisms. Patient information and education is vital. Women on the contraceptive pill should be advised to stop it 4 weeks before elective surgery. Patients should be advised that immobility before or after surgery increases the risk. Before surgery, they should be give verbal and written information on the risk of DVT and effectiveness of prophylaxis.

Physical methods of prophylaxis include early mobilisation, graduated compression stockings and intermittent pneumatic compression (e.g. Flowtron boots). Graduated compression stockings reduce the incidence of DVT by 50%. The stocking profile should be:

- 18 mmHg at the ankle
- 14 mmHg at the mid-calf
- 8 mmHg at the upper thigh

Staff should be trained in the use and fitting of the stockings. Stockings should be worn from the time of admission until the resumption of normal mobility. Intermittent pneumatic compression devices should also be used during surgery.

Pharmacological methods invariably include the use of heparin. Heparin is an acidic mucopolysaccharide. Unfractionated heparin has a molecular weight of 15 kDa. Low molecular weight heparin (LMWH) has a molecular weight of 5 kDa. Both potentiate antithrombin III activity by inactivating activated clotting factors. LMWH does not have a significant effect on the APPT. Side effects of unfractionated heparin include osteoporosis and idiosyncratic thrombocytopenia. Unfractionated and low molecular weight heparin are equally effective at reducing the risk of venous thromboembolism.

Clinical features

The clinical presentation of a DVT can be very non-specific. Many are asymptomatic. The clinical features depends on site of the venous occlusion. The classical clinical features of a calf DVT are calf pain and tenderness, pyrexia and persistent tachycardia. Homan's sign is pain on passive dorsiflexion of the ankle and is non-specific. Occlusion of the ileofemoral vein can result in venous gangrene (phlegmasia cerulea dolens).

Investigation

D-dimers are a fibrin degradation product that can be assayed in plasma. Levels are raised in the presence of recent thrombus. A negative result almost excludes the presence of venous thrombosis. Compression ultrasound is the imaging modality of choice. The decision whether to proceed to ultrasound is often based on D-dimer results. The technique has three components – all operator dependent.

- Venous compressibility
- Detection of Doppler flow
- Visualisation of clot

In the femoro-popliteal segment it has a sensitivity and specificity of 95% and 100%, respectively. In the calf veins, both the sensitivity and specificity are less. However, ultrasound is able to exclude femoro-popliteal or major calf DVT in symptomatic patients.

Management

The aims of treatment of venous thrombosis are prevention of pulmonary embolus and restoration of venous and valvular function to prevent the post-thrombotic limb. Anticoagulation is the main component of treatment, initially with LMWH followed by oral anticoagulation. The treatment of isolated calf DVTs is of unproven benefit and the optimal duration of treatment unknown. There is no proof that treatment beyond 3–6 months is required. Thrombolysis is of unproven benefit.

Surgical thrombectomy should be considered in massive ileo-femoral thrombosis associated with phlegmasia cerulea dolens. The early results are good with 60% complete and 40% partial clearance of thrombus from the ileo-femoral segment. Unfortunately, re-occlusion commonly occurs.

Pulmonary embolism

Acute pulmonary embolism is a common and often fatal disease. Mortality can be reduced by prompt diagnosis and therapy. Pulmonary embolism accounts for 10% of hospital inpatient deaths. Untreated, it has a mortality of up to 30%. With treatment, the mortality can be reduced to about 2%. Only 10% patients presenting with pulmonary embolus have clinical signs of a DVT.

Clinical features

The challenge in diagnosing a pulmonary embolism is that patients rarely display the classic presentation of abrupt onset of pleuritic chest pain, shortness of breath and hypoxia (**Table 17.2**). Studies of patients who died unexpectedly from pulmonary embolism have shown that patients often had symptoms for several weeks before their death.

Investigation

Investigation of a possible pulmonary embolus should include:

- Arterial blood gases – hypoxia, hypocarbia but may be normal
- ECG – Signs of right heart strain – classically $S_1Q_3T_3$
- Chest x-ray – show oligaemia and excludes other pathologies
- CT pulmonary angiogram
- Ventilation/Perfusion scanning
- Lower limb investigations for a DVT

Management

The management of a pulmonary embolus depends on the degree of suspicion and whether the patient is haemodynamically stable. If there is high degree of suspicion but the patient is stable the patient should be anti-coagulated with LMWH, oxygen given and analgesia administered. The patient should be warfarinised for at least 3 months.

Clinical presentation of pulmonary embolus

Symptoms	Signs
Dyspnoea	Low-grade pyrexia
Pleuritic chest pain	Central cyanosis
Haemoptysis	Tachycardia
	Tachypnoea
	Hypotension
	Neck vein distension
	Pleural rub
	Increased pulmonary second sound

Table 17.2 Clinical presentation of pulmonary embolus

If the patient is haemodynamically unstable consideration should be given to a pulmonary thrombolysis via a pulmonary artery catheter. If thrombolysis is contraindicated, a pulmonary embolectomy may be required.

Inferior vena caval filters are inserted percutaneously usually via the femoral vein. They present a physical barrier to emboli. They are indicated if recurrent pulmonary emboli occur despite adequate anticoagulation or there is extensive proximal venous thrombosis and anticoagulation is contraindicated.

Lymphatics and spleen

Lymphoedema

Lymphoedema presents with gradual, often bilateral, limb swelling (**Table 17.3**). It is due to progressive failure of the lymphatic system. Primary lymphoedema has no obvious cause and is classified as:

- Congenital (age less than 1 year) – familial or non-familial
- Praecox (age less than 35 years) – familial or non-familial
- Tarda (age more than 35 years)

Secondary lymphoedema can be due to:

- Malignant disease
- Surgery – axillary surgery or groin dissection
- Radiotherapy
- Infection – parasitic (e.g. filariasis)

Pathology

Primary lymphoedema is more common in women and is usually bilateral. It is the result of a spectrum of lymphatic disorders. It can be due to aplasia, hypoplasia or hyperplasia of lymphatics. In 80% of patients, obliteration of the distal lymphatics occurs. A proportion of patients have a family history (Milroy's disease). In 10% of patients, proximal occlusion of the lymphatics in the abdomen and pelvis is seen. In 10% of patients, lymphatic valvular incompetence develops. Chronic lymphoedema results in subcutaneous

Causes of lower limb swelling

Bilateral pitting oedema	Painful unilateral oedema	Painless unilateral oedema
Heart failure	Deep venous thrombosis	Post-phlebitic limb
Renal disease	Superficial thrombophlebitis	Extrinsic compression of the deep veins
Proteinuria	Cellulitis	Deep venous incompetence
Cirrhosis	Trauma	Lymphoedema
Carcinomatosis	Ischaemia	Immobility
Nutritional		

Table 17.3 Causes of lower limb swelling

fibrosis. The fibrosis can be worsened by secondary infection.

Clinical features

The initial presentation is usually with peripheral oedema worse on standing. It begins distally and progresses proximally. The affected limb usually feels heavy. With secondary lymphoedema the underlying cause if often apparent. Examination shows non-pitting oedema. The skin often has hyperkeratosis, fissuring and secondary infection. Ulceration is rare.

Investigation

Chronic venous insufficiency should be excluded with Doppler ultrasound. Lymphoedema and its cause can be confirmed with lymphoscintigraphy and CT or MRI scanning. Lymphangiography is painful and rarely required. Normal lymphoscintigraphy essentially excludes a diagnosis of lymphoedema.

Management

The aims of treatment are to reduce the limb swelling, improve limb function and reduce the risk of infection. General skin care will reduce the risk of infection. Swelling can be reduced by elevation. Physiotherapy and manual lymphatic drainage may help. External pneumatic compression will also reduce swelling. Once the swelling is reduced, compression stockings should be applied. Antibiotics should be given at the first sign of infection. Drugs (e.g. diuretics) are of no proven benefit. Surgery consists of two approaches – debulking and bypass procedures.

Debulking operations include:

- Homan's operation – excision of skin and subcutaneous tissue with primary closure
- Charles' operation – radical excision of skin and subcutaneous tissue with skin grafts

Both produce good functional results however cosmesis is often poor. Bypass operations include:

- Skin and muscle flaps
- Omental bridges
- Enteromesenteric bridges
- Lymphaticolymphatic anastomosis
- Lymphaticovenous anastomosis

The spleen

The normal spleen weighs about 150 g. It lies within the anterior leaf of the dorsal mesogastrium, parallel to 9th to 11th ribs. It is closely related to the:

- Tail of pancreas
- Greater curvature of stomach
- Left kidney and lienorenal ligament
- Greater omentum

The blood supply is from splenic artery and short gastric arteries. The splenic artery divides within the hilum to form four or five end arteries. The spleen is an important component of the lympho-reticular system. It is a site of haemopoesis in the fetus and in patients with bone marrow pathology. It is a site of maturation and destruction of red blood cells. It is an important component of both the humoral and cell-mediated immune systems. Antigens are trapped and IgM is produced in the germinal centres. It produces opsonins for the phagocytosis of encapsulated bacteria. Causes of splenomegaly include:

- Chronic myeloid leukaemia
- Myelofibrosis
- Portal hypertension
- Lymphoma
- Leukaemia
- Thalassaemia
- Glycogen storage diseases
- Polycythaemia rubra vera
- Haemolytic anaemias
- Infections – infectious mononucleosis, malaria
- Connective tissue disorders
- Infiltrations – amyloid, sarcoid

Indications for splenectomy

Indications for splenectomy include:

- Trauma
- Spontaneous rupture
- Hypersplenism
- Neoplasia
- Hydatid cysts
- Splenic abscesses

Physiological effects of splenectomy

Following splenectomy, both the white cell and platelet counts are raised and peak at about 7 days. There is an increased proportion of abnormal red cells in the circulation. IgM levels are reduced and IgA levels are raised. There is a reduced ability to opsonise encapsulated bacteria.

Ruptured spleen

Splenic rupture should be suspected in any patient with abdominal trauma and shock, especially if there is shoulder tip pain, lower rib fractures and left upper quadrant bruising. Patients require prompt resuscitation. An abdominal CT will confirm the diagnosis and identify other pathology. Non-operative management is acceptable if the splenic injury is isolated and patient is stable. Patients should be closely monitored.

Splenectomy is required if that patient is cardiovascularly unstable. A long midline incision and full laparotomy is required. The spleen is drawn medially and the left leaf of lienorenal ligament is divided. The mobilised spleen is displaced in to the wound. Vascular control can be obtained by compression of the vascular pedicle. If total splenectomy is required, the short gastric arteries are divided and ligated avoiding damage to the stomach. The splenic artery and vein are divided and ligated avoiding damage to the tail of the pancreas. Repair with preservation of the spleen should be considered, if possible. Alternatives to total splenectomy include:

- Topical applications
- Microfibrillar collagen
- Cyanoacrylate adhesive
- Diathermy
- Packing
- Splenorrhaphy

Overwhelming post splenectomy infection (OPSI)

Overwhelming post splenectomy infection (OPSI) is due to encapsulated bacteria. About 50% of cases are due to *Streptococcus pneumoniae*. Other organisms that can lead to OPSI include *Haemophilus influenzae* and *Neisseria meningitidis*. It occurs in about 4% of post splenectomy patients without prophylaxis. The mortality of OPSI is approximately 50%. The greatest risk is in the first 2 years after surgery.

Prevention

Antibiotic prophylaxis should be given with penicillin or amoxycillin. Little consensus exists over the duration of prophylaxis. Immunisation against *Pneumococcus* and *Haemophilus* should also be given. It should be administered 2 weeks prior to a planned splenectomy and given immediately postoperatively following emergency surgery.

Lymphadenopathy

Lymphadenopathy can result form neoplastic or inflammatory processes (**Table 17.4**). In the Western adult population, 50% of cases are neoplastic and 50% are inflammatory. In children, only 20% of cases are due to neoplasia.

Clinical assessment

Clinical assessment should include:

- Duration of symptoms
- Distribution of lymphadenopathy
- Presence of pain
- Associated symptoms – fever, malaise, weight loss
- Examination – firm or rubbery, discrete or matted
- Presence of hepatosplenomegaly

Investigation

Fine needle aspiration cytology may be useful if there is suspicion that the lymphadenopathy maybe be due to metastatic solid tumours. Excision or incision biopsy is usually required if there is suspicion of a haematological disorder. The risks of a node biopsy (e.g. damage to accessory nerve) should be appreciated. Specimens should be sent 'dry' to the laboratory. This will allow samples for imprint cytology or microbiological culture to be obtained.

Hodgkin's lymphoma

Hodgkin's lymphoma was first described by Sir Thomas Hodgkin in 1832. The disease can present at any age but is most commonly seen in young adults. There are 1500 new cases per year in the UK and it accounts for 1 in 5 of all lymphomas. The male:female ratio is 2:1.

Causes of lymphadenopathy	
Neoplastic	Solid tumours – melanoma, breast, head and neck cancers
	Haematological – lymphoma, leukaemia, myeloproliferative diseases
Inflammatory	Infection – bacterial, viral, fungal, tuberculosis
	Autoimmune – rheumatoid arthritis, systemic lupus erythematosis, tuberculosis
	Miscellaneous – angiofollicular hyperplasia, dermatopathic lymphadenitis

Table 17.4 Causes of lymphadenopathy

Clinical features

Hodgkin's lymphoma usually presents as painless lymphadenopathy in superficial lymph nodes. The cervical, axillary and inguinal nodes are affected in 70%, 20% and 10% of cases, respectively. Splenomegaly occurs in 50% of patients. Cutaneous involvement occurs as a late complication in 10% of patients. Constitutional symptoms occur in those with widespread disease and include:

- Fever (Pel–Ebstein)
- Pruritus
- Alcohol-induced pain

Investigation

The diagnosis can be confirmed with a lymph node biopsy. Reed–Sternberg cells are diagnostic of the disease. There are four histological types:

- Lymphocyte predominant (7%)
- Nodular sclerosing (64%)
- Mixed cellularity (25%)
- Lymphocyte depleted (4%)

Staging investigations should include:

- Chest x-ray
- Bone marrow trephine biopsy
- Abdominal and chest CT scan
- Staging laparotomy – often not required

The staging of Hodgkin's lymphoma is as follows:

- Stage I – Confined to one lymph node region
- Stage II – Disease confined to two or more nodal regions on one side of the diaphragm
- Stage III – Disease involving nodal regions on both sides of the diaphragm

- Stage IV – Extra-nodal disease – usually liver or bone marrow

The disease can be sub-staged by the absence (A) or presence (B) of the constitutional symptoms – unexplained fever above 38ºC, night sweats or loss of more than 10% body weight in the past 6 months.

Management

Management of Hodgkin's lymphoma depends on the stage of the disease. Stage I and II disease is often managed with radiotherapy alone. Stage III and IV disease is often treated with chemotherapy and radiotherapy. The prognosis is good. Stage I and IV disease have a 5-year survival of 90% and 60%, respectively.

Raynaud's disease

Raynaud's phenomenon refers to symptoms of digital ischaemia. About 80% of patients with Raynaud disease are women and the onset is usually before the age of 35 years. The population prevalence may be as high as 5%. Most patients have primary disease and have normal arteries. Symptoms are due to an abnormal but reversible physiological response. Secondary Raynaud's disease occurs in patients with an underlying systemic disorder.

Primary Raynaud's disease

Primary Raynaud's disease is due to excessive vasoconstriction of the digital arteries. The vessels are normal between episodes. Cooling of the hands results in intense vasoconstriction and a drop in skin temperature (**Figure 17.9**). Flow in the digital arteries ceases at the critical closing

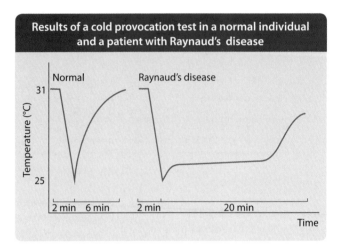

Figure 17.9 Results of a cold provocation test in a normal individual and a patient with Raynaud's disease

temperature. Reopening of blood vessels requires a rise in perfusion pressure. Possible pathophysiological mechanisms include:

- Increased sympathetic activity
- Increased sensitivity to adrenergic stimuli
- Increased number of α-receptors in the vessel wall

Secondary Raynaud's disease

Secondary Raynaud's disease is due to conditions associated with abnormal vessel walls or increased blood viscosity. These include connective tissue, haematological and arterial diseases. It also may result from neurovascular compression and drugs. Raynaud phenomena is seen in:

- 90% of patients with scleroderma
- 30% of patients with rheumatoid arthritis
- 30% of patients with primary Sjögren's syndrome

Clinical features

The diagnosis can usually be made from the clinical history. It consists of a triphasic response provoked by exposure to cold:

- Phase 1 – pallor due to intense vasoconstriction
- Phase 2 – cyanosis due to desaturation of haemoglobin
- Phase 3 – erythema due to hyperaemia and restoration of the circulation

Primary disease is usually bilateral, symmetrical and involves all the fingers.

Secondary disease is usually patchy and asymmetrical. Symptoms are often milder in primary disease. Examination often shows the peripheral pulses to be normal. Features of thoracic outlet syndrome or connective tissue disorders may be present.

Investigation

Investigations should be guided by the clinical features. Serology should include – FBC, ESR, anti-nuclear antibodies. Electrophoresis, cold agglutinins and fibrinogen levels may identify hyperviscosity states. A chest x-ray and thoracic outlet views may show a cervical rib. Duplex ultrasound or arteriography may be indicated if there is suspicion of arterial disease.

Management

Preventative measures include warm clothing, the use of hand warmers and to stop smoking. Occupational factors may need to be taken in to consideration. Sympathetic stimulants should be avoided. Drugs have a limited role. Surgery for thoracic outlet syndrome may be required.

Renal failure and transplantation
Chronic renal failure

Chronic renal failure is defined as a glomerular filtration rate of less than 60 mL/min. Causes of chronic renal failures include:

- Chronic glomerulonephritis
- Chronic pyelonephritis
- Diabetic nephropathy
- Chronic interstitial nephritis
- Chronic obstructive uropathy
- Hypertensive nephrosclerosis
- Polycystic disease
- Amyloid
- Myeloma

The stages of renal dysfunction are shown in **Table 17.5**.

Management

There are three basic stages in the treatment of chronic renal failure:

- Preserve remaining nephrons
- Conservative treatment of uraemic syndrome
- Renal dialysis and transplantation

Remaining nephrons can be preserved by controlling hypertension and heart failure and treatment of superimposed urinary tract infection. Correction of salt and water depletion is important along with careful prescribing of drugs that are potentially nephrotoxic. Dietary protein should be restricted. Conservative management of uraemic syndrome involves a reduce protein intake and the use of aluminium hydroxide to reduce intestinal phosphate absorption. Vitamin D and calcium supplements can be given to increase the serum calcium and allopurinol can be used to reduce the serum uric acid. Erythropoietin may be necessary to correct anaemia. Renal dialysis

or transplantation may be necessary once all conservative treatments have been exhausted.

Renal dialysis

Dialysis depends on diffusion – the passage of a solute through a membrane down a concentration gradient and ultrafiltration – the passage of a solvent through a membrane due to hydrostatic or osmotic pressure. The indications for renal dialysis include:

- Patients aged 5–70 years without significant systemic disease or neoplasia
- Clinical deterioration despite good conservative management
- Uraemic pericarditis
- Severe renal bone disease
- Peripheral neuropathy
- Creatinine more than 1200 mmol/L
- Glomerular filtration rate less than 5 mL/min

Peritoneal dialysis

In peritoneal dialysis, the dialysis membrane is the peritoneum. Dialysis fluid is low in urea and creatinine. It is a hypertonic solution due to a high glucose concentration. Dialysis thus occurs as a result of both diffusion and ultrafiltration. A Tenckhoff catheter is inserted below the umbilicus. Cuffs on the catheter prevent leakage and infection. Dialysis is performed on either an intermittent or continuous basis. In continuous ambulatory peritoneal dialysis (CAPD) fluid is changed four times per day. Indications for CAPD include:

Stages of renal dysfunction			
Stage	Description	Creatinine clearance (mL/min/1.73 m²)	Metabolic consequences
1	Normal	More than 90	
2	Early renal insufficiency	60–89	Increase serum parathyroid hormone
3	Chronic renal failure	30–59	Increase calcium absorption, anaemia
4	Pre-end stage failure	15–29	Increased serum PO_4 and K^+ Acidosis
5	End stage renal failure	Less than 15	Uraemia

Table 17.5 Stages of renal dysfunction

- Diabetics
- Children
- Patients with poor vascular access
- Patients unable to tolerate haemodynamic instability of haemodialysis
- Patients in whom the wait for transplantation will be short

Contraindications for CAPD include:

- Severe intraperitoneal adhesions
- Sepsis of the anterior abdominal wall
- Inflammatory bowel disease
- Abdominal wall hernias
- Stomas
- Extensive diverticular disease

Complications of CAPD include:

- Intraperitoneal bleeding
- Perforated viscus
- Obstruction and displacement of the catheter
- Dialysate leak
- Pericatheter hernias
- Sclerosing peritonitis

Haemodialysis

With haemodialysis, the dialysis membrane is an artificial membrane. Blood is moved on either side of the membrane in countercurrent directions and solutes move across the membrane by diffusion. Vascular access can be obtained by:

- Arteriovenous shunt with prosthetic graft
- Arteriovenous fistula between artery and vein
- Vascular catheters in large central veins

Arteriovenous fistulas take 4 to 6 weeks to mature. Indications for haemodialysis include a slow deterioration in renal function. It is not a suitable method of dialysis for patients who present with an acute deterioration in renal function. The upper limb is usually used for vascular access and possible sites of vascular fistulas include radiocephalic, ulnobasilic and brachiobasilic. Patency rates vary with the type of fistula. Brachiocephalic fistulae usually have an 80% patency at 2 years. Brachiobasilic fistulae have a 60% 2 year patency. Synthetic grafts have a 50% two year patency.

Contraindications for haemodialysis include:

- Obesity

- Venous stenosis/thrombosis
- Arterial disease
- Subclavian vein stenosis
- Prothrombotic disorders

Complications of haemodialysis include:

- Bleeding
- Thrombosis
- Vascular steal
- Aneurysm formation
- High-output cardiac failure
- Venous hypertension

Renal transplantation

About 1500 renal transplants are performed each year in the UK. Overall, 50% of patients on dialysis are on the transplant waiting list with 5000 patients waiting for a transplant. Of the donor kidneys, 80% are from beating-heart organ retrievals, 10% are from non-beating heart donors and 10% are from live donors. Transplant recipients are usually less than 75 years old with no history of recent neoplasia, no major infections (e.g. tuberculosis) and good cardiovascular status. Potential donors are usually aged 5–75 years with no significant renal disease, no major infections, are hepatitis B and C and HIV negative and have no history of malignancy. The outcome from renal transplantation is improving with 95% of patients alive at 1 year and 87% of patients alive at 5 years.

Complications of renal transplantation include:

- Vascular – haemorrhage, renal artery or vein thrombosis
- Urological – bladder leak, ureteric stenosis
- Lymphocele
- Infection – cytomegalovirus, herpes simplex, pneumocystis
- Post transplant neoplasia – lymphoma, Kaposi's sarcoma

Immunosuppression

Immunosuppression is classically achieved with a combination of:

- Cyclosporin A
- Azathioprine
- Prednisolone

Newer dugs include:

- Tacrolimus
- Mycophenolate mofetil

- Basiliximab
- Daclizumab
- Sirolimus

Basiliximab and daclizumab are anti-interleukin-2 receptor antibodies. Newer drugs are associated with fewer side effects. The incidence of hypertension and hyperuricaemia are reduced. The rate of adverse lipid profiles is lessened. Newer drugs may have a reduced incidence of chronic allograft nephropathy.

Rejection

About 1–2% of patients undergoing renal transplantation develop acute rejection. Acute rejection is characterised by pyrexia, graft tenderness and increasing creatinine. The diagnosis can be confirmed by a renal biopsy. Management is with high dose steroids and OKT3, a monoclonal antibody against the T cell receptor-CD3 complex and anti-T cell monoclonal antibodies.

Chapter 18

Otorhinolaryngology and head and neck surgery

Applied basic sciences
Salivary gland anatomy

Parotid gland

The parotid gland is found overlying the ramus of the mandible (**Figure 18.1**). It lies anterior and inferior to the external ear and occupies the parotid fascial space. It extends from the zygomatic arch to the angle of the mandible. The facial nerve and its branches pass through the gland. The external carotid artery also passes through the gland and gives off its two terminal branches, the maxillary artery and the superficial temporal artery within the gland. Posteriorly, it is related to the posterior belly of the digastric, the stylohyoid and the sternocleidomastoid muscles. The gland has four surfaces superior, superficial, anteromedial and posteromedial. The surfaces are separated by three borders, anterior, posterior and medial. The parotid duct (Stenson duct) drains into the buccal cavity opposite the upper second molar. The parotid papilla mark's the opening of the duct.

Although the facial nerve runs through the gland, it does not supply its parasympathetic innervation. Secretion of saliva is controlled by postsynaptic parasympathetic fibres originating in the inferior salivary nucleus. These leave the brain via the tympanic nerve branch of glossopharyngeal nerve, travel through the tympanic plexus, and then form the lesser petrosal nerve before reaching the otic ganglion. After synapsing in the otic ganglion, the postganglionic fibres travel as part of the auriculotemporal nerve to reach the parotid gland. Sympathetic nerves originate from the superior cervical ganglion, giving rise to the external carotid nerve plexus and reaching the gland by traveling along the external carotid arterial branches. Parasympathetic stimulation produces a water rich, serous saliva. Sympathetic

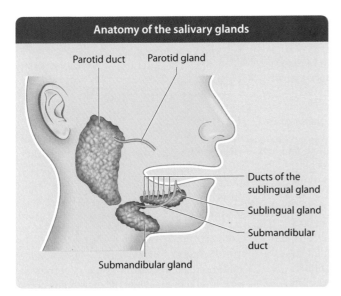

Anatomy of the salivary glands

Parotid duct   Parotid gland

Ducts of the sublingual gland

Sublingual gland

Submandibular duct

Submandibular gland

Figure 18.1 Anatomy of the salivary glands

stimulation leads to the production of a low volume, enzyme-rich saliva. There is no inhibitory nerve supply to the gland.

Submandibular gland

The submandibular glands lie superior to the digastric muscles. Each submandibular gland is divided into superficial and deep lobes, separated by the mylohyoid muscle. The superficial portion is larger and the mylohyoid muscle runs below it. Secretions are delivered into Wharton's ducts on the superficial portion. The gland hooks around the posterior edge of the mylohyoid muscle. The submandibular ducts are crossed by the lingual nerve and drain into the sublingual caruncles on either side of the lingual frenulum. This occurs along with the major sublingual duct.

The parasympathetic innervation to the submandibular glands is provided by the superior salivary nucleus via the chorda tympani, a branch of the facial nerve that synapses in the submandibular ganglion. It follows the lingual nerve leaving it as it approaches the gland. Increased parasympathetic activity promotes the secretion of saliva. The sympathetic nervous system regulates the submandibular secretions through vasoconstriction of the arteries that supply it. Increased sympathetic activity reduces glandular blood flow and decreases salivary secretions, producing an enzyme-rich serous saliva.

Salivary gland physiology

Saliva

About 1500 mL of saliva is secreted each day under the control of parasympathetic system. Parasympathetic stimulation promotes secretion. Saliva is formed in the acini of salivary glands. This initial production is similar to intestinal secretions and is isotonic. As it passes through the ducts, sodium and chloride are reabsorbed and potassium and bicarbonate are secreted. This is more pronounced during low salivary flow rates. Water is not reabsorbed. Saliva is thus hypotonic and has a pH between 7 and 8. Saliva is low in sodium and chloride and rich in potassium and bicarbonate. It contains amylase, small amounts of lipase, mucin, antibodies, lysozyme and lactoferrin. The composition varies between the types of salivary glands.

Ear, nose and throat disease
Inflammatory conditions of the ear, nose and throat

Otitis externa

Inflammatory disorders of the external ear are common. They can be either an acute or chronic disorder and are often associated with generalised skin disorders. Common pathogens include staphylococcal species and *Pseudomonas aeruginosa*. Fungi, candida and aspergillus may also be involved. The condition is often bilateral. Treatment is with topical antibiotics and steroids. Debris should be suctioned under direct vision. Systemic antibiotics are rarely required.

Acute suppurative otitis media

Acute suppurative otitis media is a common disorder in childhood. The commonest pathogens are *Streptococci pneumoniae* and *Haemophilus influenzae*. It usually presents with severe ear ache. The child is usually systemically unwell. The tympanic membrane is often red and bulging. Pain may be relieved when rupture of the tympanic membrane occurs. Treatment is with oral antibiotics. Complications of acute suppurative otitis media include:

- Chronic suppurative otitis media
- Adhesive otitis media
- Tympanosclerosis
- Ossicular destruction
- Acute mastoiditis
- Intracranial complications

Chronic suppurative otitis media

Chronic suppurative otitis media (CSOM) is classified into two types. The tubotympanic disease is associated with perforation of the pars tensa. The atticoantral disease is associated with a retraction pocket of the pars flaccida.

Tubotympanic CSOM

Tubotympanic CSOM usually follows acute otitis media or trauma. It results in chronic perforation of the tympanic membrane and presents with an intermittently discharging ear. It is associated with a conductive hearing loss. Treatment is with antibiotics, steroids and suction. If conservative treatment fails, a myringoplasty may be necessary. The temporalis fascia is usually used as the graft material.

Atticoantral CSOM

Atticoantral CSOM is a more dangerous condition and is associated with cholesteatoma formation. Squamous epithelium proliferates in the attic of the middle ear. The expanding 'ball' of skin causes a low-grade osteomyelitis. It presents with purulent aural discharge and conductive hearing loss. Complications of atticoantral CSOM include:

- Vestibular symptoms
- Facial nerve palsy
- Meningitis
- Intracranial abscess

Treatment is surgical and requires either an atticotomy or modified radical mastoidectomy.

Acute tonsillitis

Acute tonsillitis is a common condition. Approximately 60% cases are bacterial, often due to Group A streptococcal infection. It is characterised by a sore throat, fever and malaise. Cervical lymphadenopathy usually occurs. The tonsils are usually enlarged and coated with pus. Treatment is with simple analgesia and penicillin. Tonsillectomy is rarely required.

Quinsy

A quinsy is a peritonsillar abscess. It usually follows an episode of acute tonsillitis and presents with severe tonsillar pain and trismus. Examination shows swelling of the soft palate above the involved tonsil. The uvula is usually displaced. Treatment is with intravenous antibiotics. The abscess can be aspirated or drained under local anaesthetic. Following resolution, consideration should be given to an elective tonsillectomy. The indication for a tonsillectomy are shown in **Table 18.1**.

Acute paediatric stridor

The causes of stridor in a child can be either congenital or acquired.

Congenital causes include:

- Laryngomalacia
- Laryngeal web
- Subglottic stenosis

Acquired causes include:

- Angioneurotic oedema
- Impacted foreign body
- Epiglottitis
- Laryngotracheobronchitis
- Vocal cord palsy
- Benign laryngeal papillomatosis

Acute epiglottitis

Acute epiglottitis occurs in both adults and children. In children, it is a life-threatening disease and in young children symptoms can progress rapidly. It is due to *Haemophilus influenzae* infection. It presents with stridor and drooling. Insertion of spatula to examine the pharynx may precipitate complete airway

Indications for tonsillectomy	
Absolute	**Relative**
Sleep apnoea	Recurrent tonsillitis
Suspected tonsillar malignancy	Chronic tonsillitis
	Peritonsillar abscess (Quincy)
	Diphtheria carriers
	Systemic disease due to β-haemolytic streptococcus

Table 18.1 Indications for tonsillectomy

obstruction and should be performed with caution if acute epiglottis is a possible diagnosis. Patients should be managed with humidified oxygen and antibiotics. If there is potential compromise of the airway then intubation or tracheostomy should be considered.

Tracheostomy

A tracheostomy may be required to:

- To relieve upper airway obstruction
- To improve respiratory function
- To support long-term ventilation

Tracheostomy technique

The patient is positioned supine with a sandbag between the scapulae (**Figure 18.2**). A transverse cervical skin incision is made 1 cm above the sternal notch. The incision should extend to the sternomastoid muscles laterally. The fascial planes are dissected and the anterior jugular veins and strap muscles are retracted. The thyroid isthmus is divided and oversewn to prevent bleeding. A cricoid hook is placed on the 2nd tracheal ring. The stoma is fashioned between 3rd and 4th tracheal rings and the anterior portion of tracheal ring removed. There is no advantage in creating a tracheal flap. The endo-tracheal tube should be withdrawn to the level of the sub-glottis and the tracheostomy tube is inserted using an obturator. When it is confirmed that the tracheostomy tube is in the correct position, the endotracheal tube can be removed. The tube is secured with tapes.

Postoperative tracheostomy care

The postoperative management of a tracheostomy requires frequent atraumatic suction, humidification of the inspired air and oxygen, physiotherapy and occasional bronchial lavage. Infection and complications can be minimised by aseptic tube suction, handling and tube changing, by deflating the cuff on the tracheostomy tube for 5 minutes every hour and by avoiding the tube impinging on the posterior tracheal wall. The complications associated with a tracheostomy are shown in **Table 18.2**.

Percutaneous tracheostomy

Percutaneous tracheostomy is usually performed at the bedside in an intensive care unit. It is performed using a guide-wire and dilators. Bronchoscopic guidance may reduce the complication rate. Compared with an open operation it has a reduced risk of bleeding and infection.

Figure 18.2 Tracheostomy technique

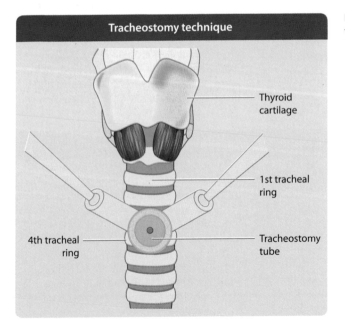

Tracheostomy technique

Thyroid cartilage

1st tracheal ring

4th tracheal ring

Tracheostomy tube

Complications of tracheostomy		
Immediate	**Intermediate**	**Late**
Haemorrhage	Tracheal erosion	Persistent tracheo-cutaneous fistula
Surgical trauma – oesophagus, recurrent laryngeal nerve palsy	Tube displacement	
	Tube obstruction	Laryngeal and tracheal stenosis
Pneumothorax	Subcutaneous emphysema	Tracheomalacia
	Aspiration and lung abscess	Tracheo-oesophageal fistula

Table 18.2 Complications of tracheostomy

Foreign bodies in the aerodigestive tract

Children ingest foreign bodies whilst playing. Adults ingest foreign bodies either when intoxicated or for perceived gain. Most foreign bodies in the aerodigestive tract are innocuous and may require no active treatment. Others may warrant urgent removal.

Oesophagus

Objects that stick in the oesophagus do so at the sites of anatomical narrowings. The commonest sites for them to arrest are at the level of the cricopharyngeus, the aortic indentation and the diaphragm. They usually present with acute dysphagia and drooling. The diagnosis may be confirmed with a plain x-ray. If the object is radiolucent and diagnostic uncertainty exists, consider a water-soluble contrast study. Foreign bodies can usually be removed by rigid oesophagoscopy. Occasionally difficultly is found with removing sharp objects (e.g. open safety pins). If removal proves difficult, then advancement into the stomach is often a safer option. Neglected objects can result in oesophageal perforation and mediastinitis. They can also result in fatal haemorrhage from an aorto-oesophageal fistula.

Pharynx

Sharp objects (e.g. fish bones) can stick in the pharynx. The commonest sites for them to be found are in the tonsils, pyriform fossa and post-cricoid region. The objects often result in a 'scratch' and symptoms can persist after the object has passed. The diagnosis can often be confirmed by indirect or fibreoptic laryngoscopy. Fish bones may be seen on a soft-tissue x-ray of the neck. They may require removal under general anaesthetic and can often be extracted by the anaesthetist before any planned surgical procedure starts!

Bronchus and lung

Due to the anatomical differences between the two main bronchi, inhaled foreign bodies usually pass down the right main bronchus. Radio-opaque objects can often be seen on chest x-ray. Radiolucent objects (e.g. peanuts) are more dangerous and more difficult to diagnose. Organic materials produce an inflammatory reaction. If neglected, they can result in bronchiectasis and a lung abscess. A bronchoscopy should be considered if there is clinical suspicion of an inhaled foreign body.

Stomach

If a foreign body reaches the stomach it will usually pass spontaneously through the remainder of the gastrointestinal tract. Ingested foreign bodies do not require the prescription of emetic or cathartic agents. Sharp objects may result in gastrointestinal perforation often in the 3rd or 4th part of the duodenum. The only objects that require urgent retrieval are button batteries that contain silver oxide, lithium and sodium hydroxide. If they leak they can cause major caustic injuries.

Epistaxis

The main blood supply to the nose is the sphenopalatine artery. It is a terminal branch of the external carotid artery. The incidence of epistaxis has a bimodal distribution. It is most commonly seen in childhood and old age. Causes are different in the two age groups. Epistaxis may be classified as either anterior or posterior. About 80% of cases are anterior and arise on the lower part of nasal septum (Little area). About 80% of cases are idiopathic. Causes of epistaxis include:

- Trauma
- Rhinitis
- Neoplasia – squamous carcinoma, juvenile angiofibroma
- Hypertension
- Haematological abnormalities
- Anticoagulation

Management

Initial clinical assessment may allow the site of bleeding to be identified. If there is a significant epistaxis, the patient may need a full blood count, clotting screen and cross match. Volume resuscitation may be required. Management depend on the site of the bleeding.

Anterior nasal haemorrhage may be controlled by direct pressure alone. If this fails, 1 : 1000 adrenaline solution can be applied to the Little area. Consideration may also be given to cautery of the retrocolumellar veins. This can usually be achieved with a silver nitrate stick. Anterior nasal packing should be considered if bleeding persists. This can be carried out with a nasal tampon or formal nasal pack. Prophylactic antibiotics should be used if the pack is to be left in place for more than 48 hours.

Posterior nasal haemorrhage requires a layered Bismuth iodoform paraffin paste (BIPP) ribbon gauze pack and occasionally the use of a postnasal balloon. If this fails to control bleeding, surgery should be considered. Endoscopic electrocautery can be attempted. Ligation of maxillary and anterior ethmoidal arteries may be required.

The facial nerve

Anatomy

The facial nerve arises at junction of pons and medulla and its course and branches are shown in **Figure 18.3**. It traverses the following structures:

- Posterior cranial fossa
- Internal auditory meatus
- Temporal bone in the facial canal
- Stylomastoid foramen
- Parotid gland

The terminal motor branches are the:

- Temporal
- Zygomatic
- Buccal
- Marginal mandibular
- Cervical

Function

The facial nerve is motor to the muscles of facial expression and provides a parasympathetic secretomotor supply to the lacrimal glands via the greater petrosal nerve. The parasympathetic supply is also secretomotor to the submandibular and sublingual salivary glands is via the chorda tympani. Taste to the anterior two-thirds of the tongue is via the chorda tympani and lingual nerve. It also supplies a somatic sensory supply to an area of skin around the external auditory meatus via fibres from the geniculate ganglion.

Facial nerve palsy

The causes of a facial nerve palsy are shown in **Table 18.3**. Lower motor neurone deficits of the facial nerve affect the whole of one side of face. With upper motor neurone deficits the forehead is spared.

Clinical features

The clinical features of a facial nerve palsy include:

- Facial asymmetry
- Eyebrow droop
- Loss of forehead and nasolabial folds
- Drooping of the corner of the mouth
- Inability to close the eye
- Inability to hold the lips tightly closed
- Facial muscle atrophy

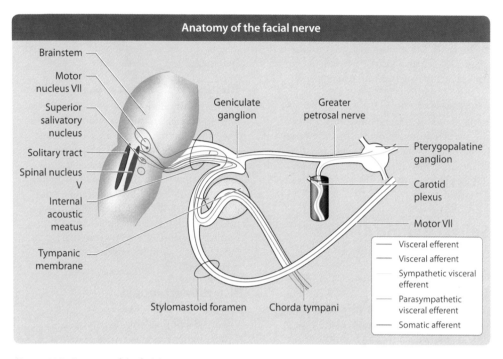

Figure 18.3 Anatomy of the facial nerve

Causes of facial nerve palsy		
Intracranial	**Intratemporal**	**Infratemporal**
Brainstem lesions	Otitis media	Parotid tumours
Cerebrovascular accident	Ramsay Hunt syndrome – herpes zoster oticus	Trauma
Multiple sclerosis	Trauma – temporal bone fracture	Surgery
Acoustic neuroma	Iatrogenic	
Cholesteatoma		

Table 18.3 Causes of a facial nerve palsy

Bell's palsy

Bell's palsy is the most common cause of facial paralysis. It accounts for 40% of facial nerve palsies. It is idiopathic and usually self-limiting. It may result from a viral infection. Bell's palsy is more common in adults, in people with diabetes and in pregnant women. The symptoms of Bell's palsy usually develop very quickly, often within a few hours and are at their worst within 2 days. About 75% of people with Bell's palsy recover completely. However, some people are left with long-lasting effects.

Ramsay Hunt syndrome

Ramsay Hunt syndrome was first described in 1907. It is an acute facial nerve palsy associated with a vesicular rash of the skin of the ear canal, auricle or mucous membrane of the oropharynx. It is due to infection of the geniculate ganglion by the varicella-zoster virus. Otalgia is usually a prominent feature. There may also be vertigo, tinnitus, a unilateral hearing loss and nystagmus.

Management

In patients with a facial palsy, protection of the eye is required and a tarsorrhaphy may be necessary if the palsy persists. In a Bell palsy, steroids may be beneficial. Patients with Ramsey Hunt syndrome may benefit from acyclovir.

Salivary gland disease
Neoplastic salivary gland disease

Pathology

Approximately 75% of salivary gland tumours occur in the parotid gland where 15% are malignant. 10% of tumours occur in the submandibular gland where 30% are malignant and 15% of tumours occur in the minor salivary glands where 50% are malignant. The pathological classification of salivary gland tumours is shown in **Table 18.4**.

Clinical features

Parotid tumours usually present as a lump in the parotid region. Most are slow-growing even if malignant. Pain is suggestive of malignancy but is not a reliable symptom. A facial nerve palsy is highly suspicious of a malignant tumour.

Investigation

The extent of the lesion can often be confirmed by CT or MRI scanning. Open biopsy is contraindicated. Fine needle aspiration cytology may confirm the diagnosis. It has a poor sensitivity but a high specificity.

Pleomorphic adenoma

Pleomorphic adenomas accounts for 75% of parotid and 50% of submandibular tumours. They are sometimes described as a 'mixed' tumour' as they were believed to have both epithelial and mesothelial elements. They are now believed to arise from ductal myoepithelial cells. The male:female ratio is approximately equal. They may undergo malignant change but the risk is small. They require excision with a 5-10 mm margin as local implantation of cells can lead to local recurrence.

Warthin's tumour

Warthin's tumour is also known as an adenolymphoma. They usually occurs in elderly patients and the male:female ratio is approximately 4:1. They account for 15% of parotid tumours. About 10% of tumours are bilateral. They are rare in other salivary glands and they do not undergo malignant change.

Intermediate salivary tumours

Acinic cell and mucoepidermoid carcinomas account for 5% of all tumours. They have low malignant potential, do not require radical therapy and can be treated similar to benign tumours.

Malignant salivary tumours

Adenoid cystic, adenocarcinomas and squamous cell tumours are rare. All are usually high-grade tumours and the prognosis is often poor regardless of

Pathological classification of salivary tumours		
Benign	**Intermediate**	**Malignant**
Pleomorphic adenoma	Mucoepidermoid tumours	Adenoid cystic carcinoma
Warthin's tumours	Acinic cell carcinoma	Adenocarcinoma
Haemangioma in children	Oncocytoma	Squamous cell carcinoma
Lymphangioma in children		

Table 18.4 Pathological classification of salivary tumours

treatment. Adenoid cystic tumours have a tendency for perineural spread into the brain and also develop distant metastases to the lung. Cannon-ball metastases may be present for years without symptoms. The overall 5-year survival is approximately 50%.

Management of salivary tumours

All tumours require partial or complete excision of the affected gland. Enucleation of tumours often results in local recurrence. For parotid tumours, this involves either superficial or total parotidectomy. In both procedures, the facial nerve is preserved. For malignant salivary tumours, consideration should be given to postoperative radiotherapy and neck dissection if there is evidence of nodal involvement.

Non-neoplastic salivary gland enlargement

Causes of non-neoplastic salivary gland enlargement include:

- Acute sialadenitis – viral, bacterial
- Recurrent acute sialadenitis
- Chronic sialadenitis – tuberculosis, actinomycosis
- Calculi
- Cysts – mucous retention, ranula
- Systemic disease – pancreatitis, diabetes, acromegaly
- Sjögren's syndrome
- Sarcoidosis
- Mikulicz's syndrome
- Drug induced – phenothiazines
- Allergic

Acute sialadenitis

Mumps

Mumps is the commonest cause of acute, painful swelling of the parotid gland in children. It is due to a paromyxovirus infection. A flu-like illness is followed by acute bilateral painful parotid swelling which resolves spontaneously over 5–10 days. Sometimes the parotid swelling may be unilateral. Occasionally it may affect the submandibular glands. A similar clinical picture may occur with Coxsackie A or B or parainfluenza virus infection.

Bacterial sialadenitis

Acute ascending bacterial sialadenitis usually affects the parotid glands due to *Staphylococcus aureus* or streptococcus viridans infection. The incidence of this condition is decreasing. It used to be seen in dehydrated postoperative patients with poor oral hygiene. It presents with painful tender swelling of the parotid gland. Pus can often be expressed from the parotid duct. A sialogram is contraindicated. Treatment is with parenteral broad-spectrum antibiotics. Late presentation can cause a parotid abscess to develop.

Sialolithiasis

Of all salivary gland stones, 80%, 10% and 7% occur in the submandibular, parotid and sublingual glands, respectively. About 80% of submandibular stones are radio-opaque. Most parotid stones are radiolucent. The clinical presentation of a submandibular stone is usually with pain and swelling prior to or during a meal. Symptoms arise due to complete obstruction of the submandibular duct. In partial obstruction, the swelling may be mild with chronic painful enlargement of the gland. If there is diagnostic doubt then the stone can be demonstrated by a sialogram (**Figure 18.4**). Treatment is by either removal of the stone from the duct or excision of the gland. The stone can be removed if it is palpable and there is no evidence of chronic infection. The gland should be excised if the stone lies posterior in the gland or if the gland is chronically inflamed.

Sjögren's syndrome

Sjögren's syndrome was first described by Henrich Sjögren in 1933. It is an autoimmune condition affecting the salivary and lacrimal glands. The female:male is approximately 10:1. Patients present with:

- Dry eyes – keratoconjunctivitis sicca
- Dry mouth – xerostomia
- Bilateral parotid enlargement

Sjögren's syndrome is often associated with other connective tissue disorders. Primary Sjögren's syndrome has no connective tissue disorder. Secondary Sjögren's syndrome is

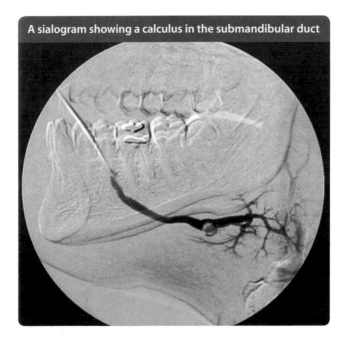

A sialogram showing a calculus in the submandibular duct

Figure 18.4 A sialogram showing a calculus in the submandibular duct

usually associated rheumatoid arthritis or systemic lupus erythematosis. The risk of B-cell lymphoma is increased. A sialogram shows characteristic sialectasis and parenchymal destruction. The diagnosis can be confirmed by labial gland biopsy. Treatment is symptomatic. No treatment will reverse the keratoconjunctivitis and xerostomia.

Common neck swellings

There are many causes of lumps in the neck. The most common cause is lymphadenopathy as a result of bacterial or viral infections or malignancy. A lump can also arise in either the salivary or thyroid gland. In children, most neck lumps are caused by treatable infections. In adults the likelihood of malignancy increases.

Pharyngeal pouch

A pharyngeal pouch is a posteromedial pulsion diverticulum through Killian's dehiscence (**Figure 18.5**). It occurs between thyropharyngeus and cricopharyngeus muscles, both of which form the inferior constrictor of the pharynx. The male:female ratio is approximately 5:1. It is usually seen in the elderly. The aetiology is unknown but upper oesophageal sphincter dysfunction may be an important aetiological factor. A carcinoma can develop within the pouch.

Clinical features

The commonest symptoms are dysphagia, regurgitation of undigested food and a cough. Recurrent aspiration can result in pulmonary complications. Clinical signs are often absent. A cervical lump may be present that gurgles on palpation.

Investigation

Indirect or fibreoptic laryngoscopy may show a pooling of saliva within the pyriform fossa. A barium swallow may show a residual pool of contrast within the pouch (**Figure 18.6**).

Management

Management depends on the size of the pouch and the age of the patient. Options include a diverticulectomy or Dohlman's procedure.

Diverticulectomy

Following rigid endoscopy, the pouch is packed with gauze. A bougie is placed within

Anatomy of a pharyngeal pouch

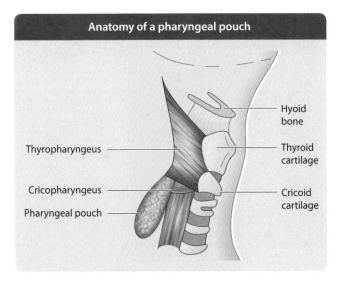

- Thyropharyngeus
- Cricopharyngeus
- Pharyngeal pouch
- Hyoid bone
- Thyroid cartilage
- Cricoid cartilage

Figure 18.5 Anatomy of a pharyngeal pouch

A barium swallow showing a pharyngeal pouch

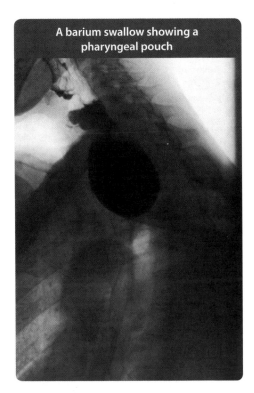

Figure 18.6 A barium swallow showing a pharyngeal pouch

the oesophagus and a collar incision is made at the level of the cricoid cartilage. The fascia at the anterior border of sternomastoid is divided and the pouch is identified anterior to the prevertebral fascia. The pouch is then excised and the defect closed. A cricopharyngeal myotomy is performed to prevent recurrence. The patient should be fed via a nasogastric tube for a week postoperatively. Complications include:

- Recurrent laryngeal nerve palsy
- Cervical emphysema
- Mediastinitis
- Subcutaneous fistula

Dohlman's procedure

A Dohlman's procedure is performed endoscopically. A double-lipped oesophagoscope is used and the wall between the diverticulum and oesophageal wall is exposed. The hypopharyngeal bar is divided with diathermy or laser. This minimally invasive techniques allows a:

- Shorter duration of anaesthesia
- More rapid resumption of oral intake
- Shorter hospital stay
- Quicker recovery

Applied basic sciences

Paediatric anatomy and physiology

Children are not small adults. They have different body proportions and marked differences in both their anatomy and physiology that have implications for both the assessment and management of surgical disease.

Thermoregulation

Thermoregulation in neonates is inefficient and to maintain a stable temperature they need a higher ambient temperature with little variation. They are susceptible to a labile body temperature due to:

- High body surface area:volume ratio
- Reduced subcutaneous fat
- Poor peripheral vasomotor control
- Inability to shiver or sweat
- Inability to voluntarily control their own environment

Cardiovascular system

The cardiovascular system undergoes significant changes at birth. The right and left side of the fetal circulation become separated by a combination of circulatory and mechanical events. These include:

- Gas exchange changes from placental to pulmonary
- The foreman ovale closes
- Closure of the fetal vessels within the umbilical cord

The neonatal heart rate is rapid and peaks at about 1 month of age. There is beat-to-beat variation and sinus arrhythmia is common. The heart rate declines to adult levels at puberty. In the first few months of life, oxygen carriage is impaired by the persistence of fetal haemoglobin. The oxygen dissociation curve is shifted to left. The total blood volume and haemoglobin levels are increased. The neonatal myocardium is relatively

non-complaint. Left ventricular filling is unable to increase cardiac output which, as a result, is increased by an increase in heart rate.

Respiratory system

Following birth, the lungs adapt rapidly to extrauterine life. There are several differences between the respiratory system in adults and children. In neonates, airway management can be difficult due to:

- Large occiput tends to flex neck and can cause obstruction
- Neonates are obligate nasal breathers
- Large tongue with small mandible
- Large epiglottis
- Short trachea
- Airway diameters are small and can be blocked by secretions

Neonates increase respiratory rate rather than tidal volume in response to increased oxygen demand. Respiratory muscles are immature and easily fatigued.

Renal system

The kidneys in neonates have a lower glomerular filtration rate and reduced ability to concentrate urine compared with adults. High solute loads require an obligatory urine volume which can lead to dehydration and hyponatraemia. The water content of a neonate is very high and the extracellular fluid volume is twice that of an adult (40% vs. 20%). There is a high turnover of fluid which can be rapidly lost, contributing to dehydration.

Paediatric trauma

Trauma is the commonest cause of death in childhood. Road traffic accidents and falls account for 80% of injuries. Thoracic and abdominal injuries usually result from blunt trauma. Penetrating injuries are uncommon. In children, significant injuries can occur without overlying fractures.

Assessment

Assessment should follow the same principles as in adults. It is important to know or estimate the weight of the child to calculate fluid volumes and drug doses. Weight can be estimated from age or the head-to-toe length.

Airway and breathing

Airway management in a child can be difficult due to the large head size relative to the size of the body, a small oral cavity with a large tongue and large angle of the jaw. The larynx is cephalad and the trachea is short. Infants less than 6 months are obligate nose breathers. Uncuffed endotracheal tubes should be used in children before puberty.

Circulation

Normal values for pulse and blood pressure vary with age. Less than 1 year, the pulse is 120 to 140 and systolic BP is 70–90 mmHg. Between 2 and 5 years, the pulse is 100–120 and systolic BP is 80–90 mmHg. Between 5 and 12 years, the pulse is 80–100 and systolic BP is 90–110 mmHg. Venous access in a child can be difficult and femoral or external jugular access may be required. If percutaneous cannulation fails, then consideration needs to be given to a medial cephalic venous cut down, long saphenous venous cut down or intraosseous infusion. Initial resuscitation should be with a 20 mL/kg crystalloid bolus.

Occult chest injuries in children

Chest injuries may be occult in children and dependent on the mechanism of injury, the following should be suspected:

- Pulmonary contusion
- Pulmonary laceration
- Intrapulmonary haemorrhage
- Tracheobronchial tear
- Myocardial contusion
- Diaphragmatic rupture
- Partial aortic or other great vessel disruption
- Oesophageal tears

Child protection

A number of high profile child abuse cases and subsequent enquires have reinforced the importance of having systems in place to detect and managed suspected child abuse. The incidence of child abuse in the UK is about 3 per 1000 with over 80 deaths per year. Abuse can be :

- Physical
- Sexual
- Neglect
- Emotional

Risk factors include:

- Preterm and infants less than 1 year of age
- Teenage mothers
- Single parents
- Parental mental health problems
- Drug and alcohol abuse
- Domestic violence

Diagnostic criteria for non-accidental injury

Non-accidental injury should be suspected if the following are seen:

- Delay in seeking medical advice
- Vague or inconsistent account of the accident
- Discrepancy between the history and degree of injury
- Abnormal parental behaviour or lack of concern for the child
- Interaction between child and parents is abnormal
- Finger tip bruising over upper arm, trunk, face or neck
- Bizarre injuries – bites, cigarette burns or rope marks
- Sharply demarked burns in an unusual site
- Perioral injuries – torn frenulum
- Retinal haemorrhages
- Ruptured internal organs without a history of major trauma
- Perianal or genital injury
- Long bone fractures in children less than 3 years
- Injuries of differing ages

Correctable congenital abnormalities

Approximately 2% of live births have major congenital abnormalities. The incidence is increased in pre-term and small for gestational age infants. A malformation can be defined as a disturbance of growth during embryogenesis. A deformation can be defined as a late change in a previously normal structure due to intrauterine factors. Causes of deformations include:

- Primigravidity
- Oligohydramnios
- Abnormal presentation
- Multiple pregnancy
- Uterine abnormality

Malformations can occur because of genetic abnormalities or exposure to teratogens (**Table 19.1**). In many cases the cause remains obscure. The commonest systems affected are the heart, urogenital and central nervous systems.

Teratogenesis

A teratogen as a drug, chemical or virus that can cause fetal malformations. They act during critical periods of fetal development which varies between different organs:

- Brain: 15–25 days
- Eye: 25–40 days
- Heart: 20–40 days
- Limb: 24–36 days

Drugs know to be teratogens include:

- Hormones – progestogens, diethyl stilbestrol, male sex hormones
- Antipsychotics – lithium, haloperidol, thalidomide
- Anticonvulsants – sodium valproate, carbamazepine, phenobarbitone
- Antimicrobials – tetracycline, chloramphenicol, amphotericin B
- Antineoplastics – alkylating agents, folic acid antagonists
- Anticoagulants – warfarin

- Antithyroid agents – carbimazole, propylthiouracil
- Others – toluene, alcohol, marijuana, narcotics

Microbial agents know to be teratogens include:

- Rubella
- Toxoplasmosis
- Syphilis
- Cytomegalovirus
- Coxsackie B virus

Cleft lip and palate

Cleft lips and palates are a diverse and variable congenital abnormality. They are the commonest congenital abnormalities of the orofacial structures. Cleft lip and palate occurs in 1:600 live births. Isolated cleft palate occurs in 1:1000 live births. They usually occur in isolation but can be associated with other anomalies (e.g. congenital heart disease). Cleft lip and palate predominates in males. Isolated cleft palate is more common in females.

Aetiology

Cleft lip and palate is believed to have both a genetic and environmental component. Cleft palate may be inherited as an autosomal dominant condition with variable penetrance. A family history in a first-degree relative increases the risk by a factor of 20. Important environmental factors include maternal epilepsy, drug exposure (steroids, diazepam, phenytoin) and possibly folic acid deficiency. Cleft lip

Causes of malformations	
Cause	**Percentage**
Mendelian genetic aberration	20
Chromosomal	10
Teratogens	10
Multiple factors	30
Unknown	30

Table 19.1 Causes of malformations

and palate also occur as part of over 100 syndromes including:

- Pierre Robin syndrome
- Stickler syndrome
- Down's syndrome
- Treacher Collins syndrome

Embryology

The cleft lip deformity is usually established in the first 6 weeks of life due to failure of fusion of the maxillary and medial nasal processes. It may be due to incomplete mesodermal ingrowth into the processes. The extent of the deficiency determines the extent of the cleft. Palatal clefts result from failure of fusion of the palatal shelves of the maxillary processes.

Clinical features

The typical distributions of cleft types are:

- Cleft lip alone (15%)
- Cleft lip and palate (45%)
- Isolated cleft palate (40%)

Cleft lips are more common on the left.

Management

Antenatal diagnosis of a cleft lip may be possible. The degree of functional and aesthetic deficit is related to the type and severity of the cleft. Feeding is rarely a difficulty. Breast feeding may be achieved or modified teats for bottle feeding may be required. Major respiratory obstruction is uncommon. Speech may be affected by the altered anatomy of the lip and soft palate and dysfunction of the palatal muscles. Hearing may be affected as the abnormal palate interferes with eustachian tube function. Dentition is abnormal if the alveolus is involved.

The aims of surgery for cleft lips and palate are:

- To achieve a normal appearance of the lip, nose and face
- To allow normal facial growth
- To allow normal speech

Many different techniques have been advocated. Cleft lip repair is usually performed between 3 and 6 months of age. Cleft palate repair is usually performed between 6 and 18 months. Two or more operations may be required. A multidisciplinary team approach is essential. Other aspects that need to be addressed included:

- Hearing
- Speech therapy
- Dental
- Orthodontics

Congenital heart disease

The commonest classification of congenital heart disease is into:

- Septal defects
- Obstructive defects
- Cyanotic defects

The commonest congenital heart defects are shown in **Table 19.2**.

Classification of congenital heart disease		
Septal defects	**Obstructive defects**	**Cyanotic defects**
Atrial septal defect	Aortic stenosis	Tetralogy of Fallot
Ventricular septal defect	Pulmonary stenosis	Transposition of great vessels
	Coarctation of the aorta	Pulmonary atresia
		Truncus arteriosus
		Total anomalous pulmonary venous connection
		Hypoplastic left heart syndrome

Table 19.2 Classification of congenital heart disease

Atrial septal defect

With an atrial septal defect (ASD) a communication between the right and left atria creates a shunt. The degree of left-to-right shunt is dependent on the ventricular compliance and the size of the defect. There are four main types:

- Ostium secundum defect (70%)
- Ostium primum defect (20%)
- Sinus venous defect (10%)
- Coronary sinus defect (<1%)

Ventricular septal defect

Ventricular septal defects (VSD) are the commonest congenital heart defect. The classification is based around the division of the septum into membranous and muscular components. Perimembranous defects are the most common (70%) and are situated between the inlet and outlet portions of the septum. The size of the VSD rather than its location has the greatest bearing on outcome.

Tetralogy of Fallot

Tetralogy of Fallot is the commonest cyanotic heart defect (**Figure 19.1**). It occurs in approximately 5 per 10,000 live births and represents 5–7% of congenital heart defects. Its cause is thought to be due to both environmental and genetic factors. It is associated with chromosome 22 deletions and di George syndrome. It occurs slightly more often in males than in females. It has four components:

- Right ventricular outflow tract obstruction (pulmonary stenosis)
- Ventricular septal defect
- Aorta overrides VSD
- Right ventricular hypertrophy

The VSD and pulmonary stenosis determine the pathophysiological features. Untreated, 25% of infants die in the 1st year of life. The risk of death is greatest in the 1st year, then constant until about 25 years of age.

Clinical features

Cyanosis is usually constant but may be intermittent with hypoxic spells. Infants with severe infundibular and pulmonary stenosis are deeply cyanosed from birth. They have a moderate systolic ejection murmur which disappears during a cyanotic spells. Patients are polycythaemic and develop clubbing.

Figure 19.1 Tetralogy of Fallot

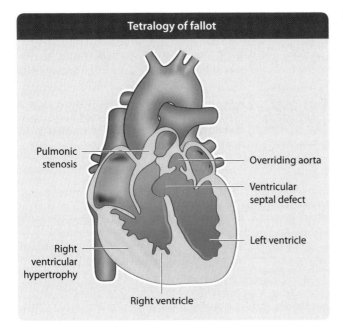

Tetralogy of fallot

Pulmonic stenosis

Overriding aorta

Ventricular septal defect

Left ventricle

Right ventricular hypertrophy

Right ventricle

Investigation

A chest x-ray shows a 'boot-shaped' heart and is more common in older infants and children. An ECG shows right ventricular hypertrophy and right axis deviation. Echocardiography shows the VSD and right ventricular outflow tract obstruction. It can also delineate coronary artery anatomy, AV valve morphology and the central pulmonary arteries.

Management

The majority of patients have adequate oxygen saturation and can undergo elective repair. Progressive hypoxaemia (oxygen saturation 75–80%) is an indication for surgery. Occurrence of cyanotic spells is also an indication for surgery. Asymptomatic children with uncomplicated morphology should have an elective repair between 3 and 24 months of age. Very young infants with complicated morphology can be managed with a staged shunt (usually modified Blalock–Taussig procedure). The goal is to repair the defect and provide blood flow from the right ventricle to as many pulmonary segments as possible. Perioperative mortality is 2–5% and survival at 5 years is about 90%.

Transposition of the great vessels

Transposition of the great vessels presents in the immediate neonatal period, particularly if no VSD is present. Infants can present shocked and severely acidotic. The infant is invariably cyanosed. No murmur is present, unless there is a VSD or some other structural cardiac lesion. Radiologically, the lungs appear to have increased blood flow and increased pulmonary vascular markings. The mediastinum is narrow, as the great arteries are running in parallel. The diagnosis is made by echocardiography. Cardiac failure may be apparent in the presence of a large VSD. In the short-term, a prostaglandin infusion should be commenced to ensure continued patency. A balloon atrial septostomy is usually performed within the first day or two of life to assist with mixing at the atrial level. An arterial switch procedure is usually required within the first week of life.

Patent ductus arteriosus

Patent ductus arteriosus (PDA) is persistence of a functioning lumen in the fetal ductus arteriosus. This connects the proximal descending aorta to the left pulmonary artery. The normal neonatal ductus arteriosus is closed by smooth muscle contraction within hours of birth. Over the following weeks this is made permanent by fibrous obliteration of the lumen to form the ligamentum arteriosus.

Coarctation of the aorta

Coarctation is a narrowing of the proximal descending thoracic aorta. The coarctation is usually juxtaductal but can be pre- or post-ductal. It is a form of left ventricular outflow obstruction and pressure overload on the left ventricle eventually leads to left ventricular hypertrophy and cardiac failure.

Exomphalos and gastroschisis

Exomphalos and gastroschisis are two different congenital anomalies. They differ markedly in their clinical appearance. The overall incidence is approximately 1:3000 live births. They are usually diagnosed prenatally on ultrasound and can usually be differentiated prior to birth.

Exomphalos

An exomphalos or omphalocele is more common in male infants. It always has a sac but the sac may be intact or ruptured. The sac has three layers – peritoneum, Wharton jelly and amnion. The umbilical cord arises from the apex of the sac. The sac contains intestinal loops, liver, spleen and bladder. It is often associated with other major congenital anomalies (e.g. Beckwith–Wiedemann syndrome) and prognosis depends on these associated anomalies. Mortality is approximately 40%.

Management

No consensus exists on the optimal management of a large unruptured exomphalos. Treatment depends on the size of the lesion. The aim of treatment are to reduce the contents into the small abdominal cavity and, if the bowel is covered, there is no urgency to do this. Treatment options are both surgical or conservative and include:

- Biological dressings
- Polymer films

- Direct surgical closure
- Skin flap closure

Small defects can usually be closed surgically but closure of large defects may require staged procedures. Overzealous reduction can result in caval compression. After conservative treatment, a ventral hernia repair may be required at about 1 year of age.

Gastroschisis

Gastroschisis also has a male preponderance. A gastroschisis never has a sac. The umbilical cord arises from the normal place in the abdominal wall, usually to the left of the abdominal wall defect. The evisceration usually only contains intestinal loops. It is rarely associated with other major congenital anomalies, but may be associated with intestinal atresia. Infants have better a prognosis than those with an exomphalos. Mortality is approximately 10%.

Management

A gastroschisis can often be treated by direct full-layer closure of the abdominal wall. If direct closure is not possible, then staged reduction within a silo maybe preferable. Surgery is often associated with postoperative gut dysfunction and patients usually require postoperative nutritional and ventilatory support.

Congenital diaphragmatic hernia

A congenital diaphragmatic hernia occurs in 1 in 4000 live births. It results from failure of closure of the pleuro-peritoneal canals. Approximately 95% occur through the posterior foreman of Bochdalek. Less than 5% occur through the anterior foreman of Morgagni. About 90% occur on the left. The midgut herniates into the chest impairing lung development. It is often associated with gastrointestinal malrotation.

Clinical features

Patients often present with cyanosis and respiratory distress soon after birth. The prognosis is related to the time of onset and degree of respiratory impairment. Examination often shows the abdomen to be flat and air entry is reduced on the affected side. The heart sounds are often displaced. A chest x-ray will confirm the presence of gastrointestinal loops in the chest. Occasionally, patients present later in life with respiratory distress or intestinal obstruction.

Management

Respiratory support with intubation and ventilation is usually required. A nasogastric tube should be passed. Gas exchange and acid–base status should be assessed. Any acidosis may need correction with a bicarbonate infusion. Surgery should be considered early after resuscitation. The hernial contents are usually reduced via an abdominal approach. The hernial sac is excised and the diaphragm repaired with non-absorbable suture or a Gortex patch. A Ladd's procedure may be required for malrotation. A chest drain is usually not required. Early respiratory failure is associated with a poor prognosis.

Oesophageal atresia

Oesophageal atresia affects 1 in 3000 live births. The aetiology is unknown but the incidence is increased in first degree relatives. It is often associated with a trachea-oesophageal fistula (TOF – **Figure 19.2**). The various presentations include:

- Oesophageal atresia with TOF – 85%
- Isolated oesophageal atresia – 8%
- Isolated TOF – 4%
- Oesophageal atresia with proximal and distal TOF

About 50% of patients have other congenital abnormalities usually involving the cardiovascular, urogenital or anorectal systems.

Clinical features

Prenatally, oesophageal atresia may be diagnosed by the finding of polyhydramnios. The stomach is empty on ultrasound. Postnatally, the diagnosis should be suspected by the neonate drooling, being unable to swallow and cyanosed during feeding. Unrecognised, the patient usually develops aspiration pneumonia. A 10 Fr

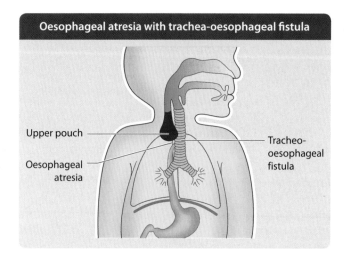

Figure 19.2 Oesophageal atresia with trachea-oesophageal fistula

nasogastric tube can not be passed more than 10 cm. On a chest x-ray, if there is gas in the stomach, there must be a distal TOF.

Management

Feeding should be withheld and suction applied to the oesophageal pouch. The patient should be nursed in an upright position. The presence of other associated congenital abnormalities should be assessed. Surgery is required within the first 24 hours of life. The operation involves a right thoracotomy and an extrapleural approach. The azygos vein and any TOF are divided. The oesophagus is mobilised and a primary anastomosis is usually achieved. If an anastomosis is impossible, then a staged procedure is required. With the latter approach, a gastrostomy is performed and the fistula divided at the initial operation. The oesophagus can be replaced by colon or stomach after a few months. Complications following surgery for oesophageal atresia include:

- Oesophageal dysfunction
- Dilated proximal pouch
- Gastro-oesophageal reflux
- Anastomotic stricture
- Recurrent fistula

Neonatal intestinal obstruction

Neonatal intestinal obstruction can be due to a variety of causes. The presenting clinical features are often similar. Bile-stained vomiting is never normal in a neonate and implies obstruction. Approximately 95% of normal babies pass meconium within the first 24 hours of life. Failure to pass meconium should be regarded also as a feature of obstruction until proved otherwise. The degree of abdominal distension is variable.

Duodenal atresia

Duodenal atresia occurs in 1 in 10,000 live births. The site of the obstruction is most commonly in the 2nd part of the duodenum. The proximal the duodenum become hypertrophied. About 50% cases are associated with polyhydramnios and 60% of such pregnancies are complicated or end prematurely. Approximately 30% of babies with duodenal atresia have Down's syndrome. Other associated abnormalities are cardiac anomalies, intestinal malrotation and biliary atresia. Duodenal atresia can often be diagnosed by antenatal ultrasound. Postnatally, it presents with bilious or non-bile stained vomiting. An abdominal x-ray may show a 'double-bubble' and no gas within the bowel distal to the obstruction (**Figure 19.3**).

Management

A nasogastric tube should be passed. Intravenous fluid resuscitation should

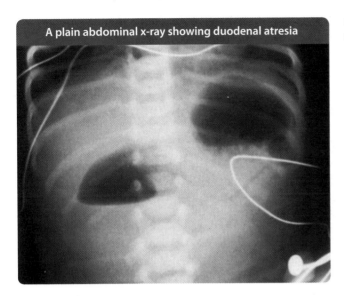

A plain abdominal x-ray showing duodenal atresia

Figure 19.3 A plain abdominal x-ray showing duodenal atresia

be given and major cardiac and other defects should be excluded. A duodenoduodenostomy should be performed once the patient is resuscitated.

Other atresias

Atresias of the small bowel and colon are less common but again, are often associated with polyhydramnios. Bilious vomiting and distension are key features. An abdominal x-ray will show dilated bowel and a gas-free rectum. A nasogastric tube should be passed and intravenous fluid resuscitation should be given. At operation, dilated proximal bowel should be resected or tapered and a primary anastomosis may be possible.

Meconium ileus

Meconium ileus is the commonest cause of neonatal intraluminal intestinal obstruction. About 80% cases are associated with cystic fibrosis. Cystic fibrosis occurs in 1 in 2000 live births and is inherited as an autosomal recessive condition. Viscid pancreatic secretions cause autodigestion of pancreatic acinar cells. The resulting meconium is abnormal and 'putty-like' in consistency. Meconium becomes inspissated in the lower ileum. There is a microcolon. It presents with bilious vomiting and distension usually on first day of life. The passage of meconium is

delayed. Meconium filled loops of bowel may be palpable. An abdominal x-ray may show a 'ground-glass' appearance, especially in the right upper quadrant.

Management

The administration of a gastrografin enemas may be successful in 50% of patients. If unsuccessful, surgery will be needed. A limited resection and stomas may be required.

Malrotation

Between 4 and 10 weeks of development, the intestines herniate into the umbilical cord. During normal development, when returned to abdomen, they rotate 270° anticlockwise. As a result, the duodenojejunal (DJ) flexure lies to the left of the midline and the caecum lies in right iliac fossa. The transverse colon lies anterior to the small bowel mesentery. Partial failure of rotation results in malrotation. The commonest abnormality results in the caecum lying close to DJ flexure. The resulting midgut mesentery is abnormally narrow and liable to undergo a volvulus. Fibrous bands may be present between the caecum and DJ flexure (Ladd bands).

Clinical features

There are two principal clinical presentations. Malrotation can present early with collapse and acidosis due to intestinal infarction. It can present late with intermittent bile-stained vomiting and distension. Radiological investigations are often unhelpful.

Management

After resuscitation, an early laparotomy is required. Any volvulus should be reduced. Resection may be required if there has been small bowel infarction. Any Ladd bands should be divided. The base of the mesentery should be elongated. The colon should be placed on the left of the abdomen. The small bowel should be placed on the right. An inversion appendicectomy should be performed to prevent future diagnostic uncertainty.

Hirschsprung's disease

Hirschsprung's disease is due to absence of the autonomic ganglion cells in Auerbach's plexus of the distal large intestine. It commences at the internal anal sphincter and progresses for a variable distance proximally. It affects 1 in 5000 live births and the male:female ratio is 4:1. It accounts for 10% of cases of neonatal intestinal obstruction. Some cases appear to be due to autosomal dominant inheritance. About 75% cases are confined to the recto-sigmoid but 10% cases have total colonic involvement.

Clinical features

Approximately 80% of cases present in the neonatal period with delayed passage of meconium. This is followed by increasing abdominal distension and vomiting. The child is at increased risk of enterocolitis and perforation. It occasionally presents with chronic constipation in infancy.

Diagnosis

A plain abdominal x-ray will confirm intestinal obstruction. A contrast enema may show a contracted rectum, cone shaped transitional zone and proximal dilatation. Anorectal manometry may show a recto-sphincteric inhibition reflex on rectal distension. The diagnosis is confirmed by a rectal biopsy which will show absence of ganglion cells in the submucosa, increased acetylcholinesterase cells in the muscularis

mucosa and increased unmyelinated nerves in the bowel wall.

Management

An initial defunctioning stoma should be fashioned to relieve the obstruction. Definitive treatment involves either a bypass of the affected segment (Duhamel or Soave bypass) or excision of the aganglionic segment and anastomosis (Swenson procedure).

Anorectal anomalies

Anorectal malformations comprise a wide spectrum of abnormalities. They affect 1 in 5000 live births and are often associated with other congenital malformations. Prognosis depends on the severity of the malformation and the extent of other anomalies. Early treatment of neonates with anorectal anomalies is required.

Clinical assessment

Clinical inspection of the perineum is important. In 80% of patients, clinical examination and urinalysis allows a decision to be made as to whether a colostomy is required. A flat perineum and absence of anal dimple suggest poor perineal muscle development. These features are associated with high anorectal malformations. Meconium at the perineum and a skin tag associated with an anal dimple or membrane suggests a low malformation. Even if a perineal fistula is present, meconium may not be passed for 24 hours.

Approximately 50% of all patients with anorectal malformations have an associated urogenital anomaly. Renal abnormalities include:

- Renal agenesis
- Vesicoureteral reflux
- Neurogenic bladder
- Renal dysplasia
- Megaureter
- Hydronephrosis
- Ectopic ureter

Investigation

If the clinical signs are unclear, than radiological investigations may be useful. A cross-table lateral x-ray with the baby prone, with a marker on the perineum, is a useful initial study. The presence of air in the distal rectum, within 1 cm of the perineum, suggests primary repair may be possible. Ultrasound may show features of co-existent obstructive uropathy. If a colostomy is fashioned, distal colography may demonstrate a fistula to the urinary tract. A plain x-ray of the spine and sacrum may show associated abnormalities. Urinalysis may indicate the presence of a fistula to the urinary tract.

Management

Important issues to consider in the management of anorectal anomalies are:

- Is there any other associated life threatening abnormality?
- Should the patient undergo primary repair with covering colostomy?
- Should the patient undergo defunctioning colostomy and later definitive repair?

Intravenous fluids are required. A nasogastric tube should be inserted. A colostomy should be considered if there is:

- Recto-bulbar urethral fistula
- Recto-prostatic urethral fistula
- Rectovesical fistula
- Imperforate anus without fistula
- Rectal atresia

A posterior sagittal anoplasty may be possible if there is a low abnormality with a rectoperineal fistula. This avoids the need for colostomy.

Surgery

Repair of any anorectal malformation requires a meticulous and delicate technique. The posterior sagittal approach is an ideal method of defining and repairing anorectal anomalies. Patients are placed in the prone position with the pelvis elevated. Anorectal abnormalities in 90% of male patients can be repaired with a posterior sagittal approach alone. The external sphincter is mobilised to bring the anus back to the center of the external sphincter. This can be performed in the neonatal period without a protective colostomy. An electrical stimulator helps identify the location of the sphincteric mechanism and postoperative anal dilatation is required.

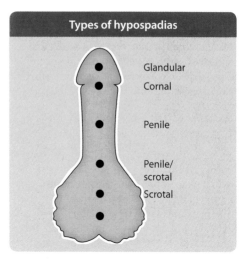

Figure 19.4 Types of hypospadias

Postoperative constipation is common and if unrecognised can result in a megarectum. About 25% of patients have faecal incontinence. Urinary incontinence may also occur. Severe bowel disturbances and urinary incontinence are often associated with sacral defects.

Hypospadias

Hypospadias affects approximately 1 in 500 boys (**Figure 19.4**). It is due to incomplete fusion of genital folds and the glandular urethra. The urethra is found on the ventral surface of penis and is replaced distally by a fibrous chordee. The deformity consists of a malpositioned meatus, chordee and abnormal foreskin. Hypospadias is classified as glandular, coronal, penile or scrotal. About 70% are glandular or coronal, 10% are penile and 20% are scrotal. Perineal hypospadias is associated with intersex conditions and anorectal anomalies.

Management

If any degree of hypospadias is present, circumcision is contraindicated. Treatment is required to improve the urinary stream and allow sexual intercourse. Surgery is usually performed between 2 and 4 years of age. Glandular hypospadias requires a glandular meatotomy. Coronal hypospadias requires a meatal advancement and glanduloplasty.

Proximal hypospadias without a chordee can be treated by a skin flap advancement. If a chordee is present it should be excised and an island flap urethroplasty performed. Complications of hypospadias surgery include a urethral fistula and stricture formation.

Neural tube defects

Embryology

The central nervous system develops from the dorsal ectoderm. The lateral edges of the neural plate fold to form the neural groove. Fusion of the edges of the neural groove generates the neural tube. Fusion starts cranially and progresses caudally. Both the caudal and cranial ends of the tube remain temporarily open. The anterior neuropore usually closes at about 25 days. The posterior neuropore usually closes at about 27 days.

Spina bifida

The term spina bifida covers a range of vertebral and neural tube defects. It results from failure of the posterior vertebral arch to fuse and most commonly occur in lumbo-sacral region (**Figure 19.5**).

Spina bifida occulta

Spina bifida occulta is the commonest form of spina bifida. Its true prevalence is unclear. Isolated laminar defects are seen on about 5% of lumbar spine x-rays. The spinal cord is usually normal. The only clinical sign is often a tuft of hairs or skin dimple at the site of the defect. Neurological deficit is rare. It may present with subtle neurological abnormalities such as enuresis or incontinence.

Meningocele and myelomeningocele

If the meninges bulge through vertebral defect, it results in either a meningocele or myelomeningocele. A meningocele does not contain spinal cord elements (**Figure 19.6**). A myelomeningocele contains the spinal cord and nerve routes and may be associated with caudal displacement of medulla and cerebellum. This can result in hydrocephalus (Arnold–Chiari malformation). It may also be associated with other congenital abnormalities.

Clinical features

A myelomeningocele occurs in 2–3 per 1000 live births. It can be detected prenatally by increased maternal serum α-fetoprotein. The spinal defect is clinically obvious and can result in various degrees of limb weakness, sensory loss, joint dislocation and contractures and urinary disorders. Of all patients with a myelomeningocele, one-third have complete paralysis and loss of sensation below the level of the defect, one-third have preservation of distal segments below the level of the defect and one-third have an incomplete lesion. About 90% of children develop urinary problems.

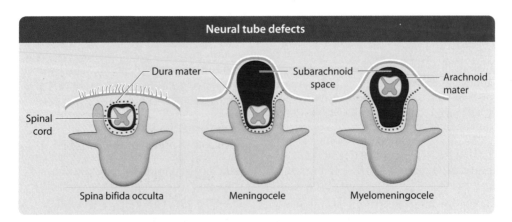

Figure 19.5 Neural tube defects

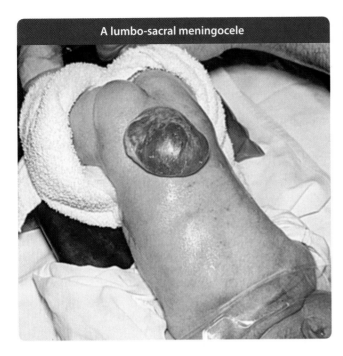

A lumbo-sacral meningocele

Figure 19.6 A lumbo-sacral meningocele

Management

Management is complicated and should involve a multidisciplinary team. The team should include a paediatrician, orthopaedic surgeon, neurologist and physiotherapists. Treatment depends on the level and severity of the defect. Patients with high defects and gross neurological defects many not be candidates for surgery. If the prognosis is good, the aim of treatment should be to achieve skin closure with 48 hours of birth. Ventriculo-caval shunting may be required in the first week. Early treatment of orthopaedic abnormalities is by physiotherapy. Surgical intervention (e.g. osteotomies) may be required in the first few years of life.

Common paediatric surgical disorders
Infantile hypertrophic pyloric stenosis

Infantile hypertrophic pyloric stenosis is often described as congenital hypertrophic pyloric stenosis but is not truly a congenital disorder. It results from hypertrophy and hyperplasia of pyloric sphincter in the neonatal period and mainly affects the circular muscle fibres. The pylorus becomes elongated and thickened, possibly due to failure of nitric oxide synthesis. It results in gastric outflow obstruction, vomiting and dehydration. It has a multifactorial inheritance with a strong genetic factor. It affects 3 per 1000 live births. The male:female ratio is 4:1. It is most common in first born males.

Clinical features

Infantile hypertrophic pyloric stenosis usually presents between 3 and 6 weeks of age but late presentation up to 6 months can occur. The main clinical feature is rapidly progressive projectile vomiting without bile. The child is usually hungry and often feeds immediately after vomiting. Dehydration and alkalosis are other clinical features. The clinical signs of dehydration include:

- Sunken eyes
- Depressed anterior fontanelle
- Reduced skin turgor
- Dry mucous membranes
- Increased capillary refill time
- Lethargy

A palpable 'tumour' in right upper quadrant of the abdomen is best felt from left during a test feed. Visible peristalsis is often seen.

Investigation

The diagnosis can be confirmed by abdominal ultrasound by assessment of the length, diameter and thickness of the pylorus. A wall thickness of great than 3 mm supports the diagnosis. Serum electrolytes and capillary gases should be measured. Biochemically a hypochloraemic alkalosis is usually present.

Management

Dehydration should be corrected over a 24 to 72 hour period prior to surgery. A nasogastric tube is often required. Ramstedt described his pyloromyotomy in 1911. The operation can be performed via either a transverse right upper quadrant or circumumbilical incision. A longitudinal incision should be made in the pylorus down to the mucosa. The incision should extend from the duodenum proximally on to the gastric antrum. Mucosal perforation should be avoided. Feeding is re-established within 12–24 hours of surgery. Recurrence rarely occurs. Complications are rare and mortality is negligible. Persistent postoperative vomiting may be due to delayed return of normal gastric motility, gastro-oesophageal reflux or an inadequate pyloromyotomy. The operation has been described using a laparoscopic approach but no clear benefit has been demonstrated over a circumumbilical approach.

Intussusception

Intussusception occurs when one part of the bowel invaginates (the intussusceptum) into an adjacent section (the intussuscipiens) resulting in intestinal obstruction and venous compression. If uncorrected, it can progress to arterial insufficiency and necrosis. It is the commonest abdominal emergency in infants between 3 months and 2 years. The peak incidence is 6 to 9 months. Most are idiopathic with the lead point due to enlarged Peyer's patches as a result of a viral infection. About 5% of cases are due to a polyp, Meckel's diverticulum, duplication cyst or tumour. The commonest site involved is the ileocaecal junction.

Clinical features

Intussusception usually presents with intermittent colicky abdominal pain and vomiting. Each episode classically last 1–2 minutes and recurs every 15–20 minutes. There may be the passage of blood, described as 'red currant jelly', per rectum. A sausage-shaped abdominal mass may be palpable.

Investigation

The diagnosis can be confirmed with water soluble contrast enema or ultrasound.

Management

Resuscitation with intravenous fluids and nasogastric tube is required. In the absence of peritonitis, reduction with air or contrast enema under radiological guidance can be attempted. If there is clinical evidence of peritonitis, shock or a failed reduction then surgery is required. The intussusception should be reduced. If there is necrosis of the bowel, then resection with primary anastomosis should be performed.

Necrotising enterocolitis

Necrotising enterocolitis affects about 1 per 1000 live births. The aetiology is unknown but bacterial infection and hypoxia appear to be important. It occurs in premature or low birth weight infants and is associated with premature rupture of membranes, prolonged labour and respiratory distress. It is also well recognised following umbilical artery catheterisation. It usually affects the terminal ileum and colon to a variable extent and is characterised by mucosal necrosis with progression to intestinal infarction and perforation.

Clinical features

Necrotising enterocolitis usually occurs in the first week of life. The child is lethargic and apathetic with vomiting and increasing abdominal distension. Bloody diarrhoea is a late feature. Abdominal examination may show peritonitis or a mass.

Investigation

An abdominal x-ray may show distended bowel with mucosal oedema, intramural gas (pneumatosis intestinalis) and portal venous or free intraperitoneal gas. The extent of pneumatosis is not proportional to the severity of the illness. The presence of pneumatosis per se is not an indication for surgical intervention. Portal venous gas is a poor prognostic sign.

Treatment

Initial treatment involves vigorous resuscitation and medical management. The placement of a nasogastric intubation and use of antibiotics are important. Parenteral nutrition should be considered. Indications for surgery include:

- Increasing peritonitis
- Failure of stabilisation with medical treatment
- Development of an abdominal mass
- Persistent loop or free gas on an abdominal x-ray

Surgical treatment will involve resection with possible primary anastomosis. Overall, the prognosis is poor. The mortality of those undergoing medical treatment is about 20%. The mortality of those coming to surgery is about 30%. Amongst survivors, about 30% develop ischaemic colonic strictures.

Abdominal masses in children

The identification of an abdominal mass in a child is a cause for concern because of the possibility of malignant disease.

Even benign conditions can be serious and warrant prompt evaluation and treatment. The assessment of a child with an abdominal mass involves a number of diagnostic considerations dependent on the age and sex of the patient, the location of the mass, and the presence or absence of other potentially related clinical features. The common causes of abdominal masses in children is shown **Table 19.3**.

Nephroblastoma

A nephroblastoma (Wilms' tumour) originates from the embryonal kidney. Pathologically, it contains renal tissue with various degrees of differentiation. It affects about 1 in 10,000 live births. Approximately, 60% present before the age of 3 years and 10% of tumours are bilateral. The presentation is with an:

- Abdominal mass (90%)
- Abdominal pain (20%)
- Haematuria (30%)

The diagnosis can be confirmed by an abdominal CT scan. About 40% of patients have metastatic spread at presentation but this does not prevent cure. Treatment is with nephrectomy and postoperative chemotherapy and radiotherapy. Stage 1 disease (localised to the kidney) has a 3-year survival of more than 80%. Stage 4 disease (haematogenous spread) has a 3-year survival less than 30%.

Neuroblastoma

Neuroblastomas arises from neural crest tissue, usually the adrenal medulla or

Common causes of abdominal masses in children			
Gastrointestinal	**Liver**	**Genitourinary**	**Other**
Congenital hypertrophic pyloric stenosis	Biliary atresia	Hydronephrosis	Neuroblastoma
	Choledochal cysts	Nephroblastoma	Splenomegaly
Crohn's disease	Hepatitis	Urethral valves	Retroperitoneal sarcoma
Intussusception	Hepatoblastoma		Teratoma
Constipation			

Table 19.3 Common causes of abdominal masses in children

sympathetic ganglia. They show a range of malignancy from benign ganglioneuroma to malignant neuroblastoma. They affects about 1 in 8000 live births and usually occur in first 5 years of life. Tumours in children are usually malignant. About 75% are abdominal and 25% arise in the thorax, pelvis or neck. Clinical presentation depends on the site of the tumour and the presence or absence of metastases. Bone and pulmonary metastases are relatively common. Symptoms are often due to metastatic spread and include:

- Pallor, weight loss, irritability (40%)
- Limb pain and hypertension (15%)
- Abdominal mass or pain (30%)

About 90% of patients have increased urinary VMA and HVA levels. A plain abdominal x-ray often shows diffused speckled calcification. The diagnosis can be confirmed by an abdominal CT scan. Treatment is with surgery and postoperative radiotherapy. Prognosis is best in children presenting before 2 years. Stage 1 disease (localised to kidney) has a 3-year survival of more than 90%. Stage 4 disease (haematogenous spread) has a 3-year survival less than 30%.

Choledochal cysts

Choledochal cysts are localised cystic dilatations of all or part of the common bile duct (**Figure 19.7**). About 80% of choledochal cysts present in childhood. There is a large regional variation in incidence. They are most commonly seen in Japan (1 in 1000 live births) and are relatively rare in Western Europe (1 in 100,000 live births). The male:female ratio is 1:4 and the aetiology is unknown.

Pathology

The cyst wall consists of fibrous tissue without muscle and the cyst may contain a large volume of bile. The cyst is often associated with distal common bile duct stenosis. If undiagnosed, the condition can progress to biliary fibrosis, cirrhosis and liver failure. Three types of choledochal cysts are described.

Clinical features

Choledochal cysts may be diagnosed prenatally on ultrasound. About 25% present in neonates with prolonged jaundice and cholestasis. The other 75% present later in childhood with the triad of abdominal pain, abdominal mass and intermittent jaundice. The differential diagnosis includes biliary atresia and neonatal hepatitis. Complications include:

- Recurrent cholangitis
- Hepatic fibrosis
- Biliary cirrhosis and portal hypertension
- Rupture with biliary peritonitis
- Pancreatitis

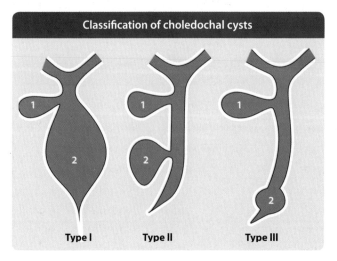

Figure 19.7 Classification of choledochal cysts. 1 = Gallbladder; 2 = Choledochal cyst.

Classification of choledochal cysts

Type I   Type II   Type III

- Hepatic abscess
- Gallstoness
- Carcinoma of the biliary tree

Investigation

An abdominal ultrasound usually reveals the cyst. Cysts can be further imaged by abdominal CT or ERCP. Radioisotope scanning may show delayed biliary excretion and accumulation of isotope within the cyst.

Management

Type I and II cysts should be resected and a hepaticojejunostomy performed. This prevents both an anastomotic stricture and malignancy in the cyst. Postoperative cholangitis is uncommon. Type III cysts should be treated by cholecystectomy and choledochojejunostomy or choledochoduodenostomy. If the diagnoses is made early, the liver fibrosis regresses and normal hepatic function can be expected. Prognosis is poor if the patient presents with advanced disease and portal hypertension.

Rectal bleeding in children

Most rectal bleeding in children is benign. However, is may signify a life-threatening disease. The likely aetiology can be determined by the patient's age and other associated clinical features (**Table 19.4**).

Anal fissures

Anal fissures can occur at any age. The child may be constipated and the fissure is often visible. They often settle with laxatives. Surgery is rarely required but the child may need a 'gentle' anal stretch.

Large bowel polyps

Large bowel polyps present with painless bleeding in an otherwise fit and well child. Juvenile polyps account for 80% of polyps in childhood and 70% of patients are less than 5 years old. Polyps are usually solitary and are often found in the rectum.

Infective enteritis

Infective enteritis can occur at any age. Causative agents include:

- Viruses – rotavirus, cytomegalovirus
- Bacteria – *Campylobacter, Shigella, Salmonella, Escherichia coli*
- Protozoa – *Amoeba, Giardia*

Fresh stool should be sent for microscopy, virology and culture.

Meckel's diverticulum

A Meckel's diverticulum is a remnant of vitello-intestinal duct, found in 2% of population. About 30% of diverticulae have heterotopic gastric mucosa that can result in ulceration and bleeding. It usually

Causes of rectal bleeding in children			
	Neonates	**Infants**	**Children**
Common	Anal fissure	Anal fissure	Anal fissure
	Necrotising enterocolitis	Intussusception	Juvenile polyp
	Viral gastroenteritis	Gastroenteritis	Meckel's diverticulum
Less common	Midgut volvulus	Meckel's diverticulum	Inflammatory bowel disease
	Intussusception	Upper GI haemorrhage	Intussusception
			Vascular malformations
			Solitary rectal ulcer
			Henoch–Schonlein purpura

Table 19.4 Causes of rectal bleeding in children

presents with painless rectal bleeding. It is best diagnosed with a radioisotope scan. Other complications include intussusception, small bowel obstruction, Meckel's diverticulitis or a gastrointestinal perforation.

Circumcision

A circumcision was first performed on Abraham at the age of 90 years! Several other references to circumcision exist in the Old Testament. It is also depicted on Egyptian tombs and murals. Each year 21,000 circumcisions are performed in the UK where 4% of boys will have had a circumcision by the age of 15 years. In Scandinavia, only 2% of boys are circumcised. Many operations are probably unnecessary.

At birth the prepuce is normally adherent to the glans penis. This produces a physiologically non-retractile foreskin. Only 4% of boys have a retractile foreskin at birth. By 5 years, in 90% of boys the foreskin will be retractile. Only 1% of boys have a true phimosis and 3% of boys have recurrent balanitis. Indications for circumcision are:

- Social and cultural
- Phimosis due to balanitis xerotica obliterans, lichen sclerosis or trauma
- Balanitis or posthitis
- Ballooning of foreskin
- Paraphimosis

Technique

All preputial adhesions should be freed. It is important to avoid excessive tension in order to preserve skin. To avoid injury to the glans, blind dissection of the foreskin is ill-advised. Sutures or bipolar diathermy should be used for haemostasis. Excessive numbers of skin sutures should be avoided. Complications are rare but include ulceration of the glans and urethral meatitis. About 1% need reoperation for bleeding or haematoma.

Neck lumps in children

Neck lumps are common in children but neoplasia is rare. Most head and neck lumps result from congenital or inflammatory processes. The position in either the anterior or posterior triangle of the neck my give an indication of the underlying pathology.

Neck lumps in the anterior triangle include:

- Lymphadenopathy – infective, neoplastic
- Thyroglossal cysts
- Dermoid cyst
- Goitre
- Branchial cyst

Neck lumps in the posterior triangle include:

- Lymph nodes
- Cystic hygroma
- Sternomastoid tumours
- Parotid swellings

Branchial remnants

Branchial cysts arise from the second branchial sinus and are found on the anterior border of sternomastoid. They are often bilateral and extend deep into the neck. An internal opening is occasionally found in the tonsillar fossa. Treatment is by surgical excision.

Cystic hygroma

A cystic hygroma is a hamartomatous lymphatic malformation resulting in a multi-cystic mass. About 60% are found in the neck region and they often present in early childhood as an expanding mass. They contain clear fluid and transilluminate brightly. Large lesions can be diagnosed prenatally and can result in obstructed labour. Surgical excision is difficult and can result in a poor cosmetic result. The use of sclerosants may be useful.

Sternomastoid tumours

A sternomastoid tumour is a mass in the middle third of the sternomastoid muscle. It results from muscle damage during labour and presents with a neck lump and torticollis away from the affected side. Treatment should involve physiotherapy to correct the torticollis. Surgery to remove the lump is rarely required.

Paediatric hernias

Inguinal hernias

An inguinal hernia is the commonest surgical condition encountered in Childhood. Approximately, 2.5% of children require an operation for a hernia. The incidence is increased in premature and low birth weight infants. The male:female ratio is 9:1. About 5% of newborn males have an inguinal hernia – 70% are right-sided and 5% are bilateral. Almost all are indirect hernias. Approximately 30% of hernias present within the first year of life and 15% present with incarceration or strangulation.

Embryology
The testis descends into the scrotum during the 7th month of gestation. It is preceded by the processus vaginalis – an outpouching of peritoneum. The processus normally begins to obliterate prior to birth and closure is normally complete during the first year of life. Persistence of all or part of the processus can result in an:

- Inguinal hernia
- Communicating hydrocele
- Hydrocele of the cord

Clinical features
Inguinal hernias usually present with an intermittent groin lump. In girls, the lump is in the upper part of the labia majora. Hernias can be difficult to detect in a quiet child but they increase in size with straining or crying. They may reach into the scrotum.

Management
Hernias presenting less than 1 year of age should be operated on as urgent elective cases. In the older child, the need for intervention is less pressing. Surgery can often be performed as a day case and inguinal herniotomy is the operation of choice. A transverse incision is made in the inguinal skin crease, Scarpa's fascia is divided and the external ring is identified. The sac is dissected off the cord and divided. Dissection is continued proximally until the peritoneal reflection is identified. The sac is then transfixed and excised. The wound is closed and the testis pulled back into the scrotum. About 20% of boys will develop a contralateral hernia at some stage in their life. Controversy exists as to whether contralateral exploration should be performed. Complications of herniotomy include:

- Wound infection
- Recurrence
- Vas injury
- Undescended testis
- Testicular atrophy

Irreducible hernias
The initial management of an irreducible hernia is to attempt reduction by taxis. It requires gentle pressure usually without sedation. Forcible reduction under general anaesthesia is contraindicated. If the hernia remains irreducible, then the child should be operated on within 24 hours.

Paediatric umbilical hernia
Paediatric umbilical hernias are present in about 10% of caucasian babies. They are seen in 90% of babies of Afro-Caribbean descent. The incidence is increased in low birth weight infants, Down's syndrome and Beckwith–Wiedemann syndrome. The hernia is usually symptomless and strangulation is extremely rare. About 95% close spontaneously by 2 years of age. Surgical repair need only be considered if the hernia persists beyond this age.

Undescended testes
The testis undergoes intra-abdominal descent up to 28 weeks gestation. It is normally found in the inguinal canal from 28 to 32 weeks and it would be expected to be found in the scrotum from about 30 weeks gestation.

Cryptorchidism is the presence of a testis in an abnormal position. In full-term infants, cryptorchidism is seen in 6% of boys. By 3 months, the incidence has fallen to 2%. A higher incidence of cryptorchidism is seen in premature infants. A 'normal' testis is scrotal or retractile testis. An 'abnormal' testis has never been seen low in the scrotum and can not be manipulated to that position. An undescended testis is found in the normal path of descent, in the inguinal canal or abdomen. A maldescended testis has exited via the superficial inguinal ring but is now in an ectopic position. The usual sites are the femoral triangle or perineum. In 80% of patients with cryptorchidism, the testis is palpable. About 90% of impalpable testes are either high in the inguinal canal or abdomen. True anorchidism is rare and is due to primary agenesis or neonatal torsion.

Cryptorchidism increases the risk of testicular tumours by ten-fold and 10% of patients with testicular tumours give a history of testicular maldescent. Cryptorchidism also increases the risk of infertility. Of patients with cryptorchidism, 30% have oligospermia and 10% azospermia.

Management

If the testis is palpable in the inguinal canal or high in scrotum, the patient requires an orchidopexy, scheduled for during the second year of life. It is usually performed via a 'groin and scrotum' incision and the testis is placed in a dartos pouch. Early orchidopexy may improve fertility but there is no evidence that it reduces the risk of malignancy.

If the testis is impalpable, laparoscopy is the best means of identifying an intra-abdominal testis, vas and vessels. If no vas, vessels or testis is present then there is primary agenesis. If vas and vessels are identified and no testis is seen, then neonatal testicular torsion must have occurred. If an intra-abdominal testis is identified, consideration needs to be given to a staged orchidopexy or microvascular transfer. If the vas and vessels are seen entering inguinal canal then the groin should be explored. A Fowler–Stephen's orchidopexy is a two-staged procedure. The gonadal vessels are divided at the first operation. This can be achieved laparoscopically. This encourages a collateral blood supply to develop via the cremasteric and vassal vessels. Six months later the testis is mobilised on these vessels and delivered through the abdominal wall into the scrotum, passing medial to the inferior epigastric vessels. Following an orchiopexy, the testis is often smaller and higher in the scrotum than normal testis. The testis may atrophy and retract to a higher position.

Orthopaedic disorders of infancy and childhood

Cerebral palsy

Cerebral palsy is a disorder of movement and posture due to a defect in the immature brain. The underlying brain pathology is non-progressive. It often presents at birth or in early childhood and is caused by birth trauma or asphyxia or disease or injury in early life. It is essentially a motor disorder that affects voluntary movements. It may also be associated with other deficits including blindness, sensory abnormalities, speech defects and learning difficulties.

Clinical features

The motor defects takes several forms in either isolation or combination and include:

- Spasticity
- Loss of coordination
- Rigidity
- Hypotonic muscles

Developmental milestones are often delayed and the paralysis can be variable in extent affecting:

- Arm and leg on one side – hemiparesis
- One limb – monoparesis
- Both legs – paraparesis
- All four limbs – quadriparesis

Spasticity is of an upper motor neurone type. The flexor muscles are often more spastic than the extensors. Tendon reflexes are exaggerated and stretch reflexes are abnormally sensitive. Deformities develop early due to muscle imbalance and several patterns are seen, including flexion of the elbow wrist and fingers and flexion and adduction of the hips.

Management

The clinical features are variable and complex and patients should be managed by a multidisciplinary team including:

- Paediatricians
- Orthopaedic surgeons
- Physiotherapists
- Psychologists
- Speech therapists
- Social workers

The mainstay of treatment is physiotherapy. Physiotherapy aims are to assist in assessment, prevent or attempt to correct musculo-skeletal deformity, train the child in posture and movement and provide suitable sensory stimulation.

Surgery

Surgery aims to correct any established deformity and involves the tendons, joint capsules, skin and bones. Muscle balance is restored and spasticity diminished by tendon lengthening, tendon transfers, partial denervation and splintage. Surgery is most valuable in the lower limb and the timing of surgery is important.

Hip disorders

Accurate diagnosis and treatment of paediatric hip disorders is important because of the potential for complications, which may lead to degenerative joint disease in adult life. Different disorders have a propensity to occur at different ages (**Table 19.5**).

Development dysplasia of the hip

This condition is often described as congenital dislocation. Developmental dysplasia of the hip is a more accurate term as common features include dysplasia of the acetabulum and femoral neck anteversion. The apparent incidence of developmental dysplasia depends on the age of the child. Approximately 20 per 1000 neonates have clinical evidence of hip instability but only 1 per 1000 have evidence of hip dislocation at 3 months.

Pathophysiology

The acetabulum develops from a triradiate cartilage and three ossification centres. Normal growth is dependent on apposition within the acetabulum and requires the presence of a normal femoral head. The female:male ratio is 5:1. Ligamentous laxity may be an important aetiological factor. Other important factors include:

- Family history
- Breech presentation
- Foot deformity
- Torticollis
- Neuromuscular disorders
- Skeletal dysplasias

Clinical features

Developmental dysplasia of the hip can present as:

- A neonate with hip instability
- An infant with limited hip abduction
- A toddler with a limp
- An adult with degenerative hip changes

All neonates should be screened for hip instability. The hips are flexed to 90° and instability detected by reduction of the dislocation by abduction and forward pressure (Ortolani's test) and dislocation of the hip by adduction and backward pressure (Barlow's test). Examination may also show limb shortening, an extra thigh skin crease and hip external rotation. At an older age, Galeazzi's sign may be elicited. It is a sign of unilateral hip displacement. The child is supine with hips and knees flexed and one

Diagnostic calendar of hip disorders	
Age at onset (years)	**Probable diagnoses**
Birth	Developmental dysplasia
0–5	Perthe's disease
	Late presentation of developmental dysplasia
	Irritable hip
5–10	Perthe's disease
	Irritable hip
10–15	Slipped upper femoral epiphysis
	Infection
	Rheumatoid arthritis

Table 19.5 Diagnostic calendar of hip disorders

leg is shown to be shorter than the other. It is important to be aware that bilateral hip dislocation can be difficult to demonstrate.

Investigation

Hip ultrasound is useful, but with a high sensitivity, can result in significant over diagnosis. Plain x-rays are unreliable until the child reaches 3 months of age. A hip x-ray will show a shallow acetabulum with an underdeveloped femoral head.

Management

The aims of treatment are to reduce the dislocation by traction or open reduction and to maintain reduction by a harness, cast, soft tissue release or osteotomy. The ultimate aim is to achieve stable congruant reduction without damaging the growth plate. The above aims can be achieved by:

- Pavlick hip harness or Von Rosen splint in a neonate
- Traction in an infant
- Open reduction, osteotomy or acetabuloplasty in an older child

Irritable hip

Causes of an 'irritable hip' in a child include:

- Perthe's disease
- Slipped upper femoral epiphysis
- Juvenile chronic arthritis
- Septic arthritis
- Osteomyelitis
- Rheumatic fever

Perthe's disease

Perthe's disease is a childhood osteochondrosis of the hip that occurs secondary to avascular necrosis of the capital femoral epiphysis. It is a self-limiting disorder with revascularisation occurring within 2 to 4 years. The femoral head may however remain deformed resulting in osteoarthritis. Four stages of the disease are recognised:

- Stage 1 – Avascular necrosis
- Stage 2 – Fragmentation of the femoral epiphysis
- Stage 3 – Regeneration and revascularisation
- Stage 4 – Healing

Clinical features

The median age of onset is 6 years and the male:female ratio is approximately 4:1. The patient presents with hip pain and a limp. Examination will show reduced movement, especially abduction and internal rotation. About 10% of patients have a fixed deformity.

Investigation

A hip x-ray will show the capital femoral epiphysis to be smaller, denser and flattened. The medial joint space is increased and the ossific nucleus is fragmented. If performed, a bone scan will show a 'cold' femoral epiphysis.

Management

The aims of treatment are to prevent deformation of the femoral head and prevent osteoarthritis. This can be achieved by a period of bed rest and reduced weight bearing. Surgical containment can be achieved by a subtrochanteric or innominate osteotomy.

Slipped upper femoral epiphysis

A slipped upper femoral epiphysis is the commonest significant hip disorder of adolescence. The femoral head 'slips' posteriorly and into varus. It tends to occur in the obese and skeletally immature child. It is a progressive disorder and therefore early diagnosis is essential. The male:female ratio is 3:1 and approximately 20% of cases are bilateral. About 5% of patients have a family history.

Clinical features

Slipped upper femoral epiphysis usually presents with a gradual onset of hip or knee pain. The initial clinical features can be minimal and the diagnosis is often missed. It occasionally presents with sudden onset of pain after exercise. Examination shows an antalgic gait. The hip initially may have a full range of movement. A severe slip results in fixed external rotation.

Investigation

A radiological diagnosis can be difficult. A 'frog lateral' radiograph is probably best at demonstrating the slipped epiphysis.

Treatment

The aims of treatment are to preserve the blood supply to the femoral head, stabilise the physis and prevent avascular necrosis and chondrolysis. This is usually achieved by in situ pinning of the epiphysis. Occasionally a reconstructive subtrochanteric osteotomy is required.

Scoliosis

A scoliosis is an apparent lateral curvature of the spine. It is a triplanar deformity with lateral, anteroposterior and rotational components. A postural scoliosis is secondary to pathology away from the spine (e.g. short leg or pelvic tilt) and the curvature disappears when patient sits down. A structural scoliosis is a non-correctable deformity. Vertebral rotation results in spinal processes swinging to the concavity of curve and secondary changes occur to counterbalance the primary deformity. Most cases of structural scoliosis are idiopathic but it can also result from bone, neurological or muscular disease.

Clinical features

A scoliosis shows a typical deformity with a 'skew back' and 'rib hump'. The hip normally protrudes on the concave side. The scapula normally protrudes on the convex side. The level and direction of the major curve convexity should be noted. Convexity of curvatures determines the nomenclature of the lesion (e.g. a right thoracic scoliosis has the thoracic spine convex to the right). A balanced deformity keeps the occiput in midline. A fixed scoliosis become more obvious on flexion. The younger the child and the greater the curvature, the worse the prognosis.

Investigation

Full length posterior–anterior and lateral films of the spine are required. The upper and lower ends of the spinal curve can be identified and the angle of curvature (Cobb's angle) can be measured either directly or geometrically (**Figure 19.8**). A lateral bending view can assess the degree of correctability. Assessment of the degree of skeletal maturity is important as a scoliosis can progress during skeletal growth.

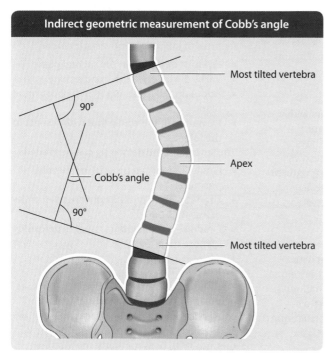

Indirect geometric measurement of Cobb's angle

- 90°
- Most tilted vertebra
- Cobb's angle
- Apex
- 90°
- Most tilted vertebra

Figure 19.8 Indirect geometric measurement of Cobb's angle

Idiopathic scoliosis

Approximately 80% of scoliosies are idiopathic. Patients often have a family history. Many patients have a trivial curvature and only about 0.2% of the population have a scoliosis with greater than 30° of curvature. The age of onset defines three groups as adolescent, juvenile and infantile.

Adolescent idiopathic scoliosis

Adolescent idiopathic scoliosis occurs with an onset older than 10 years. About 90% of patients are female and progression is not inevitable. With a curvature of less than 20°, spontaneous resolution can occur. Predictors of progression include young age, marked curvature and skeletal immaturity. The main aim of treatment is to prevent mild deformity becoming severe. If there is mild scoliosis with progression, consideration should be given to the use of a brace. If there is greater than 30° of curvature and progression occurs, then operative intervention may be required. Harrington rods are used to reduce the rotational deformity and lateral curvature.

Juvenile idiopathic scoliosis

Juvenile idiopathic scoliosis occurs with an onset between 4 and 9 years. It is a relatively uncommon condition. The prognosis is worse than in the adolescent group. Spinal fusion may be necessary before puberty.

Infantile idiopathic scoliosis

Infantile idiopathic scoliosis occurs with an onset less than 3 years. It is a rare condition and 60% of patients are boys. In 90% of patients, the deformity resolves spontaneously. In those in whom progression occurs the curvature can be severe. It is associated with a high incidence of cardiopulmonary dysfunction.

Osteopathic scoliosis

Osteopathic scoliosis is associated with hemivertebrae, wedged and fused vertebrae. The overlying tissue often shows angiomas, naevi and skin dimples. The degree of scoliosis is usually mild. Before considering surgery it is necessary to exclude a meningomyelocele.

Neuropathic/myopathic scoliosis

Neuropathic/myopathic scoliosis is associated with polio, cerebral palsy and muscular dystrophy. The scoliosis is typically long and convex towards of muscle weakness. X-rays with traction will assess the degree of correctability.

Clubfoot

Clubfoot or congenital talipes equinovarus is the commonest congenital ankle deformity in the UK. It affects about 3 per 1000 live births and the male:female ratio is 3:1. About 40% of cases are bilateral. There is a low incidence in far east Asians and Polynesians and high incidence in black South Africans. Genetic factors seem to important in its aetiology but most cases are idiopathic. It is occasionally associated with neuromuscular disorders. Aetiological factors include:

- Developmental arrest or delay
- Intrauterine moulding
- Retracting fibrosis
- Neuromuscular factors

Clinical features

Many cases are diagnosed with prenatal ultrasound but ultrasound can not assess the severity of the condition. The anatomical features of talipes equinovarus include:

- Equinus deviation in the sagittal plane
- Varus deviation in the frontal plane
- Adduction of the forefoot in the horizontal plane
- Deviation of the whole foot with respect to the talus

The severity of the deformity can be graded:

- Grade 1 – foot can be held in neutral position
- Grade 2 – fixed equinus or varus deformity of less then 20°
- Grade 3 – fixed equinus or varus deformity of more than 20°

Management

Treatment should begin within the first week of life. Initial management should be with conservative therapy involving manipulation and serial casting and continuous physical therapy. With both methods, the forefoot adduction and cavus deformity, then the whole foot varus deformity and finally the equinus deformity are addressed, in that order. False correction of the deformity can occur leading to a 'rocker-bottom foot'.

Surgery

Surgery is required in 10%, 50% and 90% of patients with Grade 1, 2 and 3 deformity, respectively. By 3 months of age, it is usually clear whether conservative management will be effective. The timing of surgery is controversial. Most surgeons recommend surgery between 9 and 12 months of age. Plaster can then be removed at the time the child begins to walk. The aim of surgery is release all the tight structures and lengthen muscles.

Structures that may need to be divided include the:

- Plantar fascia
- Tendon sheaths of tibialis posterior, flexor hallucis longus, flexor digitorum longus
- Posterior part of deltoid ligament
- Posterior part of ankle joint and subtalar joint capsules
- Fibulocalcaneal and fibulotalar ligaments
- Peroneal tendon sheaths
- Talonavicular joint capsule

Tendons that may require lengthening include:

- Achilles tendon
- Tendon of flexor digitorum longus
- Tendon of flexor hallucis longus
- Tendon tibialis posterior

Percutaneous wires may be need to maintain correction and the foot is kept in plaster for about 6 weeks. Following plaster removal, a splint is required until the child is walking normally. Late problems following surgery include dynamic forefoot adduction and varus, recurrent deformity and overcorrection. Most children undergoing surgery achieve a plantigrade foot and most can wear normal shoes.

Chapter 20

Plastic and reconstructive surgery

Applied basic sciences

Anatomy of the skin

The skin consists of three major layers:

- Epidermis – outer superficial layer
- Dermis – middle layer
- Hypodermis – deepest layer

The epidermis

The epidermis is composed of keratinised stratified squamous epithelium and is made up of four distinct cell types and five layers. The cells of the epidermis are:

- Keratinocytes – produce keratin
- Melanocytes – produce melanin
- Langerhans' cells – epidermal macrophages
- Merkel cells – touch receptors in association with sensory nerve endings

The layers of the epidermis are:

- Stratum basale (basal layer)
- Stratum spinosum (prickly layer)
- Stratum granulosum (granular layer)
- Stratum lucidium (clear layer)
- Stratum corneum (horny layer)

The dermis

The dermis is the second major skin layer containing strong, flexible connective tissue including fibroblasts, macrophages, mast cells and white blood cells. It is composed of two layers called the papillary and reticular dermis. The papillary dermis is areolar connective tissue with collagen and elastic fibres. Its superficial surface contains peg-like projections called dermal papillae. The dermal papillae contain capillary loops, Meissner's corpuscles and free nerve endings. The reticular dermis and accounts for approximately 80% of the thickness of the skin. Collagen fibres in this layer add strength and resilience to the skin. Elastin fibres provide stretch and recoil properties.

The hypodermis

The hypodermis is the subcutaneous layer deep to the skin composed of adipose and areolar connective tissue.

Sweat glands

Sweat glands are found all over the body. They have different functions at different sites. Eccrine sweat glands are found in the palms of the hand, soles of the feet and forehead. Apocrine sweat glands are found in axillary and anogenital areas. Ceruminous glands are modified apocrine glands in external ear canal and secrete cerumen. The mammary glands are specialised sweat glands that secrete milk.

Functions of skin

The functions of the skin include:

- Protection – chemical, physical and mechanical barrier
- Temperature regulation
- Cutaneous sensation – receptors sense touch and pain
- Metabolic functions – synthesis of vitamin D
- Blood reservoir – skin blood vessels store up to 5% of the body's blood volume
- Excretion – limited amounts of nitrogenous wastes are eliminated in sweat

Inflammation

Inflammation is a dynamic process that occurs in response to tissue injury. The causes of inflammation include:

- Physical injury
- Chemical injury
- Infection
- Immunological disorders

Inflammation can be acute or chronic and different mechanisms are involved in the two processes. The clinical signs of acute inflammation are:

- Redness – rubor
- Heat – calor
- Swelling – tumour
- Pain – dolor
- Loss of function

Acute inflammation

The clinical features of acute inflammation can be explained by changes at the microscopic level. Three processes are seen in acute inflammation:

- Hyperaemia
- Exudation
- Migration of leukocytes

Hyperaemia is associated with a vascular response. Following injury, initial vasoconstriction occurs followed by arteriolar dilatation This occurs in response to direct vascular injury, chemical mediators causing vasodilatation and an autonomic neurological response. This explains the redness and heat that occurs during acute inflammation. Exudation is the passage of protein rich fluid into the interstitial tissue resulting in protective antibodies entering the damaged tissue. It occurs as a result of increases capillary permeability and increased capillary pressure. This explains the swelling that occurs during acute inflammation. Increased blood viscosity reduces capillary blood flow. The loss of axial stream results in margination of polymorphs which adhere to the endothelium. These then pass between endothelial cells into interstitium with the process facilitated by chemotaxis.

Sequels of acute inflammation

There are four possible outcomes of acute inflammation:

- Resolution
- Suppuration
- Repair and organisation
- Chronic inflammation

Resolution is the restoration of normal conditions and occurs if there is minimal cell death and tissue damage, rapid elimination of the causal agent and local conditions favour removal of fluid and debris. Suppuration is the formation of pus formed by the inflammatory exudate, polymorphs and cell fragments. If pus accumulates an abscess may form. Organisation occurs when during the acute inflammatory process there is excessive exudation or necrosis. Local conditions prevent removal of exudate or debris. New vessel formation occurs and macrophage and fibroblast proliferation results in fibrosis.

Chronic inflammation

Chronic inflammation occurs if the causal agent is not removed. The cell population in the damaged tissue changes. Polymorphs are replaced by lymphocytes and plasma cells. Macrophages may form giant cells. New capillaries are formed. Fibroblasts deposit collagen resulting in fibrosis. Chronic inflammation can be primary with no prior acute inflammatory response. This occurs in tuberculosis and sarcoidosis and is characterised by the formation of granulomas.

Wound healing

The four main stages of wound healing are:

- Haemostasis
- Inflammation
- Regeneration
- Repair

These stages are not discrete but overlap.

Haemostasis

Damaged endothelium exposes platelets to sub-endothelial collagen and releases von Willebrand factor and tissue thromboplastin. von Willebrand factor facilitates platelet adhesion to sub-endothelial collagen which release ADP and thromboxane A2. This leads to further platelet aggregation. Tissue thromboplastin activates the coagulation pathways. Fibrin is the end product of the coagulation pathways which forms a plug in which platelets and red blood cells are trapped. This results in clot formation.

Inflammation

Platelets release platelet derived growth factor (PDGF) and transformation growth factor β (TGFβ). These are chemotactic to neutrophils and monocytes. Neutrophils and macrophages migrate to the site of injury and phagocytose foreign material and bacteria.

Regeneration and repair

PDGF and TGFβ are also mitogenic to epithelial cells and fibroblasts. This leads to proliferation of epithelial cells and fibroblasts. Fibroblasts produce collagen. Vascular endothelial growth factor is also mitogenic to endothelial cells. It is released by monocytes in response to hypoxia and promotes angiogenesis. Wound strength by the end of the 1st week is 10% of the original. By the end of 3rd month it reaches 70% and thereafter plateaus.

Time line of events

Within the first 24 hours of injury, neutrophils are the predominant cell type. This is the phase of acute inflammation. Epithelial cells start proliferating and migrating into the wound cavity. By the 2nd and 3rd day, macrophage and fibroblasts are the dominant cell types. Epithelial cell proliferation and migration continues. Angiogenesis begins and granulation tissue starts to appear. Collagen fibres are present but these are vertical. They do not bridge the wound gap. By the end of 5th day, fibroblasts are the predominant cell type. They synthesise collagen. Collagen now bridges the wound edges – bridging collagen. Epidermal cells continue to divide and the epidermis is now multi-layered. Abundant granulation tissue is present. During the 2nd week acute inflammation begins to reduce and collagen continues to accumulate.

Aberrations in wound healing

Keloid scar

A keloid is an overgrowth of scar tissue (**Figure 20.1**). The scar tissue extends beyond the wound margin. It is more common in coloured races and is uncommon in children. Typical sites are the sternum, back and ear lobes. Triamcinolone injections directly into the tissue is the initial treatment. Other options include excision of the overgrowth but following surgery keloid scars tend to recur.

Hypertrophic scar

Hypertrophy is overgrowth of scar tissue but it does not extend beyond wound edge. It can an occur in any race. It is more common in

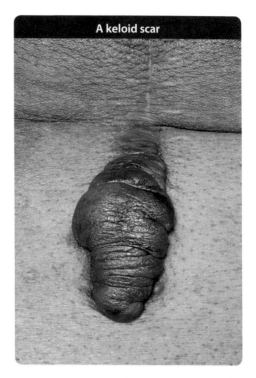
A keloid scar

Figure 20.1 A keloid scar

children. It usually subsides with time and may even regress. It is more common over flexor surfaces and after burns.

Plastic surgery trauma
Burns

Pathophysiology

A burn is defined as coagulative destruction of the skin or mucous membrane caused by heat, chemical or irradiation. Thermal damage occurs to the skin when the temperature is above 48°C. The extent of necrosis is related to both the temperature and duration of contact. Burns can result in:

- Increased capillary permeability and fluid loss
- Hypovolaemia and shock
- Increased plasma viscosity and microthrombosis formation
- Haemoglobinuria and renal damage
- Increased metabolic rate and energy metabolism

The ability of the skin to repair depends on the depth of the burn. Burns can be classified as:

- Superficial burns
- Partial thickness burns
- Full-thickness burns

Superficial burns

Superficial burns need to be differentiated from simple skin erythema. In a superficial burn, only the epidermis and papillae are involved. This results in red serum-filled blisters. The skin blanches on pressure. The burn is painful and sensitive. Healing occurs in about 10 days without scarring.

Partial-thickness burns

In partial-thickness burn, the epidermis is lost with varying degrees of dermis. The burn is usually coloured pink and white and may or may not blanche on pressure. Variable degrees of reduced sensation may be present. Epithelial cells are present in hair follicles and sweat glands resulting in regeneration and spread. Healing occurs in about 14 days. Some depigmentation of the scar may occur. A partial-thickness burn requires skin grafting.

Full-thickness burns

In a full-thickness burn, both the epidermis and dermis are destroyed. The burn appears white and does not blanche. Sensation is absent and without grafting healing occurs from the edge of the wound.

Assessment

Initial assessment of a patient with burns should be with ATLS principles. Good early management is required to prevent morbidity or mortality. In the airways assessment it is important to look for signs of inhalation injury including facial burns and soot in nostrils or sputum. When assessing breathing, there needs to be an awareness of carbon monoxide poisoning. The patient may appear 'pink' with a normal pulse oximeter reading. The fluid loss from a burn is significant and can result in hypovolaemic shock and acute renal failure.

Assessment of the extent of the burn needs an accurate measurement of the percentage of body surface area (BSA) involved. This can be calculated from either a Lund and Browder Chart or by the Wallace 'Rule of Nines' (**Table 20.1**). Also, the surface area covered by the patient's hand with fingers closed is about 1% the BSA. In a child, the body proportions are different. The head is relatively larger (19% vs. 9%) and each lower limb relative smaller (13% vs. 18%). The other body proportions are similar to adults.

Fluid replacement

Patients with extensive burns require significant fluid resuscitation. To assess fluid replacement it is necessary to know:

- Time of injury
- Patient's weight
- Percentage BSA involved

Intravenous fluid replacement needs to be given for burns affecting more than 10% BSA in a child and 15% BSA in adult. Many formulas have been devised to estimate the fluid requirement. The most widely used are the Muir and Barclay formula and the Parkland formula.

The Muir and Barclay formula provides the volume (in mL) of colloid to be given in the first 4 hours. This volume should be repeated every 4 hours for the first 12 hours, every 6 hours between 12 and 24 hours and once between 24 and 36 hours.

$$Weight\ (kg) \times \% \ BSA\big/_2 \text{ per period}$$

The ATLS formula gives the total volume (in mL) to be infused in the first 24 hours. Half

The Wallace 'Rule of Nines'	
Body area	**Percentage (%)**
Head	9
Each upper limb	9
Each lower limb	18
Front of trunk	18
Back of trunk	18
Perineum	1

Table 20.1 The Wallace 'Rule of Nines'

the volume should be given in the first 8 hours.

$$Weight\ (Kg) \times \%\ BSA \times 4$$

Metabolic water should be given in addition to resuscitation fluid. In the adult, this amounts to about 2 litres of 5% dextrose. In a child this amounts to 100 mL/Kg for the first 10 kg and 50 mL/Kg for each subsequent Kg of body weight.

The patient should be monitored to assess the adequacy of resuscitation by:

- Clinical assessment
- Vital signs – pulse, blood pressure
- Urine output (>50 mL/ hour in adult)
- Haematocrit (aim for 0.35)

Criteria for referral to burns unit
Patients should be referred to a burns unit if:

- Greater than 10% BSA in a child
- Greater than 15% BSA in an adult
- Inhalation injuries
- Burns involving the airway
- Electrical burns
- Chemical burns
- Specials areas – eyes, face, hand, perineum

Escharotomy
Deep circumferential burns of the torso can impair respiration. In a limb, they can impair the distal circulation. In both situations, escharotomies should be considered. No anaesthetic is required. The burn should be incised into subcutaneous fat and release of the underlying soft tissue should be ensured. On the chest wall, escharotomies should be performed bilaterally in the anterior axillary lines. Bleeding may be significant and a blood transfusion may be required.

Respiratory burns
Smoke inhalations should be suspected if there is:

- Explosion in an enclosed environment
- Flame burns to the face
- Soot in mouth or nostrils
- Hoarseness or stridor

Intubation may be required. Blood carboxyhaemoglobin levels can give an indication of the extent of lung injury.

Electrical burns
Most electrical burns are flash burns and are superficial. They do not occur by electrical conduction. A flash from an electrical burn can reach 4000°C. Low-tension burns are usually small but full thickness. High-tension burns usually have an entry and exit wound. The current passes along the path of least resistance (e.g. blood vessels, fascia, muscle) and the extent of tissue destruction can often be underestimated. High-tension burns can be associated with cardiac arrhythmias. Myonecrosis and myoglobinuria can also occur.

Chemical burns
The commonest acids involved in chemical burns are hydrochloric, hydrofluoric and sulphuric. Acid burns may penetrate deeply down to bone. First aid treatment involves liberal irrigation with running water. Calcium gluconate may be useful in hydrofluoric acid burns. The commonest alkalis involved in chemical burns are sodium hydroxide and cement and these also can cause deep-dermal or full-thickness burns.

Skin grafts
A skin graft is an autograft from one part of the body to another and can be partial or full thickness depending on the amount of dermis taken.

Partial-thickness skin grafts
Partial-thickness skin grafts contains epidermis and the superficial part of dermis. It is usually taken from the donor site with a dermatome or Humby knife. The donor site epithelium grows back from sweat glands and hair follicles. Grafts can be 'meshed' to increase the area that can be covered. Excess skin can be stored in a fridge and reused for up to 3 weeks. Partial-thickness grafts can not be used on infected wounds and are not suitable for covering bone, tendon or cartilage. The cosmetic result is often poor (**Figure 20.2**).

Full-thickness skin grafts
Full-thickness skin grafts contains epidermis and all of the dermis. They can only be used

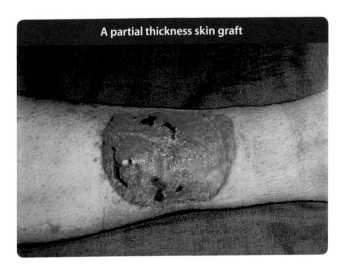

A partial thickness skin graft

Figure 20.2 A partial thickness skin graft

to cover small defects. Good cosmetic results can be obtained. The donor site needs to be closed with primary suture or a partial thickness graft. Common donor sites include the postauricular skin and supraclavicular fossa.

Skin flaps

Skin flaps are classified according to their blood supply.

Random pattern grafts

A random pattern graft receives its blood supply from a segmental anastomotic or axial artery. Examples include advancement (**Figure 20.3**) and rotation flaps (**Figure 20.4**).

Axial pattern grafts

An axial pattern graft receives its blood supply from a direct cutaneous arteries. Examples include:

- Iliofemoral island flap supplied by the superficial circumflex iliac artery
- Lateral forehead flap supplied the superficial temporal artery
- Deltopectoral island flap supplied by perforating branches of internal mammary artery

Survival of all flaps depends on it receiving an adequate blood supply. This depends on the length of flap in relationship to its base. The blood supply can be improved by

the use of 'delaying' techniques. The flap is partially raised and replaced prior to use. This encourages the flap to increase its blood supply through the pedicle.

Tube pedicle grafts

Tube pedicle grafts are frequently raised from the abdomen or inner arm. Parallel skin incisions allow a tube of skin to be formed. The skin defect is then closed. The length of the tube should not be greater than twice the base and the long axis of the tube should parallel to the direction of the cutaneous blood vessels. It is a good means of delaying tissue transfer over a long distance and can produce a good cosmetic result.

Myocutaneous flaps

In most parts of the body, the skin receives its blood supply from the underlying muscle. The muscle, fascia and overlying skin can therefore be moved as one unit and they survive on the major blood vessel supplying the muscle. Examples include:

- Latissimus dorsi flap supplied by the thoracodoral artery
- Transverse rectus abdominis supplied by the superior epigastric artery

Myocutaneous flaps allow tissue transfer to poorly vascularised areas. Bone can also be transferred for osseous reconstruction. Flaps usually have no sensation.

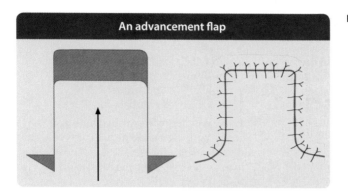

Figure 20.3 An advancement flap

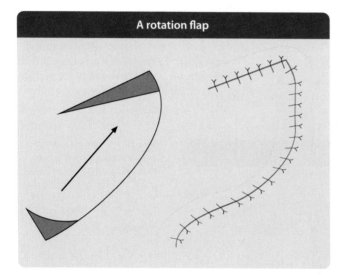

Figure 20.4 A rotation flap

Free myocutaneous flaps

Microvascular techniques allow the anastomosis of arteries and veins. Myocutaneous flaps can therefore be detached from their blood supply and can be transferred to other parts of body. Examples, include the free transverse rectus abdominis flap.

Tissue expansion

Skin can be gradually stretched to accommodate a greater area. If skin loss is anticipated, it is possible to expand adjacent skin prior to surgery. Tissue expanders can be placed subcutaneously in collapsed state. Over several weeks they can be inflated with saline through a subcutaneous port. Expanded skin can then be used to cover the defect and the tissue expander removed.

Hand tendon injuries

Hand flexor and extensor tendon injuries are common. Flexor tendon injuries are often associated with neurovascular damage. Extensor tendon injuries are often associated with articular damage. Hand injuries require careful assessment and management. Assessment should be based on knowledge of tendon anatomy. Accurate surgical repair requires meticulous surgical technique. If poorly managed, tendon injuries can lead to significant functional disability.

Anatomy of hand tendons

The flexor tendons of the hand run in fibro-osseous canals. The flexor digitorum superficialis inserts into the middle phalanx. The flexor digitorum profundus inserts into the distal phalanx. The metacarpal bones and phalanges form the dorsal wall. Synovial sheaths form the volar and lateral walls. The synovial sheath for the index to ring finger begins at the neck of the metacarpals. The synovial sheath of the little finger is continuous with the ulna bursa. Extensor tendons are extra-synovial, except at the wrist. They are surrounded by extensive paratenon with segmental arterial input. The extensor retinaculum prevents bowstringing of the extensors. The main action is extension of the metacarpophalangeal (MCP) joints.

Zones of injury

Flexor tendons are divided into five zones (**Figure 20.5**). Zone 1 is distal and Zone 5 is proximal. The five zones are:

1. Distal to the insertion of flexor digitorum superficialis
2. From insertion of flexor digitorum superficialis to the proximal edge of the A1 pulley
3. From the proximal edge of the A1 pulley to the distal edge of the carpal tunnel
4. Within the carpal tunnel
5. Proximal to the carpal tunnel

Extensor tendons are divided into eight zones. Zones 1, 3 and 5 lie over the distal interphalangeal (DIP), proximal interphalangeal (PIP) and MCP joints respectively.

Flexor tendon injuries

Assessment

An accurate history is essential. It is important to know the handedness of the patient and his or her occupation. Observation of the hand at rest may indicate which tendons are involved.

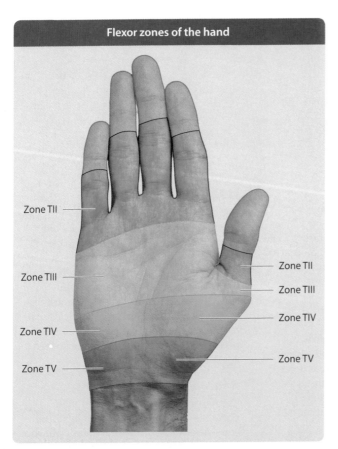

Flexor zones of the hand

Zone TII

Zone TIII

Zone TIV

Zone TV

Zone TII

Zone TIII

Zone TIV

Zone TV

Figure 20.5 Flexor zones of the hand. (Reproduced courtesy of Sam Scott-Hunter, London.)

The level of tendon injury may corresponds to the site of any laceration – but not always. If both flexor tendons are divided the finger will be extended. If the profundus tendon alone is divided then only the DIP joint will be extended. Further assessment should involve testing of individual tendons of flexor digitorum superficialis and flexor digitorum profundus. Neurovascular assessment is also required.

Management

Early exploration and repair is required and ideally surgery should be performed within 24 hours of injury. Primary repair is the gold standard but may not be possible if there has been delayed presentation or if the tendons have retracted. Antibiotic prophylaxis is required if presentation has been delayed or there is wound contamination. The ideal tendon repair requires:

- Sutures easily placed in the tendon
- Secure suture knots
- Smooth junction of the tendon ends
- Minimal gapping at the repair site
- Minimal interference with tendon vascularity
- Sufficient repair strength

Many techniques of tendon repair have been described. They invariably involve a core suture and epitendinous suture. For Zone 1 injuries, direct repair is usually possible. A periosteal flap can be raised and the tendon anchored with a core suture. For Zone 2 to 5 injuries, wounds should be excised and irrigated. They may need to be extended to retrieve and repair tendons. Incisions should be avoided that cross skin creases. Careful planning of incisions is required to prevent skin necrosis or contracture. Incisions may be required in tendon sheaths between the main pulleys. The neurovascular bundles should be identified and repaired is necessary. Tendons should be repaired using a standard technique.

Postoperative management

After repair, the hand should be placed in a back-slab with the wrist at 0–30° of flexion, the MCP joints at 60–90° of flexion and the PIP and DIP joints in full extension. The hand should be elevated to reduce swelling. Early mobilisation is required to reduce adhesion formation and improve tendon healing and the final functional outcome. This requires close supervision by a hand physiotherapist. Mobilisation can begin as early as the first postoperative day. Passive extension should be avoided.

Extensor tendon injuries

For extensor tendon injuries, open exploration and repair is required. They can often be repaired under local anaesthetic. Management depends on the zone of the injury. Proximal injuries require immobilisation with the wrist extended and the MCP joint flexed. Active movement can begin after 3 weeks. Distal injuries require longer periods of immobilisation.

Pigmented skin lesions
Malignant melanoma

Epidemiology

Malignant melanoma is a tumour of epidermal melanocytes. It accounts for less than 5% of skin cancers but more than 75% of skin-cancer related deaths. The incidence of melanoma is doubling every 10 years, especially in sunny climates. Approximately 40 and 4 cases per 100,000 population are seen each year in Queensland, Australia and the UK, respectively. In the UK it accounts for about 1000 deaths. Patient education is increasing the number of thin tumours detected but the number of thick tumours detected remains constant. It is the commonest cancer seen in 20 to 40-year-olds and is more common in women. Risk factors include:

- Giant melanocytic naevus
- Total number of naevi
- Dysplastic naevus syndrome
- History of recurrent sunburn
- Skin type
- Family history

Pathology

About 20% of melanomas arise in pre-existing naevi. Tumours have an initial radial and followed by a vertical growth phase. These determine the growth characteristics of the tumour. Malignant melanomas are classified as:

- Superficial spreading (65%)
- Nodular (20%)
- Lentigo maligna
- Acral lentiginous

Superficial spreading melanoma occurs in middle age (**Figure 20.6**). The female:male ratio is 2:1. The commonest sites are the lower leg in women and trunk in man. Nodular melanomas are a more aggressive tumour that occur in a younger age group (**Figure 20.7**). They have an early vertical growth phase. Lentigo maligna melanomas are the least malignant form and are usually found on the face of the elderly. They have a long radial growth phase. Acral lentiginous melanomas are an aggressive tumour. They are the commonest form seen in Afro-Caribbeans and Orientals. They occur on the soles of feet and palms of hand (**Figure 20.8**). Subungual melanomas are included in this group (**Figure 20.9**). Prognosis depends on:

- Tumour thickness
- Growth phase
- Epidermal ulceration
- Regression
- Lymphovascular invasion

In 5% of patients no primary tumour can be identified and the disease presents with regional or distant metastases.

Tumour thickness

Tumour thickness is the most important prognostic factor for local, distant recurrence and survival. Tumour thickness can be measured as the Clarke level or Breslow depth (**Figure 20.10**). Five anatomical or Clarke levels are recognised as follows:

- Level 1 – Melanoma confined to the epidermis (melanoma in situ)
- Level 2 – Invasion into the papillary dermis
- Level 3 – Invasion to the junction of the papillary and reticular dermis
- Level 4 – Invasion into the reticular dermis
- Level 5 – Invasion into the subcutaneous fat

The Breslow depth is determined by using an ocular micrometer at a right angle

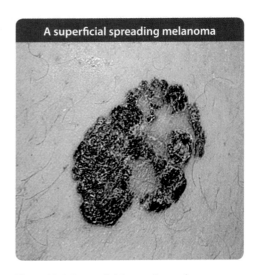

A superficial spreading melanoma

Figure 20.6 A superficial spreading melanoma

to the skin to directly measure the depth to which tumour cells have invaded the skin. It is measured from the granular layer of the epidermis down to the deepest point of invasion.

Clinical features

Superficial spreading melanomas usually present with slightly elevated lesion with variable colour. Nodular melanomas are usually uniform in colour and present with early ulceration and bleeding. Lentigo maligna melanoma presents as flat light brown macules. A lesion is unlikely to be a melanoma without at least one major sign (**Table 20.2**). When assessing a potential melanoma it is necessary to assess:

- A = Asymmetry
- B = Border irregularity
- C = Colour variegation
- D = Diameter
- E = Evolution

Suspicious skin lesions should be referred for an excision biopsy. Incisional biopsy may lead to inadequate histological assessment and should be avoided.

Management

In the absence of metastatic disease, excision with wide margins and skin grafting, as required, is the treatment of choice. The

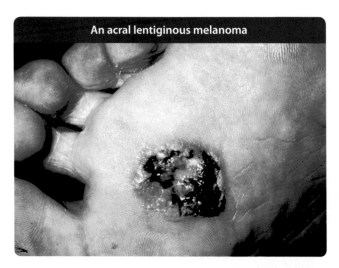

Figure 20.7 An acral lentiginous melanoma

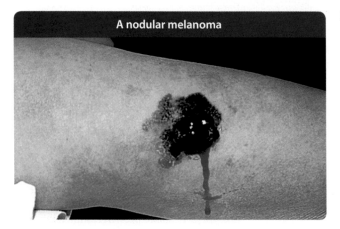

Figure 20.8 A nodular melanoma

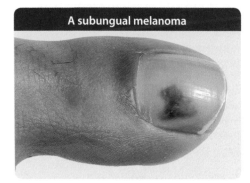

Figure 20.9 A subungual melanoma

generally accepted resection margins based on clinical appearance are:

- Impalpable lesion – 1 cm margin
- Palpable lesion – 2 cm margin
- Nodular lesion – 3 cm margin

Regional lymphadenectomy

In patients with malignant melanoma, about 20% of clinically palpable nodes are histologically negative. About 20% of palpably normal nodes have occult metastases. Patients with palpable nodes should undergo fine needle aspiration cytology. Confirmed nodal metastases in the

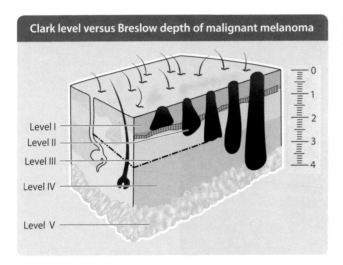

Figure 20.10 Clark level versus Breslow depth of malignant melanoma

Major and minor signs of malignant melanoma	
Major signs	**Minor signs**
Change in size	Inflammation
Change in shape	Bleeding
Change in colour	Sensory changes
Diameter >7 mm	

Table 20.2 Major and minor signs of malignant melanoma

absence of systemic spread is an indication for regional lymph node dissection. Sentinel lymph node biopsy should be considered for those with impalpable nodes.

Therapeutic lymph node dissection provides regional control and prognostic information but produces no improvement in survival. For tumours less than 0.75 mm thick about 90% are cured by local excision alone. For tumours more than 4.0 mm thick about 70% have distant metastases at presentation. For these two groups, lymphadenectomy provides no added survival benefit. The role of lymphadenectomy for 'intermediate' thickness tumours remains controversial.

The complications of lymphadenectomy include:

- Lymphoedema
- Seroma
- 'Functional deficit'
- Wound infection
- Persistent pain

Adjuvant therapy
Patients at high-risk of recurrence should be considered for systemic adjuvant therapy. High-risk patients include those with a primary tumour more than 4 mm thick and resectable positive locoregional lymph nodes. No standard adjuvant therapy exists but the use of interferon $\alpha 2b$ has shown promising results. It has been shown to increase disease-free and overall survival.

Isolated limb perfusion
Isolated limb perfusion (ILP) is the use of intra-arterial chemotherapy administered into the limb isolated from the remainder of the circulation. Commonly used agents include melphalan +/- TNF-α. It is administered with hyperoxygenation and hyperthermia at temperature of 41–42°C. Perfusion generally lasts about 1 hour. Indications for ILP include:

- In-transit metastases
- Irresectable local recurrence
- Adjuvant therapy for poor prognosis tumours
- Palliation to maintain limb function

The complications of ILP include:

- Mortality

- Limb oedema
- Persistent pain
- Neuropathy
- Venous thrombosis
- Septicaemia and thrombocytopenia

Other skin cancers

Basal cell carcinoma

Basal cell carcinoma is the commonest skin, malignancy. It occurs on sun exposed skin particularly the face above a line from the angle of mouth to the ear (**Figure 20.11**). It usually presents as a pearl-coloured nodule with rolled edges. As it enlarges, central ulceration can occur. Predisposing factors include xeroderma pigmentosa and radiotherapy. They are locally invasive and rarely metastasise.

Clinical features

The clinical types of a basal cell carcinoma are:

- Nodular or ulcerative
- Cystic
- Pigmented
- Sclerosing
- Cicatrical
- Superficial

Management

Treatment is by local excision with 0.5 cm margins and may require a full thickness graft. Other treatments modalities are radiotherapy and Mohs micrographic surgery. This is a procedure in which the tumour is excised at a 45° angle with subsequent identification of residual tumour using light microscopy. This method provides histological control of the surgical margins. It achieves the lowest recurrence rate with maximal preservation of normal tissue. The cure rate is more than 95%.

Squamous cell carcinoma

Squamous cell carcinoma is the second commonest cutaneous malignancy. The commonest sites involved are the face and the hands (**Figure 20.12**). Initially, it usually presents a red plaque. With time it invariable ulcerates and has hard and irregular edges. Predisposing factors include solar keratosis, Bowen's disease, viral warts and chronic ulceration or sinuses (Marjolin ulcers). The differential diagnosis includes:

- Keratoacanthoma
- Basal cell carcinoma
- Amelanotic melanomas
- Skin adnexal tumours

Treatment is by wide local excision, skin grafting and possible elective lymph node dissection.

Benign skin lesions and manifestations of systemic disease

Peutz–Jeghers syndrome

Peutz–Jeghers syndrome is inherited as autosomal dominant disorder. It presents with circumoral mucocutaneous pigment

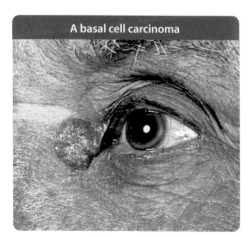

Figure 20.11 A basal cell carcinoma

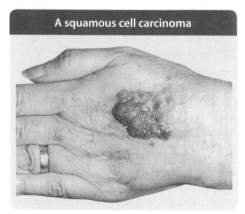

Figure 20.12 A squamous cell carcinoma

lesions on the lower lip, buccal mucosa and palate. It is associated with hamartomatous polyps in the small intestine. The polyps have fibrous and smooth muscle core with normal epithelium and may presents in childhood with gastrointestinal bleeding, anaemia or intussusception. The polyps are pre-malignant.

External angular dermoid

An external angular dermoid is a sequestration dermoid lined by epidermis. They occur on face at lines of fusion of embryonic processes. The commonest site is around eye at the site of fusion of the frontal and maxillary processes. They occasionally extend into the orbit and skull.

Tricholemmal cyst

Tricholemmal cysts are inherited as autosomal dominant condition. About 90% occur on scalp and are often multiple. They are derived from hair follicles and should not be regarded as simple epidermoid cysts.

Pyogenic granuloma

Pyogenic granulomas are neither pyogenic or granulomas. They are capillary haemangiomas often with a traumatic aetiology. They present as bright red, friable nodules characterised by contact bleeding. The commonest site affected is the hands. Treatment is by curettage or diathermy.

Cylindroma

Cylindromas are benign tumour of eccrine sweat glands. They occur on the scalp and can be solitary or multiple. Multiple tumours are often referred to as 'Turban tumours'. Treatment is by local excision.

Dermatofibroma

Dermatofibromas or benign histiocytomas are more common in women than men. They present with small firm pigmented nodules, usually pink or brown. The commonest site is the leg. Treatment is by local excision.

Keratoacanthoma

Keratoacanthomas are more common in men than women. They present as rapidly growing skin lesions over 6–8 weeks. They are usually dome-shaped with a keratin filled crater and may be up to 3 cm in diameter. If untreated, they often involute over 6 months leaving an irregular pitted scar. The differential diagnosis is a squamous cell carcinoma. Treatment is by excision biopsy.

Pigmented skin lesions

Melanocytes are of neuroendocrine origin and migrate to the skin during the first three months of intrauterine development. They produce melanin from tyrosine. Melanin is stored in melanosomes before being exported to keratinocytes. A freckle is increased melanin by a normal number of melanocytes. A naevus is a pigmented lesion due to an increased number of melanocytes. Naevi are believed to evolve from junctional via compound to intradermal lesion.

Junctional, compound and intradermal naevi

A junctional naevus usually presents as a small flat macule and often appears in childhood as a homogenous brown or black skin lesion with increased melanocytes in the rete pegs. A compound naevus presents as raised papule. It is often pale brown with a junctional component and nest of cells in the dermis. An intradermal naevus appears as a flesh coloured papule. They have an increased prevalence in middle age with no junctional activity and only intradermal nests.

Blue naevus

A blue naevus is a dome-shaped blue or black papule seen in middle-age. They are more common in women. The commonest site is the scalp and face. They have a dermal collection of spindle melanocytes with melanin in dendritic cells. They possibly arise as a result of incomplete migration of melanocytes to the epidermis.

Halo naevus

A halo naevus is a benign naevus with pale rim. It needs to be differentiated form a melanoma with regression. It results from a naevus with lymphocytic invasion and melanocyte destruction.

Juvenile melanoma

A juvenile melanoma or Spitz naevus is a benign tumour that histologically mimics a melanoma. It has regular melanocytes with a vascular stroma and epidermal hypertrophy. It is most commonly seen in young adults and is more common in women. It presents as a single pink domed-shaped nodule and is most frequently seen on the head and neck.

Nail disorders
Ingrowing toenails

Ingrowing toenails are a common problem in adolescents and young adults. They usually affects the hallux but other nails may also be affected. It is due to the lateral edge of the nail growing into the adjacent soft tissue (**Figure 20.13**). Bacterial or fungal infection may be superimposed. Attempted healing may result in over-granulation of the nail bed. Possible aetiological factors include poorly fitting shoes, poor foot care and inappropriate nail cutting.

Management

In the early stages, conservative management should be attempted. This includes regular soaking and washing of the feet, careful drying after washing and the wearing of properly fitting shoes. Patients should be taught to cut their nails transversely. The use of pledgets of cotton wool placed under the nail may encourage it to grow out.

Surgery may be required if conservative measures fail. The nail can be removed by avulsion or wedge resection. Recurrence is common. If simple avulsion fails, ablation of the nail bed should be considered. This can be achieved either chemically or surgically. Chemical ablation can be achieved with phenol. Surgical removal usually involves a Zadek procedure. Avulsion and phenolisation is more effective than surgical procedures.

Subungual haematoma

Subungual haematoma results from blunt trauma to the hallux and nail bed. Blood collects under the nail. Increased pressure causes severe pain. The nail initially appears red but becomes purple as the blood coagulates. The differential diagnosis includes a subungual melanoma, a glomus tumour or Kaposi's sarcoma. The haematoma can be evacuated by nail trephine with a heated needle or drill. Blood under pressure is released and the symptoms immediately settle.

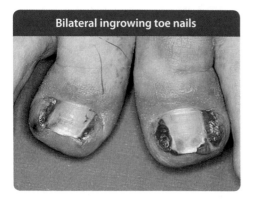

Bilateral ingrowing toe nails

Figure 20.13 Bilateral ingrowing toe nails

Chapter 21 Neurosurgery

Applied basic sciences

Neuroanatomy

The scalp

The scalp consist of five different anatomical layers that including the skin, the subcutaneous tissue, the galea aponeurotica, loose areolar tissue and the skull periosteum. The subcutaneous layer possesses a rich vascular supply that contains an abundant communication of vessels that can result in a significant blood loss when the scalp is lacerated. The relatively poor fixation of the galea to the underlying periosteum of the skull provides little resistance to shear injuries that can result in large scalp flap or scalping injuries. This layer also provides little resistance to haematomas and extensive fluid collections related to the scalp tend to accumulate in the subgaleal plane.

The skull

The adult skull is normally made up of 22 bones. Except for the mandible, all of the bones of the skull are joined together by sutures with little movement. Eight bones including one frontal, two parietal, one occipital bone, one sphenoid, two temporal and one ethmoid form the neurocranium,

a protective vault surrounding the brain. Fourteen bones form the face. The skull is a protector of the brain. The bones of the skull have three distinct layers with hard internal and external tables and a thin cancellous middle layer, or diploë. The thickest area is usually the occipital bone and the thinnest is the temporal bone. The cranium is covered by periosteum on both the outer and inner surfaces. On the inner surface, it fuses with the dura to become the outer layer of the dura.

The meninges

The meninges are the protective coverings of the brain and spinal cord consisting of three layers of membranous connective tissue (**Figure 21.1**) The dura mater is the tough outer layer lying just inside the skull and vertebrae. In the skull, there are channels within the dura mater, the dural sinuses, which contain venous blood. In the spinal cord, the dura mater is often referred to as the dural sheath. A fat-filled space between the dura mater and the vertebrae, the epidural space, acts as a protective cushion to the spinal cord. The arachnoid mater is the middle layer. Projections from the arachnoid, called arachnoid villi, protrude through one layer of the dura mater into the dural

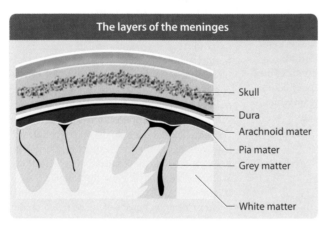

The layers of the meninges

- Skull
- Dura
- Arachnoid mater
- Pia mater
- Grey matter
- White matter

Figure 21.1 The layers of the meninges

sinuses. The arachnoid villi transport the CSF from the subarachnoid space to the dural sinuses. Two cavities border the arachnoid: the subdural space is outside the arachnoid and the subarachnoid space is within the arachnoid. This space contains blood vessels and circulates CSF. The pia mater is the innermost layer. It tightly covers the brain and carries blood vessels that provide the nervous tissues.

The brain

There are three major divisions of the brain. They are the forebrain, the midbrain, and the hindbrain. The forebrain is responsible for a variety of functions including receiving and processing sensory information, thinking, perceiving, producing and understanding language, and controlling motor function. There are two major divisions of forebrain: the diencephalon and the telencephalon. The diencephalon contains structures such as the thalamus and hypothalamus which are responsible for such functions as motor control, relaying sensory information, and controlling autonomic functions. The telencephalon contains the largest part of the brain, the cerebrum. Most of the actual information processing in the brain takes place in the cerebral cortex. The midbrain and the hindbrain together make up the brainstem. The midbrain is the portion of the brainstem that connects the hindbrain and the forebrain. This region of the brain is involved in auditory and visual responses as well as motor function. The hindbrain extends from the spinal cord and is composed of the metencephalon and myelencephalon. The metencephalon contains structures such as the pons and cerebellum. These regions assist in maintaining balance and equilibrium, movement coordination, and the conduction of sensory information. The myelencephalon is composed of the medulla oblongata which is responsible for controlling autonomic functions.

Neurophysiology

Cerebrospinal fluid

There are four cavities in the brain, called ventricles. The ventricles are filled with cerebrospinal fluid (CSF) which absorbs physical shocks to the brain, distributes nutrients to and removes wastes from the nervous tissue. It provides a chemically stable environment. The two lateral ventricles are found in the cerebral hemispheres. The third ventricle is connected by a passage (interventricular foramen) to each of the two lateral ventricles. The fourth ventricle is connected to the third ventricle (via the cerebral aqueduct) and to the central canal of the spinal cord. Additional openings in the fourth ventricle allow CSF to flow into the subarachnoid space.

A network of capillaries called the choroid plexus projects into each ventricle. Ependymal cells surround these capillaries. Blood plasma entering the ependymal cells from the capillaries is filtered as it passes into the ventricle, forming CSF. Any material passing from the capillaries to the ventricles of the brain must do so through the ependymal cells. Tight junctions linking these cells prevent the passage of plasma between them. Thus, the ependymal cells maintain a blood–CSF barrier, controlling the composition of the CSF.

Intracranial pressure

As the cranial vault is essentially a closed, fixed bony structure, its volume is constant. The contents are the brain, CSF and blood. All these components are non-compressible and as a result any increase in one of the components must be at the expense of the other two. This relationship is known as the Monro–Kellie doctrine. Once the cranial vault is filled, pressure rises dramatically.

Normal intracranial pressure (ICP) is 5–10 mmHg. Due to autoregulation, cerebral perfusion pressure (CPP), the pressure of blood flowing to the brain, is normally fairly constant. A rise in ICP reduces cerebral blood flow by reducing the cerebral perfusion pressure. Some compensation is possible as CSF and blood move into the spinal canal and extracranial vasculature, respectively. There is however a point where further compensation is impossible and ICP rises dramatically (**Figure 21.2**), CPP falls and cerebral ischaemia occurs. Common causes of raised ICP include:

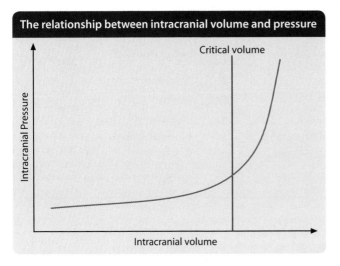

The relationship between intracranial volume and pressure

Critical volume

Intracranial Pressure

Intracranial volume

Figure 21.2 The relationship between intracranial volume and pressure

- Head injury
- Intracranial haematoma
- Subarachnoid hemorrhage
- Brain tumour
- Encephalitis
- Hydrocephalus (increased fluid around the brain)
- Cerebrovascular accident

Neurosurgical trauma
Head injuries

Epidemiology

Approximately, 1 million patients attend emergency departments each year in the UK with a head injury.

- 80% are minor (GCS 13–15)
- 10% are moderate (GCS 9–12)
- 10% are severe (GCS less than 8)

Severe head injuries account for 50% of trauma-related deaths.

Pathophysiology

Primary brain injury is damage caused at time of impact. It can be focal or diffuse. Diffuse axonal injury is due to deceleration and shearing forces. It is dependent on the extent of the initial injury and is not amenable to treatment. Secondary brain injury is any neurological insult imposed after the primary injury. It can be due to hypoxaemia, hypercapnia, hypotension and intracranial

haematoma or hypertension. The early treatment of head injured patients is aimed at the detection and prevention of secondary brain injury. Following major head injuries, autoregulation of cerebral blood flow is lost.

Clinical features

Patients with head injuries should be managed according to ATLS protocols to prevent secondary brain injury. All patients presenting to an emergency department with a head injury should be assessed by a trained member of staff within a maximum of 15 minutes of arrival. This assessment should establish whether they are at high or low-risk for clinically important brain injury. Full assessment requires:

- Glasgow Coma Scale (**Table 21.1**)
- Pulse, blood pressure
- Assessment of pupil diameter and response
- Assessment of limb movement

Depressed conscious level should be ascribed to intoxication only after a significant brain injury has been excluded.

Signs of a basal skull fracture are:

- Blood or cerebrospinal fluid from nose or ear
- Periorbital haematoma
- Mastoid haematoma (Battle sign)
- Haemotympanum
- Radiological evidence of intra-cranial air
- Radiological evidence of fluid levels in the sinuses

Glasgow Coma Scale					
Eye opening		**Motor response**		**Verbal response**	
Spontaneous	4	Obeys	6	Orientated	5
To speech	3	Localises	5	Confused	4
To pain	2	Withdraws	4	Inappropriate	3
None	1	Abnormal flexion	3	Incomprehensible	2
		Extensor response	2	None	1
		None	1		

Table 21.1 Glasgow Coma Scale

About 5% patients with a severe head injury have a cervical spine injury. Patients who have sustained a head injury and present with any of the following risk factors should have full cervical spine immobilisation:

- GCS less than 15 on initial assessment by the healthcare professional
- Neck pain or tenderness
- Focal neurological deficit
- Paraesthesia in the extremities
- Any other clinical suspicion of cervical spine injury

Investigation

CT is the primary investigation of choice for clinically significant brain injury. Indications for an immediate CT in an adult are:

- GCS less than 13 at any point since the injury
- GCS equal to 13 or 14 at 2 hours after the injury
- Suspected open or depressed skull fracture
- Any sign of a basal skull fracture
- Post-traumatic seizure
- Focal neurological deficit
- More than one episode of vomiting
- Amnesia for greater than 30 minutes of events before impact
- If LOC in patients older then 65 years, coagulopathy or dangerous mechanism of injury

Indications for an immediate CT in a child are:

- Loss of consciousness lasting more than 5 minutes

- Amnesia (antegrade or retrograde) lasting more than 5 minutes
- Abnormal drowsiness
- Three or more discrete episodes of vomiting
- Clinical suspicion of non-accidental injury
- Post-traumatic seizure but no history of epilepsy
- GCS less than 14, or for a baby under 1 year GCS less than 15
- Suspicion of open or depressed skull injury or tense fontanelle
- Any sign of a basal skull fracture
- Focal neurological deficit
- Dangerous mechanism of injury

Plain x-rays of the skull should not be used to diagnose significant brain injury without prior discussion with a neuroscience unit. Skull x-rays have a role in the detection of non-accidental injuries in children.

Management

Criteria for admission and observation after a head injury are:

- Altered level of consciousness
- Skull fracture
- Neurological symptoms or signs
- Difficult assessment – drugs or alcohol
- No responsible carer

Observations should be performed and recorded on a half-hourly basis until a GCS equal to 15 has been achieved. The minimum frequency of observations for patients with GCS equal to 15 should be as follows:

- Half-hourly for 2 hours
- Then 1-hourly for 4 hours
- Then 2-hourly thereafter

Should a patient with GCS equal to 15 deteriorate at any time after the initial 2-hour period, observations should revert to half-hourly and follow the original frequency schedule.

Indications for referral to neurosurgeon are:

- Persistent coma (GCS <8) after initial resuscitation
- Unexplained confusion persisting for more than 4 hours
- Deterioration in GCS after admission
- A seizure without full recovery
- Progressive focal neurological signs
- Definite or suspected penetrating injury
- CSF leak

Indications for intubation and ventilation following a head injury are:

- GCS less than or equal to 8
- Loss of protective laryngeal reflexes
- Ventilatory insufficiency as judged by blood gases
  - PaO_2 less than 9 kPa
  - $PaCO_2$ greater than 6 kPa

- Spontaneous hyperventilation
- Respiratory arrhythmia
- Bilateral fractured mandible
- Copious bleeding into mouth
- Seizures

Antibiotics and anticonvulsants are of no benefit in uncomplicated head injuries. Both may be used in compound depressed fractures and penetrating brain injury.

Complications of head injuries

Acute extradural haematoma

An extradural haematoma is a complication of low velocity injuries. The classic presentation is with transient loss of consciousness with rapid recovery followed by a lucid interval and then rapid deterioration in the level of consciousness. This may be associated with an increased blood pressure, falling pulse rate, contralateral limb weakness and ipsilateral pupillary dilatation. Treatment is by emergency burr holes (**Figure 21.3**).

Acute subdural haematoma

A subdural haematoma is a complication of high velocity injury (**Figure 21.4**).

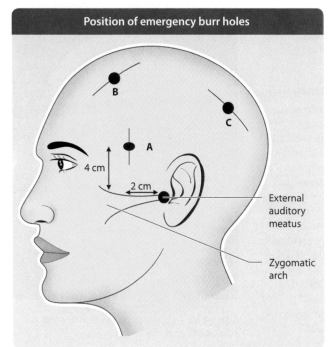

Position of emergency burr holes

B

C

A

4 cm

2 cm

External auditory meatus

Zygomatic arch

Figure 21.3 Position of emergency burr holes. A = Temporal; B = Frontal; C = Parietal burr holes.

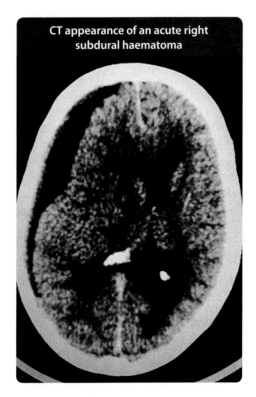

CT appearance of an acute right subdural haematoma

Figure 21.4 CT appearance of an acute right subdural haematoma

The patient is usually unconscious from the time of injury with deteriorating level of consciousness. Treatment is by decompressive craniotomy.

Chronic subdural haematoma

Chronic subdural haematoma is one of the commonest neurosurgical emergencies. It occurs when blood expands in the subdural space over a period of weeks. The incidence increases with age and is more common in men. The majority occur after an initial minor head injury. About 40% of patients are unable to recall the injury and in 30% of patients the haematomas are bilateral. Risk factors include cerebral atrophy, coagulation disorders and arachnoid cysts. The bleeding results from rupture of the small bridging veins between the dura and cranium. The subdural space is progressively filled by extravasated blood. With time, the liquefying haematoma contains a high protein content that leads to osmotic swelling. The haematoma may reach a size to cause and mass effect and raised intracranial pressure.

Clinical features
The classical presentation is of an elderly patient with a history of falls who presents with deteriorating neurological function. The patient often has headaches, confusion or focal mass effect – hemiparesis or dysphasia.

Investigation
A CT scan may show a crescent-shaped mass between the inner table of the cranium and the outer surface of the cortex (**Figure 21.5**). Most haematomas are located in the fronto-parietal region. The natural history if for the clot to be initially hyperdense early after injury and then to become hypodense with time. Bilateral isodense subdural haematomas can easily be missed.

Management
Small haematomas without significant mass effect can be managed conservatively. If the

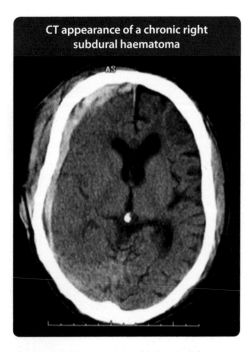

CT appearance of a chronic right subdural haematoma

Figure 21.5 CT appearance of a chronic right subdural haematoma

haematomas are large and have significant mass effect, then burr holes should be considered. Craniotomy is indicated if the clot does not completely liquify or becomes loculated. Over 90% of operated cases show residual blood on early postoperative imaging and as many as 20% of cases require further surgery.

Spinal cord injuries

All patients with multiple trauma should be suspected of having a spinal injury. Failure to detect usually results from failure to suspect. The cervical spine and thoraco-lumbar junction are the commonest site of injury. The percentage of nerve injuries seen in patients with spinal fractures are:

- Cervical spine – 40%
- Thoracic spine – 10%
- Thoraco-lumbar junction – 35%
- Lumbar spine – 5%

All injuries should be assumed to be unstable until proved otherwise.

Initial assessment

At the scene of the accident, it is vital to maintain in-line spinal immobilisation. This requires supporting of the neck with a stiff collar and sandbags. The patient should be transported on a spinal board. During the primary survey, if intubation is required in-line immobilisation should be maintained. Cervical spine injuries reduce sympathetic outflow. Therefore, in patients with spinal cord injuries, pharyngeal stimulation with an airway or endotracheal tube can cause vagal discharge and cardiac arrest. Patients may be both hypotensive and bradycardic and may require the use of atropine and inotropic support. Aggressive fluid resuscitation can induce pulmonary oedema.

Clinical features

The level of the cord lesion is conventionally defined as the most caudal location with normal motor and sensory function (**Table 21.2**). Spinal shock may mimic a complete cord lesion with total loss of motor and sensory function distal to the injury. However, if the lesion is incomplete some function will return. Almost all patients with a complete cord lesion will not show functional recovery.

Patients with a partial lesion may regain substantial or even normal neurological function even though the initial neurological deficit may be severe. The presence of the bulbocavernous reflex or anal–cutaneous reflex indicates sacral sparing and a more favourable prognosis.

Patients may develop respiratory failure due to:

- Intercostal paralysis
- Partial phrenic nerve palsy
- Impaired ability to cough
- Ventilation–perfusion mismatch
- Variable intercostal nerve paralysis
- Associated chest injuries

Respiratory failure may develop as a late feature due to ascending oedema in the cervical cord. The abdomen may be flaccid with absent sensation. Features of peritonism may be absent. Priapism may develop.

Partial cord lesions

With partial cord lesions, function may be preserved distal to the level of cord injury. The diagnosis may be missed if it does not fit the classical injury pattern. The clinical features of partial cord lesions are as follows:

- Central cord lesion – flaccid paralysis of the upper limbs
- Anterior cord lesion – loss of temperature and sensation
- Posterior cord lesion – loss of vibration sensation and proprioception
- Brown–Sequard syndrome – loss of ipsilateral power and contralateral pain and temperature

Radiological assessment

Approximately 20% patients with spinal cord injury have no radiological evidence of bony injury. Lateral cervical spine x-rays were until recently the commonest means of assessing the cervical spine. With the increasing availability of CT scanning, this is being more commonly used to assess possible cervical spine injuries.

Lateral cervical spine x-ray should be taken during the primary survey. It should ensure that the junction between C7 and T1 is seen. Anterio-posterior and odontoid peg views should be taken during the secondary

Assessment of level of spinal injury		
Muscle group	**Nerve supply**	**Reflex**
Diaphragm	C3, C4, C5	
Shoulder abductors	C5	
Elbow flexors	C5, C6	Biceps jerk
Supinators/pronators	C6	Supinator jerk
Wrist extensors	C6	
Wrist flexors	C7	
Elbow extensors	C7	Triceps jerk
Finger extensors	C7	
Finger flexors	C8	
Intrinsic hand muscles	T1	
Hip flexors	L1, L2	
Hip adductors	L2, L3	
Knee extensors	L3, L4	Knee jerk
Ankle dorsiflexors	L4, L5	
Toe extensors	L5	
Knee flexors	L4, L5, S1	
Ankle plantar flexors	S1, S2	Ankle jerk
Toe flexors	S1, S2	
Anal sphincter	S2, S3, S4	Bulbocavernosus reflex
		Anal reflex

Table 21.2 Assessment of level of spinal injury

survey. If unable to see the C7/T1 junction consider a 'swimmer's view'. On a lateral cervical spine film it is necessary to assess:

- Anterior vertebral alignment
- Posterior vertebral alignment
- Posterior facet joint margins
- Anterior border of spinous processes
- Posterior border of spinous processes
- Integrity of vertebral bodies, laminae, pedicles and arches
- Pre-vertebral space
- Retropharyngeal space should be less than 6 mm
- Retrotracheal space should be less than 22 mm
- Interspinous gaps

Radiological signs of spinal instability include:

- Compression of a vertebral body more than 25%
- Kyphotic angle of more than 10%
- Facet joint widening
- Teardrop fracture
- Base of odontoid peg fracture
- Atlanto-axial gap more than 3 mm
- Atlanto-occipital dislocation

Various reports confirm a higher sensitivity and specificity of CT sacnning versus conventional plain films in cervical spine injury The chance of finding additional information, like bony ligamentous avulsion or dorsal arch fractures is substantially higher with CT.

Management

A spinal cord injury is a medical emergency requiring immediate treatment to reduce the long-term effects. The time between the injury and treatment is a critical factor affecting the eventual outcome. Steroids may be used to reduce the swelling of the spinal cord. Decompressive surgery may be necessary to remove bony fragments or stabilise the spine.

The rehabilitation process following a spinal cord injury should begin in the acute care setting. Physiotherapists, occupational therapists, social workers, psychologists and other healthcare professionals work as a team to determine an individualised management plan. In the acute phase, management focuses on the patient's respiratory status, prevention of complications, maintaining the range of motion and muscle bulk.

Complications of a spinal cord injury include:

- Deranged blood pressure control
- Chronic kidney disease
- Deep vein thrombosis
- Pulmonary infections
- Pressure sores
- Contractures
- Urinary tract infections
- Incontinence
- Loss of sexual function
- Muscle spasticity

Neurosurgical disorders
Subarachnoid haemorrhage

Subarachnoid haemorrhage accounts for approximately 5% of cerebrovascular accidents. The outcome depends on the degree of neurological deficit. The lower the GCS on presentation, the worse the prognosis. About 70% are due to berry aneurysms. The remainder are due to arteriovenous malformations and hypertension.

Pathology

Berry aneurysms are found in 8% of individuals at post mortem. They are thin walled saccular aneurysms found at arterial bifurcations on the Circle of Willis. They occur due to turbulent flow and damage to the internal elastic lamina of the intracranial arteries. The commonest site of aneurysms are:

- Posterior communicating artery (30%)
- Anterior communicating artery (25%)
- Middle cerebral artery (25%)

Most aneurysms remain asymptomatic but they are a common cause of sudden death. About 15% of aneurysms are multiple.

Clinical features

The classic presentation of a subarachnoid haemorrhage is with a sudden onset of a severe headache often associated with nausea, vomiting, photophobia and neck stiffness. Neurological symptoms and signs may be present. The level of consciousness may be reduced. Fundoscopy may show subhyoid haemorrhages. The clinical course is unpredictable. Overall mortality is approximately 40%. Many patients die before reaching hospital.

Investigation

The diagnosis can often be confirmed by an early CT or MRI. CT has a sensitivity of 90% if performed within the first 24 hours. The sensitivity is reduced to 50% by 72 hours as blood is reabsorbed. The CT may also identify the source of haemorrhage. Fluid-attenuated inversion recovery (FLAIR) is the most sensitive MRI pulse sequence for the detection of subarachnoid hemorrhage. On FLAIR images, blood appears as high signal-intensity in normally low signal-intensity CSF spaces. MRA may be useful for evaluating aneurysms and other vascular lesions. If the diagnosis is in doubt then lumbar puncture may be indicated and will show uniform blood-staining of CSF and xanthochromia.

Complications

The major complications of a subarachnoid haemorrhage are:

- Rebleed
- Delayed ischaemic neurological deficit
- Hydrocephalus

The risk of rebleed is 4% at 24 hours, 25% at 2 weeks and 60% at 6 months. Rebleeding is associated with a 60% mortality. Delayed ischaemic neurological deficit (DIND) is due to intense vasospasm. Treatment is by maintaining cerebral perfusion with adequate hydration. Hydrocephalus results from impaired CSF reabsorption through arachnoid villi and 10% of patients will require CSF diversion or shunting.

Management

In patients fit for surgery, the aneurysm should be clipped at craniotomy. The aim is to clip the neck of the aneurysm whilst maintaining flow in the native vessel. It may also be embolised endovascularly with platinum coils. The timing of intervention is controversial. Vasospasm is usually greatest at 5 days after the bleed. Surgery has traditionally been deferred until 10 days after the initial bleed but patients may die as a result of rebleed during this period. Early surgery or coiling may be associated with reduced mortality and no increased morbidity.

Brainstem death

Brainstem death is a clinical concept, implying an unconscious patient, with irreversible apnea and loss of brainstem reflexes. The concept defines the core physiological basis for the neurological diagnosis of death in the UK. All modern neurological criteria of death are primarily met through clinical tests of brainstem function. These tests seek to ascertain that brainstem reflexes, motor responses, and respiratory drive are absent in a normothermic comatose patient with a known irreversible massive brain lesion and no contributing metabolic derangements.

Preconditions
- Diagnosis compatible with brainstem death
- Presence of irreversible structural brain damage
- Presence of apnoeic coma

Exclusions
- Therapeutic drug effects (sedatives, hypnotics, muscle relaxants)
- Hypothermia (Temp >35°C)
- Metabolic abnormalities
- Endocrine abnormalities
- Intoxication

Clinical tests
- Confirmation of absent brainstem reflexes
- Confirmation of persistent apnoea

Clinical tests should be performed by two experienced practitioners, at least one of whom should be a consultant. Neither should be part of the transplant team. The tests should be performed on two separate occasions. There is no prescribed time interval between the two tests.

Clinical tests for absent brainstem reflexes
- No pupillary response to light
- Absent corneal reflex
- No motor response within cranial nerve distribution
- Absent gag reflex
- Absent cough reflex
- Absent vestibulo-ocular reflex

Test for confirmation of persistent apnoea
- Preoxygenation with 100% oxygen for 10 minutes
- Allow $PaCO_2$ to rise above 5.0 kPa before test
- Disconnect from ventilator
- Maintain adequate oxygenation during test
- Allow $PaCO_2$ to climb above 6.65 kPa
- Confirm no spontaneous respiration
- Reconnect ventilator

Central nervous system infections

Intracranial abscess

Intracranial abscesses are rare but require prompt recognition and treatment is required. Delayed diagnosis often results in disability or death. Abscesses can be extradural, subdural or intracerebral. Most are bacterial infections that reach the central nervous system by:

- Inoculation from a penetrating wound
- Spread from adjacent infective focus (e.g. otitis media, sinusitis)
- Blood-borne spread from distant focus (e.g. endocarditis, lung abscess)

In 20% of patients, no source of infection is identified. In the UK, otitis media and sinusitis are the commonest causes of intracranial abscesses.

Pathology

From a local focus of infection, bacteria can penetrate the skull through the diploeic veins. Also, local osteomyelitis may result in venous sinus thrombosis. As the dura is normally a good barrier to the intracranial spread of infection, pus in the extradural space usually causes an extradural empyema. Subdural sepsis causes oedema and cortical venous thrombosis. Brain penetration causes an early diffuse cerebritis. A localised abscess may develop with oedema and increased intracranial pressure. The abscess usually forms in the subcortical white matter near to the septic focus. Haematogenous abscesses may be multiple.

Clinical features

Intracranial abscesses can affect any age or sex. The systemic upset is often mild. Symptoms of increased intracranial pressure include headache and vomiting, often associated with progressive clouding of consciousness. As the abscess develops, focal neurological symptoms may evolve. As a result, symptoms of increased intracranial pressure associated with focal neurological signs requires urgent neurosurgical assessment. The differential diagnosis includes meningitis or an intracranial tumour. Osteomyelitis due to frontal sinusitis or middle ear disease may produces localised swelling (Pott puffy tumour).

Investigation

MRI, with and without gadolinium enhancement, is the investigation of choice. It is more specific than CT scanning in differentiating a cerebral tumour, haematoma and abscess. On contrast enhanced CT scanning, a cerebral abscess appears as radiolucent space occupying lesion with ring enhancement of the capsule. It is often surrounded by considerable cerebral oedema. The position, size and number of abscesses may suggest the underlying pathology. Lumbar puncture is contraindicated as in the presence of raised intracranial pressure it can precipitate tentorial or tonsillar herniation.

Management

The principles of treatment of intracranial abscess are:

- Drain intracranial collection
- Administer effective antibiotic therapy
- Eliminate primary source of infection

Supratentorial abscesses can be drained via a burr hole. Pus should be aspirated and sent for culture. Clinical progress can be monitored by serial CT scans. Stereotactic drainage may be required for multiple or multiloculated abscesses. Cerebellar abscesses may require a suboccipital craniectomy and open drainage. Subdural empyemas are often diffuse and difficult to drain and may require craniectomy and open drainage. Parenteral antibiotic should be administered for at least 2 weeks. The choice of antibiotics depends on the primary pathology and antibiotic sensitivities.

Prompt treatment results in a mortality of less than 10%. Delayed treatment results in mortality greater than 50%. About 50% of survivors have neurological sequelae including hemiparesis, visual field losses and epilepsy.

Spinal abscess

Spinal abscesses are usually bacterial. Infection arises in adjacent bone or by haematogenous spread. The commonest organisms are staphylococcal and streptococcal species. Pus is usually confined to extradural space. Subdural and intramedullary infections are rare.

Clinical features

The patient is often systemically unwell and may present with severe thoracic or lumbar back pain at the level of the abscess. The pain is worse on movement and associated with marked muscle spasm and vertebral tenderness. Radicular signs are often present at the level of the lesion. Cord compression results in long tract signs. Thrombophlebitis can cause cord vessel thrombosis and cord infarction, presenting with complete paralysis, sensory and sphincter loss.

Investigation

Serum white cell count, ESR and CRP are invariably raised. X-rays are often normal but may show soft tissue swelling or vertebral collapse. MRI is the investigation of choice.

Management

A high index of suspicion is required to make the diagnosis. Once identified, prompt neurosurgical assessment is required. If vertebral body collapse occurs, consideration should be given to anterior decompression and stabilisation. If no vertebral collapse is seen then laminectomy or CT-guided aspiration may be appropriate.

Chapter 22

Trauma and orthopaedic surgery

Applied basic sciences
Bone

Bone has several functions including:

- Calcium homeostasis
- Haemopoesis
- Structure and protection of internal organs
- Movement

Compact bone

Compact bone is found in the shafts of long bones and the outside surfaces of some other bones. It makes up 80% of the total body mass. It consists of cylindrical units called osteons (**Figure 22.1**). Each osteon contains concentric lamellae of a calcified matrix with osteocytes lodged in lacunae between the lamellae. Smaller canals, or canaliculi, radiate outward from a central canal – Haversian canals. These contains blood vessels and nerve fibres. Osteocytes within an osteon are connected to each other and to the central canal by fine cellular extensions.

Through these cellular extensions, nutrients and wastes are exchanged between the osteocytes and the blood vessels. Perforating or Volkmann's canals provide channels that allow the blood vessels, that run through the central canals, to connect to the blood vessels in the periosteum that surrounds the bone.

Trabecular bone

Trabecular or spongy bone consists of thin, irregularly shaped plates called trabeculae. These are arranged in a latticework network. Trabeculae are similar to osteons in that both have osteocytes in lacunae. As in compact bone, the canaliculi present in trabeculae, provide connections between osteocytes. Each trabecula is only a few cell layers thick and each osteocyte is able to exchange nutrients with nearby blood vessels.

Microstructure of bone

Bone matrix or osteoid has both organic and inorganic components. The organic

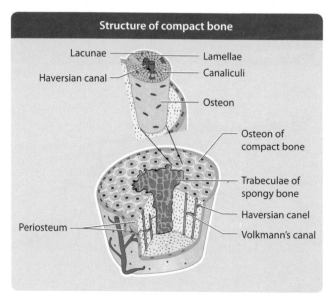

Structure of compact bone

Lacunae

Haversian canal

Lamellae

Canaliculi

Osteon

Osteon of compact bone

Trabeculae of spongy bone

Haversian canel

Periosteum

Volkmann's canal

Figure 22.1 Structure of compact bone

component is composed of Type 1 collagen and proteoglycans. The inorganic matrix is mainly made up of calcium and phosphate salts. Osteoblasts secrete organic bone matrix or osteoid. They become osteocytes when they are surrounded by the bone matrix. Osteoclasts are multinucleate cells derived from monocytes. They actively resorb bone. Periosteum covers bones and contains blood vessels, nerves and lymphatics. Its inner surface is osteogenic and contains both osteoblasts and osteoclasts.

Ossification

Bone undergoes either intramembranous or endochondral ossification. Both result in the same microstructure. Intramembranous ossification is directly from mesenchyme and occurs in flat bones such as the skull. Endochondral ossification is the development of bone through an intermediate cartilage stage and occurs in long bone.

Cartilage

Cartilaginous matrix makes up over 80% of cartilage and is primarily composed of elastin, collagen and proteoglycans. These are large molecules with a protein backbone and glycosaminoglycan side chains. Chondrocytes are mature cartilage cells and are scattered throughout the cartilage matrix. Hyaline cartilage is made up of mainly Type 2 collagen and functions as articular

cartilage in synovial joints. It is also found in the centres of ossification in growing bone. Elastic cartilage is similar to hyaline cartilage but contains more elastin bundles. It is found in the pinna, eustachian tube and epiglottis. Fibrocartilage is a tougher form of cartilage found in intervertebral discs and symphyses.

Nerves and action potential

Structure of neurones

Nerve cells are designed to respond to stimuli and transmit information over long distances. They have three parts (**Figure 22.2**). The cell body has a single nucleus and is responsible for most of nerve cell metabolism, especially protein synthesis. Proteins made in the cell body must be delivered to other parts of the nerve by an axonal transport system. The axon is designed to transmit an electrical impulse and can be several meters long. Dendrites receive impulses from other nerves.

The action potential

Neurones transmit information as action potentials. An action potential is a temporary change in the membrane potential, usually initiated in the cell body. It normally travels in one direction and is conducted in an 'all-or-nothing' fashion. If the stimulus is too low, there is no action potential. If the stimulus is above a threshold, the action potential, is always the same size. During an action

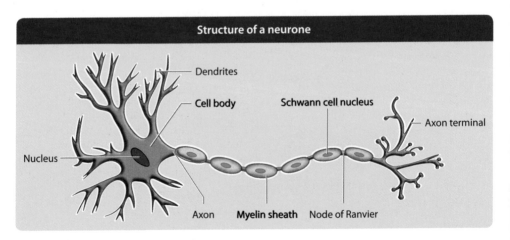

Figure 22.2 Structure of a neurone

potential the membrane depolarises and after the peak it repolarises. For a short time, the cell membrane potential becomes more negative than the resting potential before it returns to normal. Action potentials are initiated by many different types of stimuli. Sensory nerves respond to chemicals, light, pressure, touch and stretch. In the central nervous system most nerves are stimulated by neurotransmitters at synapses. Stimuli must be above a threshold level to initiate an action potential. After a nerve has fired there is a period of time during which it cannot be stimulated again. This is known as the refractory period.

Biochemical changes

The sodium pump produces gradients of both sodium and potassium ions across the cell membrane. Both ions are used to produce the action potential. Sodium concentration is high on the outside of the neurone and low on the inside. Neurones have sodium and potassium channels with gates that open and close in response to the membrane voltage. Opening of sodium channels allows sodium to rush into the cell. The spike of the action potential is caused by opening of sodium channels. The membrane recovers by closing the sodium channels and opening the potassium channels.

Myelin sheath

The conduction velocity of an action potential along an axon is increased by a myelin sheath produced by Schwann cells in the peripheral nervous system and oligodendrogliocytes in the central nervous system. Multiple layers of lipid membranes are wrapped around the nerve. Gaps are left every few millimetres and are called nodes of Ranvier. In a myelinated nerve the impulse jumps from node to node. Conduction velocities for un-myelinated neurones are about 1 m/sec. Conduction velocities for myelinated neurones are about 100 m/sec.

Synapses and neuromuscular junctions

Synapses

The junction between two nerves is called a synapse (**Figure 22.3**). At the synapse there

is a break in electrical transmission. Action potentials can not cross a synapse. Information is carried across a synapse by chemical transmitters. Chemical transmission is slower then electrical transmission. This results in a delay in transmission. Transmission is in one direction. A synapse consists of a:

- Presynaptic neurone
- Synaptic gap
- Postsynaptic neurone

Chemical transmitters are made and stored in the presynaptic terminal. Transmitters are stored in cytoplasmic vesicles.

Function of synapses

Neurotransmitters are released by an action potential and require the presence of calcium ions. The action potential arriving in the terminal axon opens calcium channels. Intracellular calcium is increased. Calcium causes vesicles to fuse to the membrane and the transmitter to be released. Transmitters diffuse across the synaptic gap and binds to post-synaptic receptors. The synaptic gap is short and the transmitter travels across it by simple diffusion.

When a transmitter binds to a receptor it produce a change in membrane potential. Depolarisation is known as an excitatory postsynaptic potential (EPSP). Hyperpolarisation is know as an inhibitory postsynaptic potential (IPSP). Most transmitters produce EPSPs – acetylcholine, adrenaline and noradrenaline. The major transmitters producing IPSPs are glycine and GABA. There are both excitatory and inhibitory nerves coming into most synapses. If there are enough EPSPs, the postsynaptic membrane will be depolarised to the threshold level. An action potential will be produced and a signal will be transmitted along the postsynaptic nerve. Once the signal has been delivered, the transmitter is removed. In some cases the transmitter is broken down by an enzyme in the synapse. In other cases, the transmitter is taken back up into the presynaptic neurone.

Neurotransmitters

Acetylcholine

Acetylcholine (ACh) is a simple molecule synthesised from choline and acetyl-CoA.

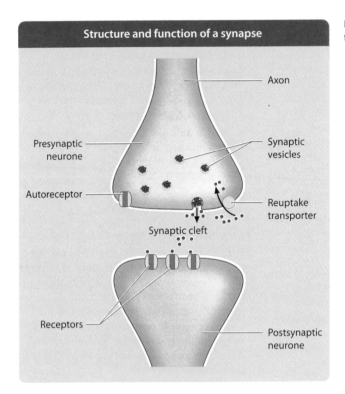

Figure 22.3 Structure and function of a synapse

This occurs through the action of the enzyme choline acetyltransferase. Neurones that synthesise and release ACh are termed cholinergic neurones. ACh receptors are ligand-gated cation channels. Two main classes of ACh receptors have been identified and are known as muscarinic and nicotinic receptors. Both receptor classes are abundant in the human brain. Nicotinic receptors are further divided into those found at neuromuscular junctions and those found at neuronal synapses. Numerous compounds have been identified that act as either agonists or antagonists of cholinergic neurones. The principal action of cholinergic agonists is the excitation or inhibition of autonomic effector cells. ACh is destroyed by hydrolysis using the enzyme acetylcholinesterase. The responses of cholinergic neurones can also be enhanced by administration of cholinesterase inhibitors.

Catecholamines

The principal catecholamines are noradrenaline, adrenaline and dopamine. These compounds are formed from phenylalanine and tyrosine. Tyrosine is produced in the liver from phenylalanine through the action of phenylalanine hydroxylase. Tyrosine is then transported to catecholamine-secreting neurones. A series of reactions convert it to dopamine, to noradrenaline and finally to adrenaline. Catecholamines exhibit peripheral nervous system excitatory and inhibitory effects. They bind to two different classes of receptors termed the α- and β-adrenergic receptors. The adrenergic receptors are coupled to intracellular G-proteins. Noradrenaline released from presynaptic noradrenergic neurones is recycled in the presynaptic neurone by a reuptake mechanism.

Serotonin

Serotonin (5-hydroxytryptamine, 5HT) is formed by the hydroxylation and decarboxylation of tryptophan. The greatest concentration of 5HT (90%) is found in the enterochromaffin cells of the gastrointestinal tract. Most of the remainder of the body's 5HT is found in platelets and the central nervous system. Neurones that secrete 5HT are termed serotonergic. The function of serotonin is exerted by its interaction with specific receptors. Several serotonin receptors have been identified and they are classified as 5HT1 to 5HT7. Some of these receptor types have subgroups. Most of these receptors are coupled to G-proteins that affect the activities of either adenylate cyclase or phospholipase C. Some serotonin receptors are presynaptic and others postsynaptic:

- 5HT2A receptors mediate platelet aggregation
- 5HT2C receptors are important in control of food intake
- 5HT3 receptors are present in the gastrointestinal tract and are related to vomiting
- 5HT6 and 5HT7 receptors are distributed throughout the limbic system
- 5HT6 receptors have high affinity for antidepressant drugs

Following the release of 5HT, some is taken back up by the presynaptic serotonergic neurones.

γ-Aminobutyric acid

Several amino acids have distinct excitatory or inhibitory effects upon the nervous system. γ-aminobutyric acid (GABA) is an inhibitor of presynaptic transmission in the central nervous system. GABA is formed by the decarboxylation of glutamate catalyzed by glutamate decarboxylase. GABA exerts its effects by binding to two distinct receptors, GABA-A and GABA-B. The GABA-A receptors form a chloride channel. The binding of GABA to GABA-A receptors increases the chloride conductance of presynaptic neurones. The GABA-B receptors are coupled to an intracellular G-protein and act by increasing conductance of an associated potassium channel.

Muscle and skeletal contraction

There are three basic types of muscle

- Skeletal muscle
- Cardiac muscle
- Smooth muscle

Skeletal muscle

Skeletal muscle is striated muscle under voluntary control. Muscle fibres are organised into motor units. When a single nerve enters a muscle it splits and activates several muscle cells. When the nerve fires, the whole motor unit is stimulated and the muscle cells contract together. Muscles with large motor units have coarse movements. Muscles with small motor units produce fine and graded movements. Muscle cells have a short refractory period.

Neuromuscular junction

Each muscle fibre is innervated by one motor neurone. Each muscle fibre has one neuromuscular junction. Each motor neurone can innervate multiple muscle fibres.

Excitation-contraction coupling

An end-plate potential is generated by a single motor neurone action potential. This is enough to depolarise the muscle and initiate a muscle action potential. This is propagated in both directions along the sarcolemma and T tubule system. The T tubular system communicates with the sarcoplasmic reticulum. Voltage-gated calcium channels open and releases calcium into the sarcoplasm, around the myofibrils. Interaction of calcium with troponin C results in muscle contraction. Muscle relaxation occurs when calcium is pumped back into the sarcoplasmic reticulum.

Muscle contraction

There are two types of muscle contraction – isotonic and isometric. In an isotonic contraction the muscle shortens, keeping a constant tension. In an isometric contraction the muscle does not shorten and tension builds up. Most muscle actions are a combination of both types of contraction.

Physiology of contraction

A single nerve impulse produces a muscle twitch. A single stimulus usually releases enough acetylcholine to produce an action potential in the muscle cell membranes. This will cause the muscle to contract after a short delay. A simple twitch usually only generates about 20–30% of the maximum tension and the muscle starts to relax before the maximum tension is reached. Muscle contractions can be added together to produce more force. If a second stimulus is given before a muscle relaxes, the muscle will shorten further. This process is known as summation. If many stimuli are given very close together the muscle will go into continuous contraction called tetanus which gives a maximum tension several times higher than a simple twitch. Another way to increase the force of contraction is to recruit more motor units. Muscle produces the greatest isometric tension at intermediate lengths. At rest, many of the body's muscles are close to their optimum lengths.

Fibre types

Within skeletal muscles, there are different types of muscle fibres. The relative proportions of the different types varies between muscles and individuals. Type 1 or red fibres have many mitochondria, contain myoglobin, contract slowly but resist fatigue. Type 2 or white fibres contain few mitochondria, rely on glycolysis to supply energy, contract rapidly but fatigue quickly.

The sarcomere

The basic unit of muscle contraction is the sarcomere (**Figure 22.4**). The striated appearance of skeletal muscle is due to the alignment of molecules in bands and lines. The most prominent are the A and I bands and the Z line. The unit between two Z lines is called the sarcomere. When muscle contracts the sarcomere shortens and the Z lines move closer together.

Actin and myosin

When muscle contracts, the protein filaments slide together. Muscle is composed of two contractile proteins:

- Thin filaments – actin, is found in both A and I bands
- Thick filaments – myosin, is found in the A band

Actin and myosin connect through crossbridges. The more crossbridges there are, the higher the tension. ATP is required for both contraction and relaxation of muscle. It is required for the sliding of the filaments, accomplished by a bending movement of the myosin heads. ATP is also required for the separation of actin and myosin which relaxes the muscle. A sudden inflow of calcium is the trigger for muscle contraction. In the resting state, the protein tropomyosin winds around actin and covers the myosin binding sites. The calcium binds to a second protein, troponin. This causes the tropomyosin to be pulled to deform, exposing the myosin binding sites. With the sites exposed, the muscle contracts.

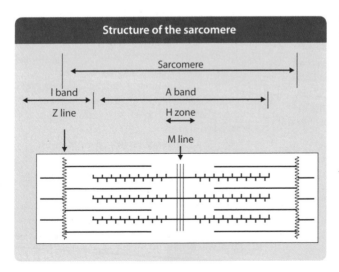

Figure 22.4 Structure of the sarcomere

Joints of the upper limb

The shoulder

The shoulder girdle is made up of a complex of five joints:

- Sternoclavicular joint
- Acromioclavicular joint
- Subacromial space
- Glenohumeral joint
- Scapulothoracic joint

The glenohumeral joint is a synovial ball and socket joint. Articulation occurs between the head of the humerus and the glenoid cavity. The articular surfaces are covered with hyaline cartilage. The surface area of the glenoid cavity is deepened by a rim of fibrocartilage – the glenoid labrum. The capsule is thin, allows a large range of movement and is strengthened by ligaments, as follows:

- Glenohumeral ligaments
- Transverse humeral ligament
- Coracohumeral ligament
- Coracoacromial ligament

The nerve supply is from the axillary and suprascapular nerves. The stability of the joint if provided by the muscles that cross it. The movements are flexion, extension, abduction, adduction lateral and medial rotation.

The rotator cuff is made up of:

- Supraspinatus
- Infraspinatus
- Teres minor
- Subscapularis

The elbow

The elbow is a synovial hinge joint. Articulation occurs between the trochlea and capitulum of the humerus and the notch of the ulna and the radial head. The articular surfaces are covered with hyaline cartilage. The capsule is strengthened by medial and lateral ligaments. The synovial membrane is continuous with that of the superior radioulnar joint. The nerve supply is from median, ulnar, musculocutaneous and radial nerves. The long axis of the extended arm is at an angle to the long axis of the arm. This is known as the carrying angle. The movements are flexion and extension.

The superior radioulnar joint

The superior radioulnar joint is a synovial pivot joint. Articulation occurs between the head of the radius and annular ligament and radial notch of the ulna. The annular ligament is attached to the anterior and posterior margins of the radial notch of the ulna and this forms a collar around the head of the radius. The synovial membrane and capsule is continuous with that of the elbow. The nerve supply is from the median, ulnar, musculocutaneous and radial nerves. The movements are pronation and supination.

Nerves of the upper limb

Brachial plexus

The brachial plexus has the following parts:

- Roots – which are from the anterior rami of the C5 to 8 and T1 nerves
- Trunks – upper, middle and lower from the joining of the roots
- Divisions – from splitting of the trunks
- Cords – from the union of the division.

The cords are lateral to the first part of the axillary artery and are mediolateral and posterior to the second part of the axillary artery (**Figure 22.5**).

Axillary nerve

The axillary nerve arises from the posterior cord of the brachial plexus (C5, C6). It passes through the quadrangular space and winds around the neck of humerus. The muscles supplied are the deltoid and teres minor. An axillary nerve palsy may occur as a result of anterior dislocation of the shoulder joint. The result is:

- Motor impairment – abduction of the arm
- Sensory impairment – sensation reduced over the deltoid muscle

Radial nerve

The radial nerve arises from the posterior cord of the brachial plexus (C5-T1). It passes along with the profunda brachial artery and travels through the radial groove on the posterior aspect of the humerus. The muscles supplied are triceps and all the muscles of the extensor compartment of the forearm. The radial nerve may be damaged in fractures of the shaft of

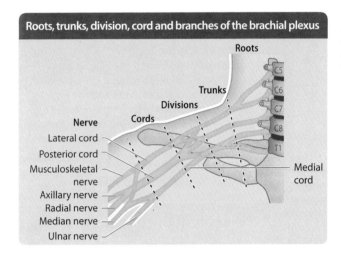

Figure 22.5 Roots, trunks, division, cord and branches of the brachial plexus. (Reproduced from Goodfellow JA. Pocket Tutor Neurological Examination. London: JP Medical Ltd, 2012.)

the humerus as it passes through the spiral groove. The results is:

- A wrist drop
- Motor impairment – inability to extend the elbow, wrists and fingers
- Sensory impairment – sensation reduced over the lower posterior part of the arm, forearm and the anatomical 'snuff box'

Median nerve

The median nerve has two roots – medial and lateral (C5–T1). The medial root arises from the medial cord of the brachial plexus. The lateral root arises from the lateral cord of the brachial plexus. It passes through the carpal tunnel. The muscles supplied are all the muscles of the forearm except for flexor carpi ulnaris and the medial half of flexor digitorum profundus and in the hand, the muscles of the thenar eminence and the lateral two lumbricals. A median nerve palsy results in:

- Thenar eminence wasting with an ape-like thumb
- Motor impairment – wrist flexion and finger flexion at the interphalangeal joints (except the 4th and 5th DIP joints). Flexion of the index and middle fingers at the metacarpophalangeal joints and inability to abduct and oppose the thumb
- Sensory impairment – sensation reduced over the lateral half of the palm and the lateral three and half fingers

Ulnar nerve

The ulnar nerve arises from the medial cord of the brachial plexus (C8, T1). It passes behind the medial epicondyle of humerus and in front of the flexor retinaculum at the wrist. The muscles supplied in the forearm are the flexor carpi ulnaris and the medial half of flexor digitorum profundus and in the hand, the hypothenar muscles, all the interossei, the 3rd and 4th lumbricals, adductor policis, and palmaris brevis. An ulnar nerve palsy results in:

- Hypothenar wasting and claw-hand deformity
- Motor impairment – wrist flexion and ring and little finger flexion at the distal interphalangeal joints. Adduction and abduction of of the fingers and adduction of the thumb
- Sensory impairment – sensation reduced over the medial half of the palm and the medial one and half fingers

Bones of the hands

The eight carpal bones (**Figure 22.6**) are made up of two rows of four.

The proximal row contains the:

- Scaphoid
- Lunate
- Triquetral
- Pisiform

Bones of the wrist and hand

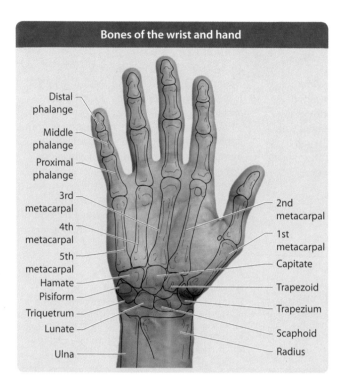

Distal phalange

Middle phalange

Proximal phalange

3rd metacarpal

4th metacarpal

5th metacarpal

Hamate

Pisiform

Triquetrum

Lunate

Ulna

2nd metacarpal

1st metacarpal

Capitate

Trapezoid

Trapezium

Scaphoid

Radius

Figure 22.6 Bones of the wrist and hand. (Reproduced from Tunstall R and Shah N. Pocket Tutor Surface Anatomy. London: JP Medical Ltd, 2012, and courtesy of Sam Scott-Hunter, London.)

The distal row contains the:

- Trapezium
- Trapezoid
- Capitate
- Hamate

Joints of the lower limb

The hip

The hip is a synovial ball and socket joint. Articulation occurs between the head of the femur and the acetabulum of the hip bone. The articular surface is horseshoe-shaped and deficient at the acetabular notch. The cavity is deepened by a rim of fibrocartilage knows as the acetabular labrum. The articular surfaces are covered with hyaline cartilage. The capsule is strengthened by ligaments as follows:

- Iliofemoral ligament
- Pubofemoral ligament
- Ischiofemoral ligament
- Transverse acetabular ligament

The nerve supply is from the femoral, obturator and sciatic nerves. The movements are flexion, extension, abduction, adduction, medial and lateral rotation.

The knee

The knee is a synovial joint but it is not a simple hinge. It has two component which are articulations between the femoral and tibial condyles and the patellofemoral joint. It is stabilised by the knee ligaments as follows:

- Anterior cruciate ligament prevents anterior translation of the tibia
- Posterior cruciate ligament prevents posterior translation of the tibia
- Medial collateral ligament provides valgus stability
- Lateral collateral ligament provides varus stability
- Posteromedial capsule resists external rotation
- Posterolateral capsule resists internal rotation

The menisci are semi-lunar shaped fibrocartilages. They increase the joint congruence and distribute the load across the joint. They are avascular and heal poorly beyond the peripheries. Knee movements are complex; the knee has dynamic stability.

The ankle

The ankle joint is a synovial hinge joint. Articulation occurs between the lower end of tibia, the two malleoli and the body of the talus. The articular surfaces are covered with hyaline cartilage. The capsule is thin and allows a large range of movement. The capsule is strengthened by ligaments as follows:

- Medial or deltoid ligament
- Anterior talofibular ligament
- Calcaneofibular ligament
- Posterior talofibular ligament

The nerve supply is from the deep peroneal and tibial nerves. The movements are dorsiflexion and plantar flexion. Important anatomical relations to the ankle include:

Structures that pass superficial to the extensor retinacula:

- Saphenous nerve
- Long saphenous vein
- Superficial peroneal nerve

Structures that pass deep to the extensor retinaculum:

- Tibialis anterior tendon
- Extensor hallucis longus tendon
- Anterior tibial artery
- Deep peroneal nerve
- Extensor digitorum longus
- Peroneus tertius

Structures that pass behind the medial malleolus deep to the flexor retinaculum:

- Tibialis posterior tendon
- Flexor digitorum longus
- Posterior tibial artery
- Tibial nerve
- Flexor hallucis longus

Structures that pass behind the lateral malleolus superficial to the superior peroneal retinaculum:

- Sural nerve
- Short saphenous vein

Structures that pass behind the lateral malleolus deep to the superior peroneal retinaculum:

- Peroneus longus tendon
- Peroneus brevis tendon

Skeletal fractures

Pathophysiology

Dislocation is total loss of congruity between two articular surfaces. Subluxation is partial loss of congruity between two articular surfaces. A fracture is a break in continuity of a bone. Fractures heal by restoration of bone continuity. The rate of healing varies with age and is quicker in children. Cancellous bone heals more quickly than cortical bone. Some movement at fractures site is required for healing to occur. It also requires an uninterrupted blood supply. Bone healing can arbitrarily be divided in to five stages (**Table 22.1**).

Principles of management

Some general principles can be applied to fracture management. For every fracture it is necessary to consider:

- Reduction of the fracture
- Immobilisation of the fracture
- Rehabilitation

Stages of bone healing	
Stage	Features
Stage 1	Haematoma formation Bone ends bleed Periosteum is stripped for variable length Surrounding soft tissues may be damaged
Stage 2	Acute inflammation Cell division begins within 8 hours Cell proliferation seen within periosteum
Stage 3	Callus formation Dead bone is resorbed Immature woven bone is laid down
Stage 4	Woven bone is replaced by lamellar bone Fracture becomes united
Stage 5	Phase of remodelling Medullary cavity is restored Bone returns to normal shape

Table 22.1 Stages of bone healing

The need for accurate reduction varies from fracture to fracture. There is usually a need to correct rotational or valgus or varus deformity. Intra-articular fractures need accurate anatomical reduction. Reduction can be performed as either an open or closed procedure. Immobilisation is required until fracture union occurs and can be performed by external or internal methods.

External methods of immobilisation include:

- Plaster casts
- Traction
- External fixation

Internal methods of immobilisation include:

- Plates
- Intramedullary nails
- K-wires

Indications for internal fixation include:

- Intra-articular fractures – to stabilise an anatomical reduction
- Repair of blood vessels and nerves – to protect vascular and nerve repairs
- Multiple injuries
- Elderly patients – to allow early mobilisation
- Long bone fractures – tibia, femur and humerus
- Failure of conservative management
- Pathological fractures
- Fractures that require open reduction
- Unstable fractures

Complications of internal fixation include:

- Infection
- Non-union
- Implant failure
- Refracture

Indications for external fixation include:

- Acute trauma – open and unstable fractures
- Non-union of fractures
- Arthrodesis
- Correction of joint contracture
- Filling of segmental limb defects – trauma, tumour and osteomyelitis
- Limb lengthening

Complications of external fixation include:

- Overdistraction
- Pin-tract infection

Union and consolidation

Fracture repair is a continuous process. The stages into which it is divided are somewhat arbitrary. Union should be regarded as an incomplete repair and is present when an ensheathing callus is formed. The fracture site is still tender. Minimal movement at the fracture site is present. Consolidation should be regarded as a complete repair. Radiologically the fracture line is obliterated. The fracture site is non-tender and no movement is possible. The time to union and consolidation depends on many factors including:

- Age
- Fracture type
- Blood supply

Fractures heal quicker in children. Upper limb fractures heal quicker than lower limb fractures. Spiral fractures heal quicker than transverse fractures.

Complications

The majority of fractures heal according to expectations. In some cases, the healing process is delayed by complications. The possible early and late complications of fractures are shown in **Table 22.2**. Early complications are often related to damage to

Early and late complications of fractures	
Early	**Late**
Infection	Delayed union
Fat embolism	Non-union
Muscle and tendon injuries	Malunion
	Avascular necrosis
Nerve injuries	Myositis ossificans
Vascular injuries	Volkmann's contracture
Visceral injuries	Stiffness and instability
	Algodystrophy
	Reflex sympathetic dystrophy

Table 22.2 Early and late complications of fractures

adjacent structures. Late complications are often related to local bone problems.

Delayed union

Delayed union is prolongation of the time to fracture union. No definite timetable to define delayed union exists. Delayed union is due to:

- Inadequate blood supply
- Infection
- Incorrect splintage
- Intact fellow bone

In delayed union, the fracture site remains tender. The bones may still move when stressed. On x-ray the fracture remains visible and little callus formation or periosteal reaction is seen. Management usually involves continuation of the previous fracture management. It may be necessary to replace casts or reduce traction. Functional bracing may promote bone union. If union is delayed more than 6 months, then it may be necessary to consider internal fixation or bone grafting.

Non-union

Non-union is failure of the fracture site to unite. It has many causes including:

- Bone or soft tissue loss
- Soft tissue interposition
- Poor blood supply
- Infection
- Pathological fracture
- Poor splintage or fixation
- Fracture distraction

Clinical assessment shows remaining movement at the fracture site. Movement is often relatively painless. Radiologically, the fracture is still visible and the bone ends on either side of the fracture are sclerosed. Non-union can be either hypertrophic or atrophic depending on the presence or absence of bone loss. Asymptomatic non-union may not require active treatment except splintage. For hypertrophic non-union, internal or external fixation may be necessary to achieve union. For atrophic non-union bone grafting is invariably required.

Myositis ossificans

Myositis ossificans is due to heterotopic ossification with a muscle. The elbow is the commonest joint involved. It is occasionally seen following a joint dislocation or muscle rupture. It also occurs without injury in unconscious or paraplegic patients. Pain is an early symptom. Joint stiffness and a reduced range of movement are late features. In the late stage of the process, a bony lump is often palpable. Early x-rays shows fluffy calcification. Late x-rays shows bone formation. Management involves joint rest in the position of function. Once pain settles, mobilisation can be begun. After several months, consideration should be given to excision of the bony mass.

Avascular necrosis

Avascular necrosis occurs when a fracture interrupts the blood supply to adjacent bone. Certain regions are prone to bone ischaemia and necrosis including the head of the femur, the proximal scaphoid and the body of the talus. Pain is the main symptom due to fracture non-union. X-ray shows an increase in bone density. Surgical intervention is required if there is a reduction in function. This may require an arthrodesis or arthroplasty.

Compound fractures

All open fractures must be assumed to be contaminated. The aim of treatment is to prevent them from becoming infected. First aid treatment is the same as for a closed fracture. Peripheral neurovascular status should be assessed. In addition, the wound should be covered with a sterile dressing. Wounds should be photographed so that repeated uncovering is avoided. Antibiotic prophylaxis should be given and the tetanus immunisation status should be evaluated.

Open fractures require early operation and ideally this should be within 6 hours of injury. The aims of surgery are to:

- Clean the wound
- Remove devitalised tissue
- Stabilise the fracture

Small clean wounds can be sutured. Large dirty wounds should be debrided and left open. Debrided wounds can be closed by delayed primary suture at about 5 days.

Pathological fractures

A pathologic fracture is one caused by a disease leading to a weakness of the bone (**Table 22.3**). This process is most commonly

Causes of pathological fractures		
Generalised	**Localised**	**Malignant**
Osteoporosis	Chronic infection	Osteosarcoma
Metabolic bone disease	Solitary bone cyst	Chondrosarcoma
Paget's disease	Fibrous cortical defect	Ewing's tumour
Myelomatosis	Chondroma	

Table 22.3 Causes of pathological fractures

due to osteoporosis, but may also be due to other pathologies such malignancy, infection, inherited bone disorders or a bone cyst. The commonest cancers that metastasise to bone and result in pathological fractures are breast, prostate, kidney, lung and thyroid. A pathological fracture usually occurs during normal activities when the underlying disease process weakens the bone to the point where it is unable to perform its normal function.

The aims of surgery for a pathological fracture are to provide pain relief and a stable bone or joint that will allow the patient to mobilise shortly after surgery and will last for the remaining life of the patient. Given the frequent large amount of bone loss, the degree of osteoporosis in the elderly, and the decreased ability of bone to heal at a tumour site, this is often difficult to achieve. The techniques used in these patients differ from those used in young trauma patients.

Principles of bone grafting

Loss of bone can occur in several situations including trauma, tumours or following the use of prostheses. The use of bone grafts may be necessary to fill the resulting defect. Bone grafts can be classified as:

- Autograft – Bone from the same individual
- Allograft – Bone from another individual of the same species
- Xenograft – Bone from another species

Autografts

Autogenous bone is the ideal graft material but it may only be available in limited amounts. Cancellous bone can be used to fill cavity defects. Cortical bone can be used to provide structural support. Both form a scaffold into which osteoblasts and osteoclasts can grow. The graft stimulates local bone growth by the process of osteoinduction. Osteoblast differentiation leads to graft resorption. Remodelling occurs as load is applied to the graft.

Bone grafts can be harvested from the iliac crest, proximal tibia and distal radius. The iliac crest is the most common donor site but its use is associated with significant morbidity. Cortico-cancellous grafts are harvested as strips. Cancellous bone can be taken from the inner or outer table. Segments of bone can be transplanted as free vascularised grafts. Local rotational bone grafts may also be used. The blood supply to the graft is maintained. They are technically difficult to perform and the results are unpredictable.

Allografts

Allograft bone is more plentiful and can be harvested from living donors or cadavers. Donor site morbidity is eliminated. Cadaveric bone and femoral heads are stored in tissue banks. Bone is frozen at −20 to −86°C. Freeze drying and storage at room temperature is occasionally used. Allografts are used in reconstruction after tumour resection or revision hip surgery. Infection is the major concern with the used of allografts. Bacterial contamination may occur, especially with cadaveric grafts but this risk can be eliminated with irradiation of the graft. Viral contamination with hepatitis or HIV is possible. Bone should be kept in quarantine and living donors tested 90 days after the bone is harvested. Allograft bone is available as morsellised bone for impaction grafting, strut grafts to cover cortical bone and massive allografts to replace significant proportions of native bone.

Bone substitutes

Interest exists in developing artificial bone substitutes that would eliminate the supply and infection problems associated with auto and allografts. Possible bone substitutes include calcium triphosphate, hydroxyapatite, calcium carbonate and glass-based cements. Unfortunately, most bone substitutes are brittle and are unable to withstand significant load bearing.

Hip fractures

In the UK, approximately 60,000 proximal femoral fractures occur each year. The mean age of patient is 80 years. The incidence increases exponentially above the age of 65 years and the main risk factors are female sex and osteoporosis. About 40% of patients with a hip fracture die within a year and 50% of survivors are less independent than before the injury. Most morbidity and mortality is related to coexisting medical conditions. The cost of managing all hip fractures in the UK is about £2 billion per year.

Clinical features

Proximal femoral fractures usually occur following a fall. Patients often have other significant co-morbidity. The main symptom is hip pain and an inability to weight bear. The leg may be shortened and externally rotated.

Investigation

The diagnosis confirmed by a anterior-posterior and lateral x-ray. However, impacted undisplaced fractures may present diagnostic difficulty. Fractures are best separated into intracapsular and extracapsular fractures. The Garden classification of hip fractures is as follows:

- Stage 1 – incomplete or impacted fracture
- Stage 2 – complete fracture with no displacement
- Stage 3 – complete fracture with partial displacement

- Stage 4 – complete fracture with significant displacement

Intracapsular fractures reduce the blood supply to the femoral head. They are at high-risk of delayed union, non-union or avascular necrosis. If the femoral head is to be preserved they need anatomical reduction. Extracapsular fractures do not interfere with femoral head blood supply and do not require anatomical reduction.

Management

All patients should be considered for surgery if fit enough for an operation. Early mobilisation is associated with improved long-term prognosis. Ideally surgery should be performed within 24 hours and postoperative rehabilitation should be by a multidisciplinary team. Multidisciplinary rehabilitation should involve mobilisation strategies, early supported discharge and intermediate care.

Intracapsular fractures

The three treatment options for intracapsular fractures are reduction and internal fixation, femoral head replacement or total joint replacement. Internal fixation is indicated in undisplaced fractures or displaced fractures in patients less than 70 years of age. Internal fixation is usually achieved with the use of three cancellous screws. Complications include non-union and avascular necrosis. Femoral head replacement is indicated in displaced and pathological fractures. The options available include:

- Cemented Thompson prosthesis
- Uncemented Austin Moore prosthesis
- Bipolar prosthesis

Total hip replacements should be considered in those with a displaced intracapsular fracture who were able to walk independently, are not cognitively impaired and are medically fit for anaesthesia and the operation. Complications of femoral head and joint replacement include:

- Dislocation
- Loosening
- Peri-prosthetic femoral fracture

Extracapsular fractures

Extracapsular fractures are usually repaired with a dynamic hip screw. This allows impaction and stabilisation of fracture. The prognosis is related to the number of bone fragments but about 90% of fractures proceed to uncomplicated fracture union.

Ankle fractures

Ankle fractures are the commonest lower limb fractures. They occur following high-energy impacts or low-energy twists. Low-energy twists cause rotation of the talus within the joint and occur if the foot is either internally or externally rotated.

Classification

The Weber classification is based on the level of any associated fibular fracture in relation to the syndesmosis:

- Type A – below the syndesmosis
- Type B – at the level (often spiral or oblique) of the syndesmosis
- Type C – above the syndesmosis

This classification does not take account of other injuries (e.g. medial malleolus). The Lauge–Hansen classification is based on the position of the foot and direction of deforming force:

- Supination–adduction
- Supination–external rotation
- Pronation–abduction
- Pronation–eversion
- Pronation–dorsiflexion

Investigation

A plain anterior-posterior and lateral ankle x-ray will show the fracture/dislocation. A motrice view (10–20°) in line with the intermalleolar line my show any diastasis – widening of the gap between the tibia and fibula.

Management

Suspected ankle fractures should be promptly assessed. Fracture-dislocations should be reduced and stabilised. This is required to prevent overlying skin necrosis. Future management depends on the fracture type and stability. Type A injuries are stable and require minimal splintage. Type B injuries

confined to the lateral part of the ankle are also stable. Type C injuries often appear undisplaced but there is often a significant ligament injury. Consideration should be given to examination under anaesthesia and fixation. The majority of displaced fractures require open reduction and fixation. The medial and posterior malleoli are fixed with lag screws. The fibular fracture is stabilised with a plate.

Other common fractures

Scaphoid fracture

Scaphoid fractures account for 75% of all carpal bone injuries and are usually caused by a fall on the outstretched hand. They usually occur in young and middle-aged adults. About 10% are associated with other fractures. Most scaphoid fractures are stable. If recognised and treated appropriately, then over 90% heal without complication. The symptoms of a scaphoid fracture include pain on the radial side of the wrist, swelling in that area, and difficulty gripping objects. The classical sign is tenderness in the 'anatomical snuff-box'. The commonest site of fracture is through the waist of the bone. The initial x-ray may be normal. If there is clinical suspicion of a fracture then the wrist should be splinted and the x-ray repeated. CT scanning is useful if their remains diagnostic doubt. Treatment of undisplaced fractures is by splinting for 6 weeks. The blood supply of the scaphoid enters the bone distally and diminishes proximally. As a result, fractures through the proximal pole are at greatest risk of complications including avascular necrosis and non-union. Internal fixation should be considered for displaced fractures.

Colles fracture

A Colles fracture is a fracture of the distal radius with dorsal displacement and angulation of the distal fragment. It was first described by the Irish surgeon and anatomist, Abraham Colles, in 1814. It is most commonly seen in post-menopausal women and usually occurs after a fall on the outstretched hand. It results in a classic 'dinner fork' deformity of the wrist. There are five components to the deformity:

- Dorsal angulation of the distal fragment
- Dorsal displacement of the distal fragment
- Radial deviation of the hand
- Supination
- Proximal impaction

In severe cases, there may be dislocation of the distal radio-ulnar joint or fracture of the styloid process of the ulna. Management depends on the severity of the fracture and the age of the patient. A minimally displaced fracture may be treated with a cast alone. The cast is applied with the distal fragment in palmar flexion and ulnar deviation. A fracture with mild angulation and displacement may require closed reduction. Significant angulation and deformity may require an open reduction and internal fixation or external fixation.

Paediatric fractures

About 50% of boys and 25% of girls will sustain a fracture during childhood. Children tend to develop a specific pattern of fractures. The commonest location of fractures is the upper extremities. The distal radius and humerus are the commonest sites of fracture.

Paediatric fractures are fundamentally different from those seen in adults. The decreased bone mineral density, proportionally stronger ligaments and tendons, increased bone flexibility and developing growth plates lead to unique fracture patterns. Greenstick fractures occur when the bone bends and partially breaks but does not extend through the width of the bone. Salter and Harris fractures (**Figure 22.7**)

occur through the growth plate and therefore they are unique to children. They are classified according to the degree of involvement of physis, metaphysis and epiphysis:

- Type I – Epiphyseal slip – no fracture
- Type II – Fracture through the epiphyeal plate with proximal fragment
- Type III – Fracture through the epiphysis extending into the epiphyseal plate
- Type IV – Fracture through both the epiphysis and shaft crossing the epiphyseal plate
- Type V – Crush injury causing obliteration of the growth plate

Classification is important as it determines both the treatment and prognosis. Overall, physeal fractures are responsible for about 30% of all long bone fractures in children. In general, the following statements hold true for Slater and Harris fractures:

- Type I involve the growth plate but growth is rarely disturbed
- Type II fractures are the most common
- Type III fractures involve the joint and can result in chronic morbidity
- Type III fractures often require surgical treatment
- Type IV fractures can also result in chronic morbidity
- Type V fractures are difficult to diagnose and can result in limb shortening

Management
Bones in children have a tremendous power for remodelling and in their management, more angulation or displacement can be

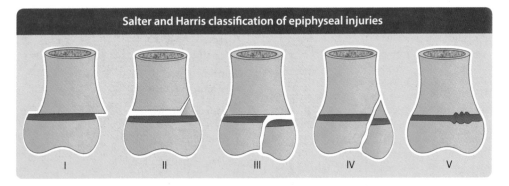

Salter and Harris classification of epiphyseal injuries

I	II	III	IV	V

Figure 22.7 Salter and Harris classification of epiphyseal injuries

accepted than in adults. Unfortunately, rotational malalignment does not remodel.

Degenerative and rheumatoid arthritis

Osteoarthritis

Osteoarthritis is the commonest condition affecting synovial joints. It is no longer considered as simple 'wear and tear'. A change in the cartilaginous matrix is probably an important aetiological factor. Primary osteoarthritis is of unknown aetiology. Secondary osteoarthritis is the result of congenital or infective joint disorders or trauma. The pathology is characterised by:

- Loss of hyaline cartilage
- Subchondral bone sclerosis
- Subchondral cyst formation
- Osteophyte formation

Several patterns of joint involvement are recognised including generalised nodular osteoarthritis and large joint osteoarthritis.

Clinical features

The joint pain associated with osteoarthritis is worse after exercise or at the end of the day and is relieved by rest. Early morning stiffness or stiffness after rest is limited. There may be bony joint swelling. Systemic features are few.

Management

The aims of treatment of osteoarthritis are to reduce joint pain and improve joint function. In the early stages, pain can often be improved with simple analgesia. Life style modification is also important. Anti-inflammatory drugs can often help and intra-articular steroid injections can reduce symptoms. If symptoms fail to improve with conservative measures, surgery may be required. The surgical options for degenerative joints are:

- Arthroscopic lavage and debridement
- Osteotomy – alteration of joint alignment
- Arthroplasty – replacement of diseased joint
- Arthrodesis – fusion of disease joint

Rheumatoid arthritis

Rheumatoid arthritis is an autoimmune inflammatory synovial disease of unknown aetiology. The worldwide prevalence is approximately 1% and the female to male ratio is about 3:1. The onset of symptoms is usually between 20 and 40 years of age. As well as the synovium of joints, it can also involve the tendon sheaths. It is seem more commonly in those with human leukocyte antigens DR4 and DW4. Pathologically, it is characterised by:

- An inflammatory process within the synovium
- Joint destruction and pannus formation
- Periarticular erosions

Clinical features

Rheumatoid arthritis, usually affects multiple joints. The commonest joints involved are the hands, elbows, knees and cervical spine. There is often prolonged early morning stiffness and stiffness after rest. The joint pain associated with rheumatoid arthritis is invariably relieved by movement. Soft tissue swelling and erythema is often marked and systemic features may be present. Extra-articular manifestations occur in approximately about 20% of patients (**Table 22.4**). Rheumatoid arthritis is seen as part of several well defined syndromes (**Table 22.5**).

In the early stages of the disease in the hands, synovitis of the metacarpophalangeal (MCP) and proximal interphalangeal (PIP) joints is often the main clinical feature. Both hands are usually affected in a symmetrical pattern. The tendon sheaths may also be inflamed. This early stage often progresses to joint and tendon erosions which prepare the ground for later mechanical derangement. Joint instability and tendon rupture results in progressive deformity and functional loss. In the late stage of the disease, the hands typically show subluxation of the MCP joints, radial deviation of the wrist joint and ulnar deviation of the fingers (**Figure 22.8**). Swan neck (hyperextension of the PIP joint with flexion of the DIP joint) and boutonniere deformities (flexion of the PIP joint and extension of the DIP joint) of the fingers may occur.

Extra-articular manifestations of rheumatoid arthritis	
System	**Manifestation**
Ocular	Keratoconjunctivitis sicca
	Episcleritis
	Scleritis
Pulmonary	Pulmonary nodules
	Pleural effusion
	Fibrosing alveolitis
Cardiac	Pericarditis/pericardial effusion
	Valvular heart disease
	Conduction defects
Cutaneous	Palmar erythema
	Rheumatoid nodules
	Pyoderma gangrenosum
	Vasculitic rashes and leg ulceration
Neurological	Nerve entrapment
	Cervical myelopathy
	Peripheral neuropathy
	Mononeuritis multiplex

Table 22.4 Extra-articular manifestations of rheumatoid arthritis

Syndromes associated with rheumatoid arthritis	
Syndrome	**Clinical features**
Felty's syndrome	Rheumatoid arthritis
	Neutropenia
	Lymphadenopathy
	Splenomegaly
Still's disease	Rheumatoid arthritis in childhood
	Rash
	Fever
	Splenomegaly
Sjögren's syndrome	Rheumatoid arthritis
	Reduced lacrimal and salivary secretion

Table 22.5 Syndromes associated with rheumatoid arthritis

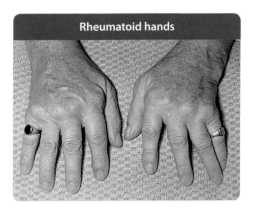

Rheumatoid hands

Figure 22.8 Rheumatoid hands

Management

Management of rheumatoid arthritis requires a multidisciplinary approach. Disease modifying drugs include:

- Non-steroidal anti-inflammatory drugs
- Methotrexate, sulphasalazine, penicillamine, gold
- Corticosteroids
- Cytotoxic drugs

Surgical intervention in patients with rheumatoid arthritis can achieve pain relief, deformity correction and functional improvement. A number of surgical procedures are available including:

- Myofascial techniques
- Excisions
- Reconstructions
- Joint fusions
- Joint replacements

The timing of surgery is a complex decision and depends on:

- Patient's age
- Stage of disease
- Level of disability
- Site of the involved joints

Early surgical intervention may be helpful in maintaining a patient's functional level. Deformities of the hand or wrist lead to loss of the ability to grip, grasp and pinch, often leaving the patient unable to perform the activities of daily living. The surgical treatments for rheumatoid arthritis of the hand and wrist include:

- Synovectomy
- Tenosynovectomy
- Tendon realignment
- Arthroplasty
- Arthrodesis

Hip replacement surgery

Hip replacement surgery was developed by Sir John Charnley in the 1960s. More than 50,000 hip replacements are performed each year in the UK and over 2 million hips have been replaced worldwide. Over 100 different types of prosthesis have been used. The 'gold standard' is the Charnley cemented prosthesis.

Principle components

The acetabular component is usually made of high density polyethylene. This is biocompatible, has a low coefficient of friction and a low rate of wear. Ceramic acetabular components have improved surface properties but are expensive and have a tendency to brittle failure. Metal cups are obsolete due to high friction, loosening and wear. The femoral component is usually made of stainless steel, titanium or cobalt-chrome alloy. It is resistant to corrosion with high endurance. Improved longevity is seen with a small femoral head.

Polymethylmethacrylate cement

Polymethylmethacrylate cement acts as a filling agent without adhesive properties. Macrolocking occurs with cement in drilled holes. Microlocking occurs with cement in the interstices of cancellous bone. It produces an exothermic reaction during preparation. Addition of barium weakens the cement. Antibiotic impregnation may increase the resistance to infection. Recently uncemented prostheses have been developed. These require a more exacting insertion technique. They are anchored by an interference fit achieved by a porous surface or hydroxyapatite coating. Uncemented prostheses have a tendency to early failure.

Indications for hip replacement surgery include:

- Osteoarthritis
- Rheumatoid arthritis
- Still's disease
- Ankylosing spondylitis
- Congenital dysplastic or dislocated hips
- Paget's disease
- Trauma or avascular necrosis
- Septic arthritis

Contraindications for hip replacement surgery:

- Uncontrolled medical problems
- Skeletal immaturity
- Active infection
- Neuropathic joint
- Progressive neurological disease
- Muscle weakness

Surgery

To justify surgery, patients should have significant pain, functional disturbance and failed conservative therapy. The principle aims of surgery are to reduce joint pain and improve joint function. The operative technique requires thorough skin preparation with sterile adhesive plastic drapes. Operating teams should wear two pairs of gloves and body exhaust suites may be worn. Laminar air flow should be provided in the operative field and antibiotic prophylaxis should be given. Specific complications include:

- Neurovascular injuries
- Leg length discrepancy
- Dislocation
- Infection
- Aseptic loosening
- Implant wear and failure
- Heterotopic ossification
- Femoral fractures
- Trochanteric non-union
- Abductor mechanism weakness

The outcome of hip replacement surgery is affected by many factors including the:

- Type of implant used
- Underlying diagnosis
- Sex of patient
- Cement type
- Cementing technique
- Surgical approach

Joint resurfacing

The outcome of hip replacement surgery of joint replacement surgery is less predictable in younger patients and those with an active life style. Metal-on-metal hip resurfacing has been developed for use in younger patients. The head of the femur is preserved and is developed into chamfered cylinder. A metal head is cemented in place and a metal cup is placed in the acetabulum. Compared to total hip replacement, joint resurfacing has a lower risk of complications, lower risk of dislocation, less bone loss and a reduced risk of component loosing. The short-term results are very encouraging but the long-term outcome remains unclear.

Infected joint replacements

Most joint replacements are carried out with few complications. When it occurs, infection is a devastating outcome. It is uncommon and occurs in approximately 1% of cases. It results in major morbidity and considerable cost. The risk can be reduced by, excluding patients who have active infection, antibiotic prophylaxis and meticulous theatre technique.

Microbiology

The commonest organisms identified in infected joint replacements are:

- Coagulase-negative staphylococcus (45%)
- *Staphylococcus aureus* (35%)
- *Streptococcal species* (10%)
- Gram-negative bacteria (<5%)

Early infection is usually a result of intraoperative contamination. Late infection usually results from haematogenous spread. Bacteria adhere to prosthetic materials and produce a biofilm which isolates the bacteria from host defences and antibiotics. Significant infection can result from a small bacterial inoculum. A low-grade inflammatory process then occurs and this leads to bone erosion and loss of bone stock.

Clinical features

Acute joint infection presents with sign of a wound infection. A purulent discharge from the wound is often present. Chronic infection presents more insidiously and pain is often the prominent symptom. The diagnosis of chronic infection can be difficult.

Investigation

The following investigations should be considered:

- Microbial culture
- Inflammatory markers
- Plain radiography
- Bone scan
- Histology
- Molecular methods

The diagnosis depends on identification of bacteria from fluid around the joint.

Management

Antibiotics should be started once the diagnosis is considered but alone they are rarely able to eradicate established infection. The antibiotic of choice should be based on culture results. In acute infection joint, debridement and washout of the joint may be appropriate. In chronic infection with a loose joint, the implant should be removed. Revision surgery can be performed as a one-stage or two-stage procedure. If insertion of new prosthesis is considered inappropriate, then excision arthroplasty or joint fusion may be required. Complications following revision joint surgery include massive bone loss, periprosthetic fracture and recurrence of infection.

Infections of bones and joints
Acute osteomyelitis

Acute osteomyelitis usually occurs in children. It is invariably a haematogenous infection from a distant focus of sepsis. Organisms responsible for acute osteomyelitis include:

- *Staphylococcus aureus*
- *Streptococcus pyogenes*
- *Haemophilus influenzae*
- Gram-negative organisms

Salmonella infections are often seen in those with sickle-cell anaemia.

Pathology

Infection usually occurs in the metaphysis of long bones. Acute inflammation results in raised intraosseous pressure and intravascular thrombosis. Suppuration produces a subperiosteal abscess that may discharge into the soft tissues. Spread of the infection into the epiphysis can result in joint infection. Within days of infection, bone death can occur. Fragments of dead bone become separated in the medullary canal (sequestrum). New bone forms deep to the stripped periosteum (involucrum). If the infection is rapidly controlled, resolution can occur. If the infection is poorly controlled, chronic osteomyelitis may develop.

Clinical features

The patient usually presents with pain, malaise and fever and is often unable to weight bear. Early signs of inflammation are often few. The bone is often exquisitely tender with reduced joint movement. Late infection presents with soft-tissue swellings or discharging sinus. The differential diagnosis includes:

- Cellulitis
- Acute suppurative arthritis
- Rheumatic fever
- Sickle-cell crisis

Metastatic infection can occur at distant sites (e.g. brain, lung). Spread into the adjacent joint can result in a septic arthritis. This complication occurs in young children in whom the growth plate is permeable, bones in which the metaphysis is intracapsular or when the epiphysis of the bone is involved by metastatic infection. Involvement of the physis can result in altered bone growth.

Investigation

Plain x-rays are usually normal during the first 3 to 5 days of the infection. In the second week, radiological signs include periosteal new bone formation, patchy rarefaction of the metaphysis and metaphyseal bone destruction. In cases of diagnostic doubt, bone scanning or MRI can be helpful. The diagnosis can be confirmed by aspiration of pus from an abscess or the metaphysis. About 50% of patients have positive blood cultures.

Management

General supportive measures should include intravenous fluids and analgesia. The painful limb often requires a splint or skin traction to relieve symptoms. Aggressive antibiotic therapy should be instituted. If the patient fails to respond to conservative treatment, surgery may be required. A subperiosteal abscess should be drained. Drilling of the metaphysis is occasionally required. Overall, about 50% of children require surgery.

Septic arthritis

Septic arthritis is an acute inflammatory condition of a joint, usually resulting from bacterial infection. Untreated, it will lead to destruction of the articular cartilage. About 50% cases occur in children less than 3 years of age. In infants less than 1 year old, the hip is the commonest joint involved. In older children the knee is the commonest joint affected. About 10% of patients have multiple joint involvement.

Pathology

The infecting organism depends on age (**Table 22.6**). Organisms can enter the joint

Infecting organisms seen in septic arthritis			
Children		Adults	
<3 years old	>3 years old	<50 years old	>50 years old
H. influenzae	S. aureus	S. aureus	S. aureus
S. aureus	H. influenzae	N. gonorrhoea	Gram-negative bacteria
Coliforms			Streptococci

Table 22.6 Infecting organisms seen in septic arthritis

via a number of routes including penetrating wounds, from the epiphysis or metaphysis or via haematogenous spread. This provokes an acute inflammatory response and a large number of neutrophils accumulate in the joint. They release proteolytic enzymes that break down the articular cartilage resulting in an effusion and reduced synovial blood supply.

Clinical features

The exact presentation depends on the age of the patient. Children are usually systemically unwell and present with pain in the affected joint. All movements of the joint are painful. They are reluctant to stand on weight-bearing joints. The affected joint is usually swollen, red and warm. Hip involvement results in flexion and external rotation. In adults, septic arthritis is usually associated with immunosuppression. Complications of septic arthritis include:

- Avascular necrosis of the epiphysis
- Joint subluxation or dislocation
- Growth disturbance
- Secondary osteoarthritis
- Persistent or recurrent infection

The differential diagnosis includes:

- Irritable hip
- Pethe's disease
- Osteomyelitis
- Gout
- Pseudogout

Investigation

The most important investigation is culture of a joint aspirate. This should be performed prior to the administration of antibiotics. Other appropriate investigations should include inflammatory markers and a plain x-ray.

Management

Antibiotics should be started after joint aspiration and empirical therapy should be based on the likely organisms, adjusted depending on antibiotic sensitivity. Antibiotics should be continued for 6 weeks. The surgical management involves joint drainage and lavage. This may be performed as either an open or arthroscopic procedure. Early joint mobilisation should be encouraged.

Pott's disease

Pott's disease is tuberculous spondylitis. It is well recognised in Egyptian mummies and was described by Sir Percival Pott in 1779. It is now rare in Western countries but is still prevalent in the developing world.

Pathology

Pott's disease usually occurs secondary to infection elsewhere and is due to a combination of osteomyelitis and arthritis. It often occurs at more than one vertebral level and usually affects the anterior part of the vertebral body. It is more common in the thoracic spine. Bone destruction leads to vertebral collapse and kyphosis. The spinal canal can be narrowed resulting in cord compression and neurological deficit.

Clinical features

Back pain is the commonest presenting symptom and may be present for several months before the diagnosis is made. The pain can be both spinal and radicular. About 50% of patients have neurological signs at presentation. Most patients have some degree of kyphosis. A cold abscess may point in the groin.

Investigation

The serum ESR is often massively raised and a tuberculin skin test is usually positive. A plain x-ray may show lytic destruction of the anterior vertebral body, anterior vertebral collapse, reactive sclerosis and an enlarged psoas shadow. A CT or MRI provides information on the disc space and neurological involvement. A CT also allows a guided biopsy to be obtained for microbiological and pathological assessment.

Management

Treatment involves both tuberculous chemotherapy and possible surgery. Nine months of combination chemotherapy should be used involving up to four drugs. Isoniazid and rifampicin should be given for the full 9 months. Pyrazinamide, ethambutol or streptomycin should be give for the first 2 months. Surgery is indicated if there is:

- Neurological deficit
- Spinal deformity with instability
- No response to medical treatment
- Non-diagnostic percutaneous biopsy

The surgical approach depends on the extent of the disease and the level of spinal involvement. It usually involves radical debridement and posterior stabilisation.

Disorders of the upper limb

Thoracic outlet compression syndrome

Thoracic outlet compression syndrome describes a collection of upper limb neurological and vascular symptoms arising as a result of proximal compression of the neurovascular structures in the region of the first rib. It usually affects middle-aged women and the male:female ratio is about 1:3. Approximately 10% of patients have bilateral symptoms. Compression can result from a bone, muscle or fibromuscular band. The compressing lesion is usually congenital. Approximately 30% of cases are precipitated by trauma (e.g. whiplash injury).

Clinical features

Neurological features are more common than vascular. Subclavian artery aneurysms and axillary vein thrombosis are uncommon. Symptoms are often worsened by carrying weights or lifting arms above the head. Differential diagnosis includes:

- Cervical spondylosis
- Distal nerve compression
- Pancoast's tumour
- Connective tissue disorders
- Vascular and venous embolic disease

Diagnosis often depends mainly on the history. Signs are few but the diagnosis may be confirmed with the reproduction of symptoms with arms flexed and abducted (Roos test) or loss of the radial pulse with head turned to the opposite side and the neck extended (Adson manoeuvre).

Investigations

The results of investigations are often normal. A chest x-ray may show a cervical rib. Nerve conduction studies may be needed to exclude a distal nerve compression. An arch aortogram may show a subclavian artery aneurysm. Duplex scanning may show arterial or venous compression and the effect of position.

Management

Symptoms may improve with physiotherapy. If symptoms are disabling, then it may be necessary to consider surgical decompression. This involves resection of most of the first rib and can be achieved through either a supraclavicular or transaxillary approach. About 10% of patients undergoing surgery will develop a pneumothorax. Following surgery, 80% report a symptomatic improvement and more than 50% of patients are symptom free. Failure to improve is often due to a double crush compression syndrome or incomplete division of the compressing structure.

Dislocation of the shoulder

The shoulder is one of the commonest joints to dislocate due to the shallowness of glenohumeral joint, the range of movement, ligamentous laxity, possible glenoid dysplasia and the vulnerability of the joint. External rotation in abduction levers the head of the humerus out of the glenoid socket. The joint capsule is often torn and the glenoid labrum may be avulsed (Bankart lesion).

Clinical features

Dislocation is usually caused by fall on the outstretched hand. It has a bimodal age distribution. The first peak occurs in young adult men after significant trauma. The second peak occurs in elderly women after minimal violence. Pain is often severe. The arm is usually held in abduction and externally rotated. All movement is restricted. The lateral outline of shoulder is flattened. A bulge may be felt below the clavicle.

Investigation

An anterio-posterior x-ray of the shoulder shows overlapping of the humeral head and glenoid fossa (**Figure 22.9**). The head of the humerus is seen below and medial to the joint. An x-ray is mandatory to exclude a humeral fracture.

Management

Numerous methods of reduction have been described. It may be reduced by simple traction and countertraction in slight abduction. Kocher method requires the elbow to be flexed to 90°; the arm to be slowly rotated laterally to 75° and the elbow lifted forward and arm rotated medially. An x-ray should be taken to confirm reduction and exclude a fracture. The arm should be rested in a sling for 2 to 3 weeks. Complications of an anterior dislocation include:

- Axillary nerve injury
- Vascular injury
- Fracture-dislocation
- Shoulder stiffness
- Unreduced dislocation
- Recurrent dislocation

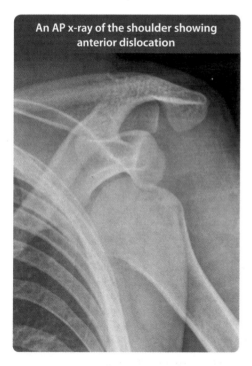

An AP x-ray of the shoulder showing anterior dislocation

Figure 22.9 An AP x-ray of the shoulder showing anterior dislocation

Posterior dislocation

Posterior dislocation of the shoulder is rare and accounts for less than 2% of shoulder dislocations. It is usually due to indirect forces resulting in internal rotation and adduction. It is occasionally seen following convulsions or electric shocks. An anterio-posterior x-ray may appear 'normal' and the injury is easily missed. If there is any doubt regarding diagnosis then a CT scan is useful.

Painful shoulder

Causes of shoulder pain include:

- Impingement syndromes
- Rotator cuff tears
- Frozen shoulder
- Calcific tendonitis

Rotator cuff impingement

Rotator cuff impingement is due to abrasion of the rotator cuff muscles on the coracoacromial arch. Impingement is usually reversible. Untreated it may lead to rotator cuff tears or degenerative changes in the glenohumeral joint. It causes a 'painful arc' between 60 and 120° of abduction. A full range of passive movement is possible. Plain radiographs may be normal. Management is by subacromial steroid injection or subacromial decompression.

Rotator cuff tears

Rotator cuff tears usually occur in the middle aged and elderly. They result from either chronic impingement or acute injury and usually present with pain and weakness. Supraspinatus and infraspinatus are usually involved resulting in weakness in abduction and resisted external rotation. An MRI should be obtained to confirm the clinical diagnosis and assess the size of the tear and the extent of retraction. Treatment options include conservative management and either open or arthroscopic repair.

Frozen shoulder

A frozen shoulder is due to chronic inflammation and fibrosis of subsynovial layer. It often occurs after minor trauma or a period of immobility. It reduces the range of active and passive movement, particularly loss of external rotation. It is associated with severe pain and recovery may be prolonged. Treatment options include physiotherapy and manipulation under anaesthetic.

Calcific tendonitis

Calcific tendonitis is due to deposition of calcium salts in the supraspinatus tendon. It produces severe pain over the anterolateral aspect of the shoulder. There is usually a full range of passive movement. Pain is aggravated by shoulder movement. Calcium deposits on x-ray are diagnostic. Treatment options include anti-inflammatory drugs, physiotherapy, subacromial injection or subacromial decompression and removal of calcium deposits.

Lateral epicondylitis

Lateral epicondylitis is often referred to as tennis elbow. It is due to inflammation at the origin of the wrist and finger extensors. It is an enthesopathy of the lateral epicondyle.

Clinical features

Lateral epicondylitis usually occurs between 30 and 50 years of age. Men and women are equally affected and 75% experience symptoms in their dominant arm. It causes pain over the lateral epicondyle radiating to the forearm. Tenderness is usually maximum 5 mm distal to the insertion of the tendon. Resisted wrist extension increases the pain. Plain x-ray may show calcification in the soft tissues.

Management

Non-surgical management involves anti-inflammatory drugs, rest and steroid injection. Surgical treatment should be considered if there is no improvement with 6 months of conservative treatment. It involves division and reattachment of the tendon. About 85% patients notice a dramatic improvement in symptoms.

Medial epicondylitis

Medial epicondylitis is often referred to as golfer's elbow. It is less common than lateral epicondylitis but occurs in the same age group. It is an enthesopathy of the pronator teres and flexor carpi radialis tendon. It is characterised by pain over the medial aspect of the elbow. Pain is exacerbated by wrist flexion. Tenderness is distal to the medial epicondyle. Management is similar to lateral epicondylitis.

Ulnar nerve entrapment at the elbow

The ulnar nerve runs behind the medial epicondyle at the elbow. It runs in a tunnel formed by the aponeurosis between the two heads of flexor carpi ulnaris. The aponeurosis is slack in elbow extension but becomes tight in elbow flexion. Disorders of the elbow joint can result in nerve compression and symptoms are often worse when elbow is flexed.

Clinical features

The main symptoms are pain and paraesthesia in the ring and little finger. This may be associated with weakness of grasp and grip and loss of manual dexterity. Wasting of the intrinsic muscles of the hand can occur.

Management

Night splints to reduce elbow flexion may improve symptoms. Surgical options include:

- Ulnar nerve decompression
- Medial epicondylectomy
- Anterior transposition

Olecranon bursitis

Olecranon bursitis is inflammation of the bursa overlying the olecranon process at the elbow (**Figure 22.10**). Inflammation may be caused by a variety of mechanisms. It is often the result of repetitive trauma but may occasionally occur as a result of infection. The patient notices a painful lump over the olecranon process with painful movement of the elbow joint. Examination will confirm a swollen bursa. Treatment is with anti-inflammatory drugs and aspiration if the swelling fails to settle.

Disorders of the hand

Carpal tunnel syndrome

The carpal tunnel is formed by the flexor retinaculum stretching across the carpus.

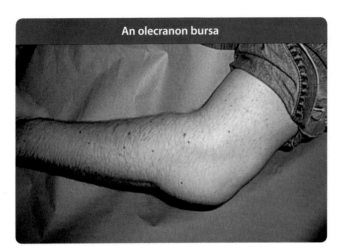

An olecranon bursa

Figure 22.10 An olecranon bursa

It forms a tight tunnel through which passes the long flexors to the fingers and thumb and the median nerve (**Figure 22.11**). Swelling within the tunnel causes nerve compression and ischaemia. Carpal tunnel syndrome affects 3% of women and 2% of men. About 30% cases are due to an underlying medical condition including:

- Hormonal – pregnancy/menopause
- Rheumatoid arthritis
- Hypothyroidism
- Diabetes

Clinical features

Carpal tunnel syndrome usually presents in middle age. The female:male ratio is approximately 8:1. Pain and parasthesia is noted in the distribution of the median nerve. Symptoms are often worse at night and signs are few. Tapping over the carpal tunnel can reproduce symptoms (Tinel sign). Flexion of the wrist for 60 seconds may precipitate symptoms (Phalen sign). Thenar wasting and loss of 2-point discrimination in the distribution of the median nerve are late features. The diagnosis is confirmed by nerve conduction studies which show slowed nerve conduction across the wrist.

Management

Nocturnal symptoms can often be controlled with night splints. Steroid injections may produce temporary symptomatic relief. Troublesome symptoms require division

of the flexor retinaculum. This may be performed endoscopically. About 70% patients are symptom-free following surgery.

de Quervain's disease

de Quervain's disease is also known as stenosing tenovaginitis. It is due to inflammation and thickening of the tendon sheaths of extensor pollicis brevis and abductor pollicis longus. It occurs where both tendons cross the distal radius.

Clinical features

It usually presents in middle age. Pain is noted over the radial aspect of the wrist and often occurs after repetitive activity. The pain is often worsened by abduction of the thumb against resistance. Passive abduction across the palm often causes the pain (Finkelstein test). The tendon sheath is thickened and tender over the radial styloid.

Management

Symptoms can often be improved with steroid injections into the tendon sheath. Persistent symptoms require surgery. The tendon sheath should be split avoiding the dorsal sensory branch of radial nerve.

Dupuytren's contracture

Dupuytren's contracture is a fibroproliferative disease of the palmar fascia. It was first described in 1614 and a detailed anatomical study presented by Dupuytren in 1831.

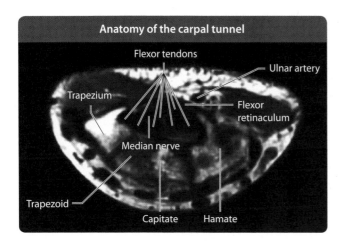

Figure 22.11 Anatomy of the carpal tunnel. (Reproduced courtesy of The Radiology Department, St George's Hospital, London.)

The aetiology is unclear but it is possibly inherited as an autosomal dominant condition with limited penetrance. It is occasionally associated with plantar fasciitis and Peyronie's disease. It is more common in northern Europe. The male to female ratio is 4:1. It affects 5% men over the age of 50 years. Risk factors include:

- Diabetes mellitus
- Alcohol excess
- HIV infection
- Epilepsy
- Trauma
- Manual labour

Clinical features

The most noticeable clinical feature is thickening of the palmar fascia with nodule formation (**Figure 22.12**). Flexion contracture occurs at the metacarpophalangeal and proximal interphalangeal joints, usually affecting the ring and little finger. In the late stage of the disease cords develop proximal to the nodules. About 65% cases are bilateral.

Management

Surgical treatment involves excision or incision of the palmar fascia. The options include fasciotomy, fasciectomy or

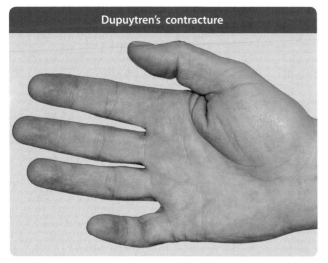

Figure 22.12 Dupuytren's contracture

dermofasciectomy. Surgery should be considered if the metacarpophalangeal contracture is greater than 30° and there is functional disability. Patients need intensive postoperative physiotherapy. Approximately 20% of patients develop complications. The recurrence rate is approximately 50%.

Ganglions

Ganglions are the commonest cause of swellings around the hand and wrist. They are cystic lesions arising from either the joint capsule or a tendon sheath. The aetiology is unknown. They are more common in women. They usually occur between 20 and 40 years of age.

Clinical features

Most ganglia present as smooth swellings 2–4 cm in diameter. Most are painless. Pain can occur due to compression of adjacent neurovascular structures.

Management

If a ganglion is asymptomatic, no specific treatment is required. The old treatment of 'hitting with the family bible' should be condemned. Aspiration can be attempted but the outcome is poor and recurrence is common. Excision is the treatment of choice. The lesion should be explored down to the joint capsule or tendon sheath. Inadequate surgery results in a high recurrence rate.

Knee injuries

Clinical features

The history of any knee injury will suggest which structures may be damaged. Direct varus or valgus forces injure the collateral ligaments. Indirect forces injure the cruciate ligaments and menisci. Twisting in flexion can damage the menisci. Immediate swelling suggests a haemarthrosis. An audible 'pop' can occur with a cruciate ligament injury. Mechanical locking is characteristic of a meniscal injury. Examination should look at joint alignment, wasting, swelling and bruising. Localised tenderness should be elicited and the range of passive and active movement should be assessed. Provocation tests include:

- Anterior and posterior draw test
- Lachman's test
- Pivot shift test
- McMurray's test

Investigation

Plain radiographs may show avulsion fractures and exclude fractures around the knee. MRI is the most useful imaging modality for assessing the integrity of the ligaments. It will show the extent of soft tissue injuries. Arthroscopy as an investigative procedure is now almost obsolete.

Management

Meniscal injuries

Mensical injuries may be traumatic or degenerative. They are classified by their position and shape. Acute peripheral injuries can be repaired. Chronic central injuries often require arthroscopic partial meniscectomy. Total meniscectomy risks later degenerative changes and should be avoided.

Anterior cruciate injuries

Acute anterior cruciate injuries result in a haemarthrosis which results in variable amounts of pain and instability. They are often associated with a medial meniscal tear. Treatment options depend on the expectation and the life-style of the patient. Options include physiotherapy and rarely or later cruciate ligament reconstruction. The most popular grafts are hamstring and bone-patella tendon-bone grafts.

Posterior cruciate injuries

Posterior cruciate injuries usually occur following dashboard injuries. They result in knee instability. Treatment is controversial due to less reliable surgical results. Surgical reconstruction is reserved for multiple ligament injuries.

Collateral ligament injuries

Medial collateral ligament injuries are common. Clinical evaluation allows injuries to be graded as follows:

- Grade 1 – Local ligament tenderness – no instability
- Grade 2 – Unstable at 20° of flexion – stable in extension

- Grade 3 – Unstable in flexion and extension

MRI is useful in evaluating the extent of injury. The management of collateral ligament injuries should be as follows:

- Grade 1 injuries require analgesia and early mobilisation
- Grade 2 injuries require a hinged knee brace
- Grade 3 injuries require surgical repair

Disorders of the foot

Hallux valgus

Hallux valgus is the commonest deformity of the foot. It results in excessive valgus angulation of the big toe. It is only seen in populations that wear shoes. Splaying of the forefoot with varus angulation of the first metatarsal predisposes to the condition. The anatomical deformity consists of increased forefoot width, lateral deviation of the hallux and prominence of the first metatarsal head. As the deformity increases, the long tendons of the hallux are shifted laterally.

Clinical features

Hallux valgus is more common in women and is often bilateral. Symptoms result from a bursa over the metatarsal head (often known as a bunion) hammer toes, metatarsalgia and osteoarthritis of the first metatarsophalangeal joint (MTPJ). The diagnosis can be confirmed by x-ray. The intermetatarsal angle should be less than 20° and the hallux angle should be less than 15°.

Management

Surgical management should be considered if the patient is symptomatic. The surgical options include:

- First metatarsal osteotomy
- Exostectomy and capsulorrhaphy
- Excision of the proximal one-third of the proximal phalanx (Keller operation)
- Arthrodesis

Hallux rigidus

Hallux rigidus is due to osteoarthritis of the first MTPJ. It affects men more often than women. It results in pain on walking,

especially on rough ground. There is no valgus deviation of the hallux. The MTPJ is swollen and enlarged and dorsiflexion of the MTPJ is reduced. A rocker-soled shoe may improve symptoms. If significant symptoms occur, then surgery may be required. The surgical options include:

- Extension osteotomy
- Cheilectomy
- Arthroplasty
- Arthrodesis

Claw toes

Claw toes result from flexion of the interphalangeal joints and hyperextension of the metatarsophalangeal joints. They are often idiopathic but can be associated with rheumatoid arthritis, poliomyelitis and peroneal muscular atrophy.

Clinical features

Claw toes result in pain in the forefoot. Symptoms are usually bilateral. Walking may be restricted. They also cause painful callosities on the dorsum of the toes or under the metatarsal heads.

Management

If the toes can be passively straightened then a 'metatarsal bar' may help. Special footwear may reduce symptoms. If non-operative management fails, then surgical options include:

- Interphalangeal arthrodesis
- Joint excision
- Metatarsal osteotomy
- Digital amputation

Plantar fasciitis

Plantar fasciitis is a self-limiting condition that occurs in middle age. It presents with intermittent heel pain. It is usually unilateral but 15% cases are bilateral. Pain is often worse early in the morning. Examination shows tenderness over the medial plantar aspect of the calcaneal tuberosity. About 50% of patients have a heel spur on plain x-ray. The differential diagnosis includes Reiter's syndrome, an entrapment neuropathy or a calcaneal stress fracture. Management should involve the use of supportive heel pads and other orthotic devices and anti-inflammatory drugs. Surgery is rarely indicated.

Morton's neuroma

Morton's neuroma is a painful forefoot disorder. It is caused by thickening and fibrosis of the interdigital nerves. The aetiology is unknown. It usually affects the second or third web space and causes plantar pain at the level of metatarsal heads. It may be associated with distal sensory loss. The differential diagnosis includes metatarsalgia, metatarsophalangeal synovitis, a stress fracture and Freiberg's infarction (osteochondrosis of the 2nd metatarsal head). Initial management is non-operative. Surgical excision of the neuroma should be considered if symptoms fail to settle.

Osteoporosis

Osteoporosis is a systemic skeletal disease characterised by low bone mass and micro-architectural deterioration. It is associated with increased bone fragility and susceptibility to fractures. It is defined as a bone mineral density less than 2.5 standard deviations below the mean. Established osteoporosis is a low bone mineral density associated with an osteoporosis-related fracture.

Pathophysiology

Bone undergoes continuous resorption and formation. About 10% of the adult skeleton is remodeled each year. Bone loss results from an imbalance between resorption and formation. The human skeleton comprises approximately 80% cortical bone and 20% trabecular bone.

Osteoporotic fractures occur at sites with more than 50% trabecular bone such as the vertebral bodies, proximal femur and distal forearm. Bone loss leads to thinning of the trabecular plates. This causes a disproportionate loss of bone strength. Peak bone mass is achieved by the age of 30 years. After skeletal maturity bone is lost at about 1% per year. Women experience accelerated bone loss after the menopause. Factors associated with increased bone loss include:

- Inactivity
- Cigarette smoking
- Poor diet
- Family history
- Early menopause
- Endocrine disease – Cushing's syndrome, diabetes, hyperthyroidism
- Drugs – steroids, thyroxine, diuretics

Clinical features

Clinical features of osteoporosis include pain, decreased mobility, deformity, loss of independence and osteoporosis-related fractures.

Investigation

Useful investigations to detect the presence of osteoporosis include:

- Dual-energy x-ray absorptionmetry
- Quantitative CT scanning
- Bone biopsy
- Biochemical markers of bone turnover

Prevention

Optimisation of peak bone mass can be achieved by exercise and supplementary dietary calcium. A reduced rate of bone loss is seen with use of hormonal replacement therapy in post-menopausal women , moderation of alcohol intake and stopping smoking.

Metabolic bone disease
Osteomalacia and rickets

Both osteomalacia and rickets result from Vitamin D deficiency. The outcome is incomplete osteoid mineralisation. In childhood, prior to epiphyseal closure, this causes rickets. In adults, it causes osteomalacia. Causes of osteomalacia include:

- Vitamin D deficiency
- Malabsorption
- Renal disease – familial hypophosphataemic rickets
- Anticonvulsant therapy
- Tumours

Clinical features

Osteomalacia is usually due to dietary deficiency in the elderly or Asian population.

Rickets is usually due to familial hypophosphataemic rickets. Rickets usually presents in early childhood with:

- Failure to thrive
- Valgus or varus long bone deformities
- Skull deformities – craniotabes
- Enlarged costochondral junctions – Rickety rosary
- Lateral indentation of the chest wall – Harrison's sulcus
- X-ray shows a widened epiphyses and cupped distal metaphysis

Osteomalacia presents in adults with:

- Bone pain and tenderness
- Proximal myopathy
- True pathological or pseudo-fractures

Investigation

In osteomalacia, the serum calcium and phosphate are low and alkaline phosphatase is increased. Skeletal x-rays may show translucent bands in the medial femoral cortex, pubic ramus or scapula (Looser's zones). In familial hypophosphataemic rickets, the serum calcium is normal and phosphate is low. A bone biopsy is rarely required but, if performed, would show increased unmineralised osteoid.

Management

Treatment is with Vitamin D replacement therapy and phosphate supplements in those with familial hypophosphataemic rickets.

Paget's disease of bone

Paget's disease of bone is named after Sir James Paget who first described *osteitis deformans* in 1877. The aetiology is unknown but it is possibly due to a viral infection. Histological features include enlarged osteoclasts. Increased bone turnover produces a mosaic pattern of lamellar bone. The disease has three phases – osteolytic, mixed and sclerotic.

Clinical features

Paget's disease is often identified as an incidental finding on an x-ray in an asymptomatic patient. If symptomatic, it usually causes bone pain. The clinical signs include characteristic skull and long bone deformities. Complications causing symptoms include:

- Pathological fractures – complete or incomplete
- Neurological effects
- Osteoarthritis
- Sarcomas
- Cardiac failure

Investigation

Skeletal x-rays in the osteolytic phase may show osteoporosis circumscripta. Bone softening can produce bowing, platybasia, protrusion of the acetabuli or greenstick fractures. In the mixed phase, radiological investigations shows generalised bone enlargement. In the sclerotic phase they show increased bone density with trabecula and cortical thickening. The serum calcium and phosphate are usually normal. The serum alkaline phosphatase is often increased. Serum uric acid levels are increased in about 30% of patients.

Management

Anti-inflammatory drugs can be used to control bone pain. Biphosphonates will reduce bone turnover. Neurological complications and fractures may require surgical intervention.

Paget's sarcomas

Most osteosarcomas that develop late in life are associated with Paget's disease. Malignant change occurs in less than 1% of patients with Paget's disease. The commonest site is the femur. The prognosis of Paget's sarcomas is poor with a median survival of 1 year and only 5% of patients are alive at 5 years.

Locomotor pain
Low back pain

Lumbar back pain is one of the commonest causes of chronic disability. It is usually due to abnormality of the intervertebral discs at the L4/5 or L5/S1 level. It can occur at any age but is most common in previously fit adults between 20–45 years.

Pathology

With age, the nucleus pulposus of the intervertebral disc dries out. The annulus fibrosus also develops fissures. Nuclear material may then herniate through annulus fibrosus. It may also perforate the vertebral end-plate to produce a Schmorl node. Flattening of the disc with marginal osteophyte formation is known as spondylosis. Osteoarthritis may develop in the facet joints. Osteophyte formation may narrow the lateral recesses of spinal canal. These can encroach on the spinal canal and result in spinal stenosis. Acute herniation of disc contents can also occur. This usually happens to one side of the posterior longitudinal ligament. Posterolateral rupture can compress nerve roots. Central posterior rupture can compress the cauda equina.

Clinical features

Acute disc rupture usually presents with sudden onset of low back pain on stooping or lifting. The pain often radiates to buttock or leg and may be associated with parasthesia or numbness in the leg. Cauda equina compression can cause urinary retention. Examination may show a 'sciatic' scoliosis. Lumbar tenderness and paravertebral spasm maybe be present and all back movements are usually restricted. Straight leg raising is often reduced. Neurological examination is essential. The neurological signs associated with an acute disc rupture depends on the nerve root compressed (**Table 22.7**).

Investigation

A lumbar spine x-ray will exclude other bone lesions. CT scanning is an effective diagnostic study when the spinal and neurological levels are clear and bony pathology is suspected. MRI is now the investigation of choice. It is most useful when the exact spinal and neurological levels are unclear, when a pathological condition of the spinal cord or soft tissues is suspected or when an underlying infective or neoplastic cause is possible.

Management

Bed rest is of unproven benefit and recovery is not hastened by traction. Anti-inflammatory drugs provide symptomatic relief. The role of epidural steroid injection is unclear. Chemonucleolysis is less effective than surgical discectomy. Surgery is required if there is:

- Cauda equina compression – neurosurgical emergency
- Neurological deterioration with conservative management
- Persistent symptoms and neurological signs

The surgical options are laminectomy and microdiscectomy. Postoperative rehabilitation and physiotherapy are essential.

Neurological signs associated with acute disc rupture	
Neurological level	**Signs**
L5 root	Weakness of hallux extension
	Loss of knee reflex
	Sensory loss over the lateral aspect of the leg and dorsum of the foot
S1 root	Weakness of foot plantar flexion
	Loss of ankle reflex
	Sensory loss over the lateral aspect of the foot
Cauda equina	Urinary retention
	Loss or perianal sensation

Table 22.7 Neurological signs associated with acute disc rupture

Facet joint dysfunction

Facet joint dysfunction usually presents with recurrent low back pain. The pain is often related to physical activity and may be referred to the buttock. It is often relieved by lying down and rest. Lumbar spine movement is often good and neurological signs are rare. Lumbar spine x-rays show narrowing of the disc space and oblique views may show facet joint malalignment. Treatment includes physiotherapy, analgesia and facet joint injections. Surgery is rarely necessary but spinal fusion may need to be considered.

Spinal stenosis

Spinal stenosis is narrowing of the spinal canal due to hypertrophy of the posterior disc margin. It may be compounded by facet joint osteophyte formation. Spinal stenosis may also be associated with achondroplasia, spondylolisthesis and Paget's disease. It usually presents with either unilateral or bilateral leg pain, initiated by standing or walking and relieved by sitting or leaning forward – 'spinal claudication'. The patient prefers to walk uphill rather than downhill. Lumbar spine x-rays often show degenerative spondylolisthesis. The diagnosis can be confirmed by MRI. It can often be treated conservatively. Surgery involves laminectomy and decompression.

Spondylolisthesis

Spondylolisthesis means forward shift of the spine. It usually occurs at L4/L5 or L5/S1 level. It can only occur if the facet joint locking mechanism has failed. It is classified as:

- Dysplastic – 20%
- Lytic – 50%
- Degenerative – 25%
- Post-traumatic
- Pathological
- Postoperative

In lytic spondylolisthesis the pars interarticularis is in two pieces (spondylolysis). The vertebral body and superior facet joints subluxate and dislocate forward. The degree of overlap is usually expressed as a percentage. The cauda equina or nerve roots may be compressed. It usually presents with back pain and neurological symptoms. Patients have a characteristic stance and the 'step' in the lumbar spine may be palpable. The diagnosis can be confirmed on a lumbar spine x-ray. Most patients improve with conservative management. Surgery may be required if:

- Disabling symptoms
- Progressive displacement more than 50%
- Significant neurological compromise

Anterior or posterior fusion may be required.

Spinal cord compression

The clinical features of a spinal cord lesion depends on its rate of development. Trauma produces acute compression with rapidly developing neurological effects. Benign neoplasms can cause substantial compression with little neurological deficit. The causes of spinal cord compression can be:

- Trauma – vertebral body fracture or facet joint dislocation
- Neoplasia – benign or malignant
- Degenerative – prolapsed intervertebral disc, osteophyte formation
- Vascular – epidural or subdural haematoma
- Inflammatory – rheumatoid arthritis
- Infection – tuberculosis or pyogenic infections

Anatomy

The spinal cord is shorter than spinal canal. The spinal cord ends at the interspace between the L1 and L2 vertebrae. Below the termination of the cord the nerve roots form the cauda equina (**Figure 22.13**). Within the cervical spine, segmental levels of the cord correspond to the bony landmarks. Below this level there is increasing disparity between levels. Spinal pathology below L1 presents with only root signs.

Clinical features

The clinical features of spinal cord compression can be variable and a high index of suspicion is required. Motor symptoms include easy fatigue and gait disturbance. Sensory symptoms include sensory loss and parasthesia. Light touch, proprioception

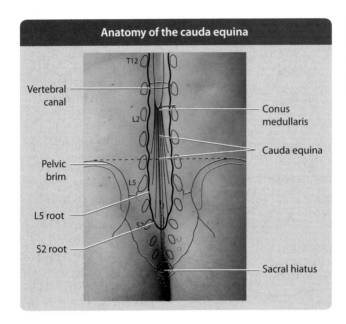

Figure 22.13 Anatomy of the cauda equina. (Reproduced from Tunstall R and Shah N. Pocket Tutor Surface Anatomy. London: JP Medical Ltd, 2012, and courtesy of Sam Scott-Hunter, London.)

and joint position sense may be reduced. Tendon reflexes are often increased below the level of compression, absent at the level of compression and normal above. Reflex changes may not coincide with sensory level.

Cervical spine disease produces quadriplegia. Thoracic spine disease produces paraplegia. Lumbar spine disease affects L4, L5 and sacral nerve roots. Sphincter disturbances are late features of cervical and thoracic cord compression. Cauda equina compression due to central disc prolapse produces:

- Loss of perianal sensation
- 'Root pain' in both legs
- Painless urinary retention

Most patients with surgically treatable causes of spinal compression have spinal pain. Movement-induced pain suggests vertebral fracture or collapse. Exquisite tenderness suggests an epidural abscess. Low-grade background pain may suggest tumour infiltration or osteomyelitis.

Investigation
Spinal x-rays may show bone or paravertebral soft tissue disease. Other features which may be seen on a plain x-ray include vertebral collapse, lytic lesions and loss of the vertebral

pedicle. The integrity of the disc may indicate the diagnosis. 'Good disc = bad news' often indicates malignancy. 'Bad disc = good news' and may indicate infection. MRI is now the investigation of choice to define the extent of any soft tissue disease. A bone scan may indicate the pattern and extent of bone pathology.

Management
Acute spinal cord compression is a 'surgical' emergency. In those with malignant disease, radiotherapy may be the treatment of choice. In general, tumour, infection and disc disease produces anterior compression and surgical decompression should be achieved through an anterior approach. The cervical spine can be approached between the larynx medially and the carotid sheath laterally. The thoracic spine can be approached through the chest by a posterior thoracotomy or costotransversectomy.

Bone tumours and amputations
Primary bone tumours

Bone and connective tissue cancers account for less than 1% of all new cancers diagnosed in the UK each year. Primary bone tumours are rare. Secondary tumours are more common, especially in the elderly. The classification of benign and malignant bone tumours is shown in **Table 22.8**.

Clinical features and investigation

Most primary bone tumours present with bone pain, a limb swelling and localised tenderness. Pain is usually worse following activity. Pain in an extremity may result in a limp. Rapid growth and associated erythema are suggestive of malignancy. The tumour may present with a pathological fracture, but this uncommon. Systemic symptoms, such as fever and night sweats, are rare. Tumours that spread to the lungs only rarely results in respiratory symptoms and this usually indicates extensive lung involvement. The diagnosis of a bone or connective tissue tumour can be confirmed by plain x-ray, CT scan, MRI and a carefully planned biopsy.

Osteoid osteoma

Osteoid osteomas are benign bone tumours. When they clinically present, they are usually less than 1 cm in diameter . They are more common in young adults. The tibia and femur are the commonest sites. Severe pain, relieved by anti-inflammatory drugs, is often the presenting complaint. A plain x-ray has characteristic appearance of a radiolucency surrounded by dense bone. Local excision is curative.

Osteochondroma

Osteochondromas are the commonest of the bone tumours. Lesions can be single or multiple. They usually appear in adolescence as cartilaginous overgrowth at the epiphyseal plate. The tumour grows with the underlying bone. The metaphyses of long bones are the commonest sites. They usually present as a painless lump or occasionally joint pain. Excision should be considered if they cause debilitating symptoms.

Chondroma

Chondromas are benign tumours of cartilage. The lesions may be single or multiple (Ollier's disease). They usually appear in the tubular bones of the hands and feet. A plain x-ray will show a well-defined osteopenic area in the medulla. The lesion can often be excised and bone grafted.

Giant-cell tumour (osteoclastoma)

Giant-cell tumours are benign, locally invasive and metastatic in equal proportions. They are found in the sub-articular cancellous regions of long bones and only occurs after closure of the epiphyses. Patients are usually between 20 and 40 years. A plain x-ray shows an asymmetric rarefied area at the end of a long bone. The cortex is thinned or even perforated.

Classification of primary bone tumours		
Cell type	**Benign**	**Malignant**
Bone	Osteoid osteoma	Osteosarcoma
Cartilage	Chondroma	Chondrosarcoma
	Osteochondroma	
Fibrous tissue	Fibroma	Fibrosarcoma
Bone marrow	Eosinophilic granuloma	Ewing's sarcoma
		Myeloma
Vascular	Haemangioma	Angiosarcoma
Uncertain	Giant-cell tumour	Malignant giant cell tumour

Table 22.8 Classification of primary bone tumours

Treatment by local excision and grafting often leads to recurrence. Wide excision and joint replacement is the treatment of choice. Amputation is required for malignant or recurrent tumours.

Osteosarcoma

Osteosarcomas occur in the metaphyses of long bones. The commonest sites are around the knee or proximal humerus. They destroy bone and spread into the surrounding tissue. Untreated, they rapidly metastasise to the lung. They usually occur between 10 and 20 years but later in life they are seen in association with Paget's disease of bone. A plain x-ray shows a combination of bone destruction and formation. The periosteum may be lifted (Codman's triangle). Soft tissue calcification produces a 'sunburst' appearance. Treatment usually involves amputation and chemotherapy. Amputation may be combined with prosthetic replacement. The 5-year survival is about 50%. The worst prognosis is seen in those with proximal and axial skeletal lesions.

Chondrosarcoma

Chondrosarcoma occurs in two forms as either 'central' tumours in the pelvis or proximal long bones or 'peripheral' tumours in the cartilaginous cap of an osteochondroma. They tend to metastasise late. Wide local excision is often possible.

Metastatic bone tumours

About 30% of patients with malignant disease will develop bone metastases and 10% of these patients will develop a pathological fracture. About 90% of skeletal metastases are multiple. Tumours spread to bone by:

- Direct invasion
- Haematogenous spread
- Lymphatic spread
- Spread via the paravertebral venous plexus

The commonest sites for bone metastases are the lumbar vertebrae, pelvis and ribs. The primary tumours which most commonly spread to bone are:

- Breast (35%)
- Prostate (30%)
- Bronchus (10%)
- Kidney (5%)
- Thyroid (2%)

Clinical features

The clinical features of bone metastases include:

- Pain or localised bone lump
- Pathological fracture
- Hypercalcaemia
- Cord compression

Investigation

Plain x-rays can be normal even in those patients with extensive bone metastases. If an x-ray is abnormal, it will show either an osteolytic or sclerotic lesion. Osteolytic metastases are encountered most frequently, especially in breast and lung carcinomas. Sclerotic metastases are typically seen in prostate cancer. Metastases usually appear in the medullary cavity, spread to destroy the medullary bone and then involve the cortex. The differential diagnosis of bone metastases on a plain x-ray includes:

- Calcified enchondroma
- Hyperparathyroidism
- Chronic sclerosing osteomyelitis
- Bone infarct
- Myeloma deposit

Isotope bone scanning has a higher sensitivity than x-rays and may identify other asymptomatic lesions. MRI is more sensitive than bone scanning and plain x-rays in the detection of bone metastases.

Management

The aims of treatment are to relieve pain and preserve mobility. If a pathological fracture occurs, consideration should be given to internal fixation for early mobilisation and pain relief. Prophylactic internal fixation to prevent a pathological fracture may be required if there is:

- Greater than 50% erosion of a long bone cortex
- A metastasis of more than 2.5 cm in diameter
- Metastasis in high-risk area (e.g. subtrochanteric femur)
- Metastasis with persistent pain

Radiotherapy is useful for the rapid relief of back pain. Spinal decompression may be needed if cord compression occurs. Percutaneous vertebroplasty involves the injection of acrylic bone cement into the vertebral body in order to relieve pain and stabilise the vertebral column. Vertebroplasty should be considered for patients who have vertebral metastases and no evidence of cord compression or spinal instability, if they have either mechanical pain resistant to analgesia or if they have vertebral body collapse.

Multiple myeloma

Multiple myeloma is a malignant disease of plasma cells in the bone marrow. It accounts for 1% of all cancers. There are about 2500 new cases each year in UK. Most patients are over 60 years of age. The disease is characterised by production of monoclonal immunoglobulins which can be detected in serum, urine or both.

Pathogenesis

The disease occurs due to the monoclonal overgrowth of one clone of plasma cells which produces either a monoclonal immunoglobulin or paraprotein. In 80% of patients, an IgG or IgA is detectable in serum. In 20% of patients, no paraprotein is detectable in the serum. Free light chains may cross the glomerulus and appear in the urine. These are known as Bence–Jones proteins.

Clinical features

The clinical features of multiple myeloma include:

- Bone pain – especially back pain
- Pathological fracture
- Spinal cord compression
- Hypercalcaemia
- Renal failure
- Anaemia
- Immunosuppression
- Amyloidosis

Investigation

The diagnosis can be confirmed by finding:

- Paraprotein in the serum or urine on electrophoresis
- Lytic lesions on plain x-rays
- Bone marrow aspirate with more than 10% plasma cells

Management

Overall, about 70% of patients respond to treatment, but complete remission is rare. The median survival is 3 years. Treatment options include:

- Melphalan chemotherapy
- Interferon-α
- Bone marrow transplantation
- Dialysis for renal failure
- Bisphosphonates for hypercalcaemia
- Radiotherapy for localised bone pain

Applied basic sciences
Anatomy of the upper renal tract

The kidneys

The kidneys are retroperitoneal structures on the posterior abdominal wall, largely covered the by the costal margins. The right kidney is slightly lower than left. The hilum lies on medial border of each kidney and transmits the ureter, renal vein and branches of the renal artery. The kidneys are surrounded by a fibrous capsule and beyond that is found perinephric fat and fascia. The upper end of each ureter expands in to the renal pelvis. The renal pelvis divides into two or three major calyces. Each major calyx divides into two or three minor calyces. The arterial supply is by the renal artery arising directly from the aorta. The venous drainage is via the renal vein into the inferior vena cava. The relations of the right and left kidney are shown in **Table 23.1**.

Structure of kidney

The substance, or parenchyma, of the kidney is divided into two major structures. Superficial is the renal cortex and deep is the renal medulla (**Figure 23.1**). These structures take the shape of about 15 cone-shaped renal lobes, each containing renal cortex surrounding a portion of the medulla called a renal pyramid. Between the renal pyramids are projections of cortex called renal columns. Nephrons, the urine-producing functional structures of the kidney, span the cortex and medulla. The initial filtering portion of a nephron is the renal corpuscle, located in the cortex. This is followed by a renal tubule that passes from the cortex deep into the medullary pyramids. Part of the renal cortex, a medullary ray, is a collection of renal tubules that drain into a single collecting duct. The components of the renal tubule are the proximal tubule, the Loop of Henle and the distal convoluted tubule and collecting duct.

The ureters

Each ureter is about 25 cm long and is lined by transitional epithelium. They are retroperitoneal structures and run down over the psoas muscle. They lie in the line of the tips of the transverse processes of the lumbar vertebrae. They cross the bifurcation of the common iliac artery and run down on the lateral wall of the pelvis to the region of ischial spine. The anatomical relations of the

Anatomical relations of the kidney		
	Right kidney	**Left kidney**
Anterior	Suprarenal gland Liver Second part of duodenum Hepatic flexure of colon	Suprarenal gland Spleen Stomach Pancreas Splenic flexure of colon
Posterior	Diaphragm Costodiaphragmatic recess of pleura Twelfth rib Psoas muscle	Diaphragm Costodiaphragmatic recess of pleura Twelfth rib Psoas muscle

Table 23.1 Anatomical relations of the kidney

Anatomy of the kidney

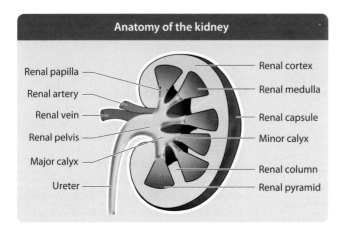

Figure 23.1 Anatomy of the kidney

left and right ureters are shown in **Table 23.2**. Three natural constrictions are found along their course where the:

- Renal pelvis joins the ureter
- Ureter crosses the pelvic brim
- Ureter enters the bladder

Anatomy of the lower renal tract

The bladder

The bladder is pyramidal in shape and, when empty, it is an extraperitoneal structure. Its superior surface is covered by the pelvic peritoneum. Anteriorly, it lies behind the pubis bone. The apex is attached to the umbilicus by the median umbilical ligament. This represents the remnant of the fetal urachus. The inferolateral surfaces are related to the levator ani and obturator internus muscles. In men, the bladder neck fuses

with the prostate and the base is related to the rectum, vas deferens and seminal vesicles. In women, the uterus lies against its posterosuperior surface. The base is related to the vagina and cervix. The ureters join the bladder at the upper lateral angles. On the interior of the bladder, the ureteric orifices are joined by the interureteric ridge. With the urethral orifice this forms a triangular area known as the trigone. As the bladder distends it strips the peritoneum off the anterior abdominal wall. The wall is made of smooth muscle and is lined by transitional epithelium.

The bladder has two sphincters. The internal sphincter is smooth muscle and is found at the bladder neck. The external sphincter is voluntary muscle distal to the internal sphincter. The blood supply is from the superior and inferior vesical branches of the internal iliac arteries. Lymphatic

Anatomical relations of the ureter

	Right ureter	Left ureter
Anterior	Duodenum Terminal ileum Right colic and ileocolic vessels Right testicular/ovarian vessels	Pelvic colon Left colic vessels Left testicular/ovarian vessels
Posterior	Psoas muscle Bifurcation of right common iliac artery	Psoas muscle Bifurcation of left common iliac artery

Table 23.2 Anatomical relations of the ureter

drainage is to the iliac and para-aortic nodes. The bladder has both a motor and sensory nerve supply. The motor supply is autonomic. A sympathetic supply arises from L1/L2 and is inhibitory. A parasympathetic supply arises from S2–S4 and is motor to the detrusor muscle. The sensory supply is parasympathetic.

The prostate

The prostate is a fibromuscular and glandular organ surrounding the proximal urethra. It has five lobes – anterior, posterior, middle and two lateral lobes. Above it is continuous with the base of the bladder. The apex sits on the sphincter urethrae in the deep perineal pouch. Posteriorly, it is separated from the rectum by Denonvillier's fascia. Anteriorly, it is separated from the pubis by extraperitoneal fat. It is surrounded by the prostatic venous plexus. Ejaculatory ducts, formed by the fusion of the vas deferens and seminal vesicles enter the upper posterior part of the prostate and open into the urethra. The blood supply is from the inferior vesical artery.

The male urethra

The male urethra is about 20 cm in length and is divided into three parts. The prostatic urethra is about 4 cm in length. The posterior wall has a longitudinal elevation known as the urethral crest. Along each side of the urethral crest is the prostatic sinus. In the middle of the crest is an elevation known as the verumontanum. The prostatic utricle opens into the verumontanum. On each side of the utricle opens the ejaculatory ducts. The membranous urethra is about 2 cm in length and is the narrowest part of the urethra. It traverses the external urethral sphincter in deep perineal pouch. The spongy urethra is about 15 cm in length. It traverses the corpus spongiosum of the penis. The external urethral orifice is the narrowest part of the urethra. Immediately within the meatus the urethra dilates into a terminal fossa.

Renal physiology

Functions of the kidney

The primary functions of the kidneys are to regulate blood volume and the chemical composition of blood. The secondary functions are the metabolism of vitamin D and the production of renin and erythropoietin.

The nephron

Each kidney contains about one million nephrons (**Figure 23.2**). There are two types of nephron. Cortical nephrons are important in regulating the chemical composition of urine. Juxtamedullary nephrons are important in concentrating urine. Each nephron is made up of a:

- Glomerulus
- Bowman's capsule
- Proximal convoluted tubule
- Loop of Henle
- Distal convoluted tubule

Several tubules enter one collecting duct. A number of ducts run through the medullary pyramids and enter the calyceal system. Blood is filtered within the nephron. The glomerular endothelium is fenestrated. Solute-rich but protein-free fluid passes into Bowman's capsule. The composition of the filtrate is modified as it passes through the renal tubule. The composition is altered by absorption and secretion from the peritubular capillaries. This mainly occurs in the proximal convoluted tubule. The loop of Henle has an important role in water balance.

Blood supply of nephron

The glomerular capillaries receive blood from afferent arterioles. The capillaries then drain into efferent arterioles. High glomerular capillary pressure facilitates filtration. Peritubular capillaries receive blood from the efferent arterioles. This is the site of resorption and secretion. Resorption is assisted by a low capillary pressure. Over 99% of the fluid filtered in the glomerulus is resorbed in the peritubular capillaries.

Juxtaglomerular apparatus

The juxtaglomerular apparatus abuts the afferent arteriole and distal convoluted tubule. It is important in regulating the content of the filtrate. Cells of the distal convoluted tubule at this point are called the macula densa. They monitor the sodium

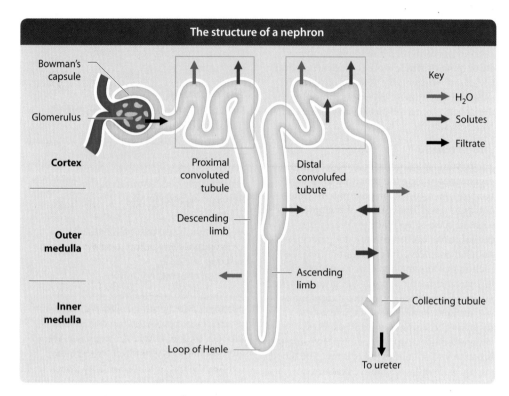

Figure 23.2 The structure of a nephron

content of the filtrate. Juxtaglomerular cells are specialised smooth muscle cells in the arteriole that act as baroreceptors and contain large amounts of renin.

Control of renal function

Filtration

About 20% of the blood that enters the glomerulus is filtered. High pressure within the glomerular capillaries favours filtration. The rate of filtration is known as the glomerular filtration rate (GFR) and is controlled by intrinsic and extrinsic mechanisms. Intrinsic mechanisms includes myogenic regulation – changes in arteriolar smooth muscle constriction and tubuloglomerular feedback – changes in response to sodium concentration in the distal convoluted tubule. Extrinsic mechanisms include sympathetic neural stimulation and the renin–angiotensin system.

Resorption

Most resorption occurs in the proximal convoluted tubule. The primary chemical that drives resorption is sodium. Sodium passively diffuses out of the proximal convoluted tubule and is actively transported in to the peritubular capillaries. Movement of sodium has three important effects:

- Creates an osmotic gradient for water resorption
- Creates an electrical gradient for negatively charged ions
- Allows secondary active transport in the the proximal convoluted tubule

Regulation of urine concentration and volume

Maintaining the concentration of body fluids is integral to homeostasis. Concentration is measured in osmolarity. A concentrated solution will have a high osmolarity. A dilute solution will have a low osmolarity. If blood osmolarity rises, the response will be for water reabsorption to increase and urine volume to decrease. If blood osmolarity falls, the response will the opposite.

Antidiuretic hormone

Blood osmolarity is measured by specialised neurones in the hypothalamus called osmoreceptors. They determine how much antidiuretic hormone (ADH) is secreted by the posterior pituitary gland. ADH increases water reabsorption in the collecting duct and decreases urine volume. When blood osmolarity rises, ADH release is increased. When blood osmolarity falls, ADH release is decreased. ADH works by increasing the permeability of the collecting ducts to water.

Aldosterone

Aldosterone is produced in the renal cortex. It increases sodium resorption and potassium excretion in the distal convoluted tubule. Release of aldosterone is stimulated by:

- Low plasma sodium
- High plasma potassium
- Low blood volume and pressure

Urological trauma
Renal trauma

In the UK, 90% of renal injuries result from blunt abdominal trauma. Isolated renal trauma is uncommon and approximately 40% of patients have other associated intra-abdominal injuries. Direct trauma crushes the kidney against the ribs. Indirect trauma can result in vascular or pelviureteric disruption.

Clinical features

The clinical features of a renal injury include:

- Loin or abdominal abrasions or bruising
- Loin tenderness
- Loss of loin contour
- Loin mass
- Macroscopic haematuria and possible clot colic

A renal pedicle injury is possible in the absence of haematuria.

Investigation

The aims of imaging in the assessment of renal trauma are to assess both the extent of injury and to determine the function of the contralateral kidney. Plain radiograph may show rib fractures, loss of the psoas shadow and the renal outline. A contrast-enhanced abdominal CT scan will detect extravasation of urine, distortion of the caliceal system and provide a crude index of renal function. Failure of radiological contrast excretion suggests a renal pedicle injury and, if the patient is cardiovascularly stable, the need for renal angiography. Ultrasound will identify haematomas and perirenal collections. Renal injuries are classified as follows:

- Class 1 – Renal contusion or contained subcapsular haematoma
- Class 2 – Cortical laceration without urinary extravasation
- Class 3 – Parenchymal lesion extending more than 1 cm into renal substance
- Class 4 – Laceration extending across cortico-medullary junction
- Class 5 – Renal fragmentation or reno-vascular pedicle injury

Management

Approximately 80% of renal injuries are minor. Class 1 and 2 injuries can be managed conservatively. Early surgical intervention is required for reno-vascular pedicle injuries, pelviureteric junction disruption and shock with signs of intraperitoneal or retroperitoneal bleeding. Surgery should be performed through a midline incision and a transperitoneal approach. Control of the renal pedicle should be obtained before the retroperitoneal haematoma is opened. The surgical priorities are to save life, remove devascularised tissue, preserve renal function and repair and drain the collecting system. Late complications of renal trauma are:

- Hypertension
- Arteriovenous fistula
- Hydronephrosis
- Pseudocyst or calculi formation
- Chronic pyelonephritis
- Loss of renal function

Lower urinary tract trauma

The management of lower urinary tract trauma is controversial and often confusing. In multiply injured patients, there are the conflicting priorities of monitoring urine output with a urethral catheter and preventing exacerbation of any possible urethral injury. Lower urinary tract injury should be suspected if the following are seen:

- Blood from urethral meatus
- Perineal bruising
- High riding prostate on rectal examination

Potentially useful investigations include CT, ascending urethrogram or cystogram.

Bladder injury

Bladder injury is often associated with pelvic fractures. It is also seen following direct blow to the abdomen with a full bladder. Rupture can be either intraperitoneal or extraperitoneal. Clinical features include lower abdominal peritonism and the inability to pass urine. An abdominal CT may show urine extravasation. The diagnosis can be confirmed by cystography. Intraperitoneal rupture of the bladder requires laparotomy, bladder repair, urethral and suprapubic drainage. Extraperitoneal rupture of the bladder can be treated conservatively with urethral drainage. Prophylactic antibiotics should be given.

Bulbar urethral injury

Bulbar urethral injury is the commonest type of urethral injury. It is usually the result of direct trauma caused by falling astride an object. Clinical features include blood from the urethral meatus and perineal bruising. If the patient is unable to pass urine then a urethral catheter should not be passed as the procedure can convert a partial tear into a complete urethral injury. If a catheter is required, it should be inserted via the suprapubic route. The diagnosis can be confirmed by an ascending urethrogram. Prophylactic antibiotics should be given. Late complications include a urethral stricture.

Membranous urethral injury

Membranous urethral injuries often occur in multiply injured patient and unless suspected can easily be missed. About 10% of men with pelvic fracture have a membranous urethral injury and the tear can be either partial or complete. Partial injuries present with urethral bleeding and perineal bruising. Complete injuries present with the inability to pass urine. On rectal examination, the bladder and prostate is displaced upwards. If a membranous urethral injury is suspected, a urethral catheter should not be passed. The diagnosis can be confirmed by ascending urethrogram (**Figure 23.3**). Treatment is with a suprapubic catheter. Urethroplasty may be

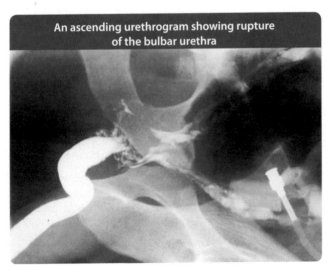

An ascending urethrogram showing rupture of the bulbar urethra

Figure 23.3 An ascending urethrogram showing rupture of the bulbar urethra

required. Late complications include urethral stricture, impotence and incontinence.

Urinary tract infections and calculi

Urinary tract infection

Bacteriuria is the presence of bacteria in the urine. Significant bacteriuria is present when more than 10^5 colony forming units are found per mL of urine. The commonest organisms causing urinary tract infections (UTIs) are:

- *Escherichia coli*
- *Proteus mirabilis*
- *Pseudomonas aeruginosa*

Pathogenesis

Urine proximal to the distal urethra is normally sterile. Most UTIs are due organisms arising from the faecal flora and they are invariably the result of ascending infection. Rarely, UTIs can arise secondary to a bacteraemia. Host defences against urinary infection include the voiding of urine, urinary antibodies, desquamation of epithelial surfaces, and antibacterial enzymes. UTIs can be uncomplicated or complicated. Uncomplicated UTIs have no underlying structural abnormality. Complicated UTIs arise secondary to a structural lesion and can result in renal damage.

Investigation

All upper UTIs require investigation. Lower UTIs in children and in adult men should also be investigated. The aims of investigation are to establish the diagnosis of a UTI, identify the organism involved and its antibiotic sensitivity and exclude a structural or pathological abnormality of the urinary tract. The diagnosis of a UTI can be suggested by dip-stick testing of urine. The presence in the urine of nitrites or leukocyte esterase is very suggestive of a Gram-negative infection. The diagnosis should be confirmed by microscopy and culture of a urine. Investigation of UTIs in adults should involve renal ultrasound and cystoscopy, supplemented by other modalities guided by the clinical presentation. Investigation of UTIs in children should be by renal ultrasound, Dimercaptosuccinic acid (DMSA) scanning to assess renal damage and micturating cystogram to evaluate vesico-ureteric reflux.

Lower urinary tract infection

Lower urinary tract infections are more common in women. Symptoms include suprapubic pain, frequency and dysuria and can be treated with increased fluid intake and antibiotics. Symptoms can be improved by alkalisation of the urine. An MSU should be repeated at 7 days to check that the infection has been cleared.

Acute pyelonephritis

Acute pyelonephritis presents with pyrexia, frequency, dysuria and loin pain. An MSU will invariably be positive for the infecting organism. Imaging in the acute situation is not required. Treatment is by parenteral antibiotics. Complications included pyonephrosis which can occur if there is coexisting upper urinary tract obstruction. Pyonephrosis requires urgent decompression usually by percutaneous nephrostomy. If inadequately treated, pyonephrosis it can result in a perinephric abscess.

Urinary tract infection in children

About 1% of boys and 3% of girls will develop a UTI. Risk factors include posterior urethral valves, neuropathic bladder and stones. UTIs in children are often associated with vesico-ureteric reflux (VUR). Reflux of infected urine can result in scarring, hypertension and renal failure. Scarring in the presence of sterile reflux is uncommon. About 50% of children with UTIs and VUR have renal scarring. Most renal scarring occurs in the first 2 years of life. The aims of treatment in children are to:

- Relieve symptoms
- Prevent recurrence
- Identify predisposing factors
- Prevent renal damage

All neonates and boys require investigation after one infection. Prophylactic antibiotics may be required for recurrent infections. Spontaneous resolution of vesico-ureteric reflux occurs in 80% of children. Indications for surgical reimplantation of the ureters are:

- Recurrent UTIs resulting from poor compliance with antibiotic prophylaxis
- Breakthrough infections despite prophylaxis
- Gross VUR with atonic ureters

Alternatives to surgery includes subendothelial injection of collagen or Teflon at the vesico-ureteric junction.

Urinary tract calculi

Pathogenesis

Urinary tract calculi form from crystalline aggregates of organic molecules. Factors favouring stone formation include increased urinary concentration of constituents, the presence of promoter substances and a reduction in concentration of inhibitors. The life time risk of developing a ureteric calculus is about 5% and recurrence rates are close to 50%. They occur most commonly in men aged between 30–60 years. About 90% are idiopathic but about 10% are due to metabolic derangement including hyperparathyroidism, vitamin D excess and primary hyperoxaluria The chemical composition of stones is as follows:

- Calcium oxalate (40%)
- Calcium phosphate (15%)
- Mixed oxalate/phosphate (20%)
- Struvite (15%)
- Uric acid (10%)

Clinical features

Ureteric calculi usually present with pain due to obstruction of urinary flow. Ureteric colic typically is severe, colicky loin to groin pain. The pain may radiate into the scrotum in men and labia in women. It may be associated with urinary frequency, urgency and dysuria. The pain may settle with the passage of the stone or if stone fails to migrate further. Abdominal examination is usually unremarkable. The different diagnosis of ureteric colic is shown in **Table 23.3**. Complications of ureteric calculi include obstruction, ureteric strictures and infection.

Investigation

Microscopic haematuria is often present. CT KUB has replaced the IVU as the investigation of choice. It has a higher sensitivity for the detection of stones and may also allow

Differential diagnosis of ureteric colic	
Non-renal causes	**Renal causes**
Appendicitis	Tumour (clot colic)
Diverticulitis	Pyelonephritis
Ectopic pregnancy	Retroperitoneal fibrosis
Salpingitis	Stricture
Torted ovarian cyst	Papillary necrosis
Abdominal aortic aneurysm	

Table 23.3 Differential diagnosis of ureteric colic

identification of other causes of loin pain. Serum electrolytes and calcium should be checked. An MSU should be obtained for microbiological evaluation. Metabolic evaluation should be considered if there is:

- Family history of urolithiasis
- Bilateral stone disease
- Presence of inflammatory bowel disease, chronic diarrhoea or malabsorption
- History of bariatric surgery
- Medical conditions associated with urolithiasis
- Nephrocalcinosis
- Osteoporosis or pathological fracture
- Stones formed from cystine, uric acid or calcium phosphate
- The patient is a child

Management

Most cases of ureteric colic can be managed conservatively with the use of adequate hydration, opiate and anti-inflammatory analgesia until resolution of symptoms when the stone is passed. Indications for urgent intervention in a patients with ureteric calculi include:

- Presence of infection with urinary tract obstruction
- Urosepsis
- Intractable pain or vomiting
- Impending acute renal failure
- Obstruction in a solitary or transplanted kidney
- Bilateral obstruction stones

Most ureteric calculi less than 5 mm in diameter will pass spontaneously. If the calculus is greater 5–10 mm in diameter and fails to pass spontaneously consideration will need to be given to intervention dependent of the position of the calculus:

- Upper third of ureter – Extracorporeal shock wave lithotripsy (ESWL)
- Lower third of ureter – Ureteroscopy (USC) + lithotripsy
- Middle third of ureter – Either ESWL or USC

Lithotripsy is the use of shock waves to break up stones. It requires an energy source – spark-gap electrode or piezoceramic array, a coupling device between patient and electrode – water bath or cushion and a method of stone localisation – fluoroscopy or ultrasound.

If large stones are present in the renal pelvis or upper ureter, consideration should be given to percutaneous nephrolithotomy, particularly if the stone is more than 3 cm in diameter or a 'staghorn calculus' is present (**Figure 23.4**). Chronic infection with urease-producing organisms (e.g. *Proteus*) precipitates stone formation. Magnesium ammonium phosphate or staghorn calculi result. Large staghorn calculi may be asymptomatic but they can lead to a deterioration in renal function. Acute infection in an obstructed kidney is a urological emergency. The patient is usually unwell with loin pain, swinging pyrexia and dysuria. Without drainage, rapid renal destruction may occur. It requires emergency percutaneous nephrostomy. Overall, less than 1% patients with stones require open surgery.

Bladder calculi

Bladder calculi are uncommon in the Western world. They are well-described in ancient medical literature. Hippocrates wrote about the management of bladder stones and operations to remove stones via the perineum were described in the centuries before Christ. Suprapubic lithotomy was described in the 15th century and transurethral lithotomy became popular in the 18th century. Lithotripsy was first described in 1822. Early surgical attempts at treating bladder calculi was often associated with significant morbidity and mortality.

Pathophysiology

Bladder calculi are usually associated with urinary stasis. Infection increases the risk of stone formation. Foreign bodies (e.g. suture material) can also act as a nidus for stone formation. However, bladder calculi can form in a normal bladder. There is no recognised

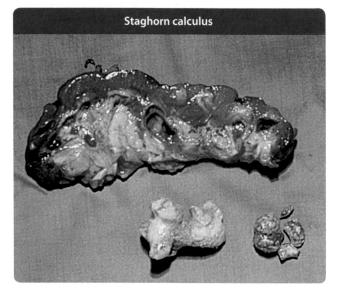
Staghorn calculus

Figure 23.4 A Staghorn calculus

association with ureteric calculi and most bladder calculi form in the bladder per se. They vary in size and can be multiple. They are more common in elderly men. Most stones in adults are formed of uric acid. Long-standing untreated bladder stones are associated with the development of squamous cell carcinoma of the bladder.

Clinical features

Many bladder calculi are asymptomatic. If they do cause symptoms they include suprapubic pain, dysuria and haematuria. Abdominal examination may be normal. Patients may present in acute urinary retention.

Investigation

Historically stones were diagnosed by the passage of urethral 'sounds'. Today they can be identified on plain abdominal x-ray, ultrasound, abdominal CT and cystoscopy. Uric acid stones are radiolucent but may have an opaque calcified layer. Any underlying bladder abnormality should be sought.

Management

Indications for surgery for bladder calculi include:

- Recurrent urinary tract infections
- Acute urinary retention
- Frank haematuria

Historically the surgical approach involved 'cutting for a stone'. This was via either a perineal or suprapubic approach. The three common approaches today are:

- Transurethral cystolitholapaxy
- Percutaneous cystolitholapaxy
- Open suprapubic cystostomy

Complications of cystolitholapaxy include:

- Infection
- Haemorrhage
- Bladder perforation
- Hyponatraemia

Extracorporeal shockwave lithotripsy is relatively ineffective for bladder calculi.

Pelviureteric junction obstruction

Pelviureteric junction (PUJ) obstruction is more common in men. It affects the left kidney more often than right and 10% cases are bilateral. The aetiology is often unknown but important factors may be aberrant lower pole vessels or persistence of a fetal urothelial fold.

Clinical features

PUJ obstruction usually presents in adolescence or early adult life and presents with loin pain, worse after alcohol intake. In late cases, a renal mass may be palpable. Haematuria is an uncommon feature. About 10% of patients develop UTIs and 3% have renal colic.

Investigation

The diagnosis can be confirmed by ultrasound or abdominal CT scanning. Isotope renography allows assessment of the percentage of renal function.

Management

The aims of treatment are to relieve symptoms and preserve renal function. This can be achieved by a pyeloplasty. The Anderson–Hynes pyeloplasty is the commonest procedure performed (**Figure 23.5**). If there is severe renal impairment (<20% function) then nephrectomy may be required.

Haematuria

Both microscopic and macroscopic haematuria are abnormal and invariably require investigation. Microscopic haematuria is defined as the presence of five or more RBCs per high-power field on urine microscopy. The prevalence of macroscopic and microscopic haematuria are approximately 1% and 5% respectively. About 50% of patients with haematuria will have an underlying abnormality. Overall, 10% and 35% of adult patients with microscopic and macroscopic haematuria respectively will have a urological malignancy. The causes of haematuria are shown in **Table 23.4**.

Investigation

All patients with haematuria should undergo investigation aimed at excluding a surgical cause. They should undergo urine microscopy and culture, urine cytology,

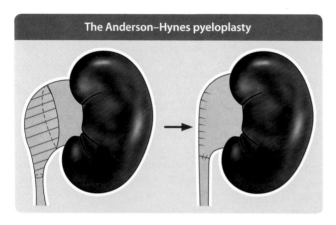

The Anderson–Hynes pyeloplasty

Figure 23.5 The Anderson–Hynes pyeloplasty

Causes of haematuria		
Surgical	**Glomerular**	**Non-glomerular**
Transitional cell carcinoma	IgA nephropathy	Urinary tract infections
Stone disease	Glomerulonephritis	Tuberculosis
Renal cell carcinoma	Systemic lupus erythematosis	Schistosomiasis
Trauma	Bacterial endocarditis	Drugs
Benign prostatic hyperplasia		Blood dyscrasias
Urethral stricture		Exercise-induced haematuria

Table 23.4 Causes of haematuria

ultrasound and cystoscopy. If the results of these investigations are normal, then the patient should be referred for a nephrological opinion.

Renal cell carcinoma

Benign tumours of the kidney are rare and all renal neoplasms should be regarded as potentially malignant. Renal cell cancer accounts for approximately 3% of all new cases of cancer diagnosed in men and around 2% of all cancers in women. There are about 8000 new cases per year in the UK. It arises from proximal tubule cells. Alternative names include hypernephroma, clear cell carcinoma and Grawitz tumour. The male:female ratio is approximately 2:1 and an increased incidence is seen in von Hippel–Lindau syndrome. Pathologically they may extend into the renal vein and inferior vena cava. Blood-borne spread can result in 'cannon ball' pulmonary metastases.

Clinical features

About 10% of patients present with the classic triad of haematuria, loin pain and a mass. Other presentations include a pyrexia of unknown origin and hypertension. Polycythaemia can occur due to erythropoietin production. Hypercalcaemia can occur due to production of a PTH-like hormone.

Investigation

The diagnosis can often be confirmed by renal ultrasound. An abdominal CT scan allows assessment of renal vein and caval spread. Echocardiogram should be considered if tumour in the inferior vena cava extends above diaphragm. The Robson staging of renal cell carcinoma is as follows:

- Stage 1 – Confined to the kidney
- Stage 2 – Involvement of perinephric fat but Gerota fascia intact
- Stage 3 – Spread into renal vein
- Stage 4 – Spread into adjacent or distant organs

Management

Unless extensive metastatic disease is present, treatment invariably involves surgery. The surgical option usually involves a radical nephrectomy. The kidney is approached through either a transabdominal or loin incision. Laparoscopic surgery may be considered. The renal vein is ligated early to reduce tumour propagation. The kidney and adjacent tissue (adrenal, perinephric fat) is excised. Lymph node dissection is of no proven benefit. Solitary (e.g. lung) metastases can occasionally be resected. Radiotherapy and chemotherapy have little role.

Bladder carcinoma

Bladder cancer is a common cancer with 10,500 new cases diagnosed each year in the UK. It is the most frequently occurring tumour of the urinary system and accounts for around 1 in every 30 new cancers. The male:female ratio is 3:1. Most bladder carcinomas are transitional cell tumours (TCCs). Superficial tumours are usually low grade and associated with a good prognosis. Muscle invasive tumours are of higher grade and have a poorer prognosis.

Pathology

Of all bladder carcinomas, 90% are TCCs, 5% are squamous cell carcinomas and 2% are adenocarcinomas. TCCs should be regarded as a 'field change' disease with a spectrum of aggression. About 80% of TCCs are superficial and well differentiated and only 20% progress to muscle invasion. Aetiological factors include:

- Occupational exposure – analine dyes, chlorinated hydrocarbons
- Cigarette smoking
- Analgesic abuse – phenacitin
- Pelvic irradiation

Schistosoma haematobium infection is associated with an increased risk of squamous carcinoma.

Clinical features

About 80% of patients present with painless haematuria. Bladder tumours can also present with treatment-resistant urinary infection, bladder irritability and sterile pyuria. Pathological staging requires bladder muscle to be included in specimen. Tumours are then staged according to depth of tumour invasion:

- T_{is} – In situ disease
- T_a – Epithelium only
- T_1 – Lamina propria invasion
- T_2 – Superficial muscle invasion
- T_{3a} – Deep muscle invasion
- T_{3b} – Perivesical fat invasion
- T_4 – Prostate or contiguous muscle

The grade of tumour is also important:

- G_1 – Well differentiated
- G_2 – Moderately well differentiated
- G_3 – Poorly differentiated

Management

Superficial TCC requires transurethral resection and regular cystoscopic follow-up. Consideration should be give to prophylactic chemotherapy if there are risk factors for recurrence or invasion. Immunotherapy may also be required. *Bacillus Calmette–Guerin* is an attenuated strain of *Mycobacterium bovis*. It reduces the risk of recurrence and progression and about a 50% response rate is seen. It is occasionally associated with development of systemic mycobacterial infection.

Carcinoma in situ is an aggressive disease and is often associated with positive cytology. About 50% patients progress to muscle invasion. Consideration should be given to immunotherapy. If this fails patient may need radical cystectomy.

For patients with invasive TCC the options are radical cystectomy or radiotherapy. Radical cystectomy has an operative mortality of about 5%. Urinary diversion can be achieved by:

- Valve rectal pouch – modified ureterosigmoidostomy

- Ileal conduit
- Neo-bladder

Complications of urinary diversions include:

- Renal and intestinal reservoir stones
- Urinary tract infections
- Metabolic derangements – hyperchloraemic acidosis
- Reservoir rupture
- Neoplasia

Local recurrence after surgery and radiotherapy occurs in about 15% and 50% of patients respectively. Preoperative radiotherapy is no better than surgery alone. The role of systemic adjuvant chemotherapy remains to be defined. Ureteric TCCs are usually managed by nephrouretectomy.

Urinary tract obstruction

Over 70% of men with lower urinary tract symptoms have proven bladder outflow obstruction. The causes of bladder outflow obstruction can be structural or functional and are shown in **Table 23.5**.

Urethral strictures

Causes of urethral stricture include:

- Congenital
- Trauma – instrumentation, urethral rupture
- Infection – gonocococcal, non-specific urethritis, syphilis, TB
- Inflammatory – balanitis xerotica obliterans
- Neoplasia – squamous, transitional cell or adenocarcinoma

The management can be with dilatation (gum-elastic bougie, metal sounds), urethrotomy (internal or external) or urethroplasty.

Benign prostatic hyperplasia

Benign prostatic hyperplasia affects 50% men older than 60 years and 90% of men older than 90 years. It results from hyperplasia of the prostatic stromal and epithelial cells, resulting in the formation of large, fairly discrete nodules in the periurethral region of the prostate. The nodules compress the urethra to cause partial, or sometimes virtually complete, obstruction interfering with normal urine flow.

Clinical features

Benign prostatic hyperplasia presents with obstructive and irritative symptoms. Obstruction causes poor urinary stream, hesitancy, dribbling and retention. Irritation causes frequency, nocturia, urgency and urge incontinence.

Investigation

Diagnosis of bladder outflow obstruction can be confirmed by uroflowmetry (**Figure 23.6**). Other investigations should include urea and electrolytes to check renal function, an ultrasound to excluded hydronephrosis and the measurement of post-micturition urine volume. A serum PSA should be measured to excluded malignancy.

Management

The aims of treatment of benign prostatic hyperplasia are to relieve symptoms

Causes of bladder outflow obstruction	
Structural	**Functional**
Urethral valves	Bladder neck dyssynergia
Urethral strictures	Neurological disease – spinal cord lesions, multiple sclerosis, diabetes
Benign prostatic hyperplasia	Drugs – anticholinergics, antidepressants
Carcinoma of the prostate	
Bladder neck stenosis	

Table 23.5 Causes of bladder outflow obstruction

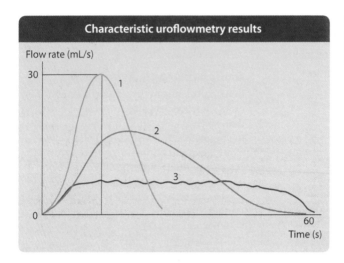

Figure 23.6 Characteristic uroflowmetry results. 1 = Normal; 2 = Benign prostatic hyperplasia; 3 = Urethral stricture.

and improve quality of life, relieve bladder outflow obstruction and to treat complications resulting from bladder outflow obstruction. Treatment options can be either pharmacological or surgical. Drugs include α-adrenergic antagonists, 5α-reductase inhibitors and LHRH antagonists. Surgical options include:

- Transurethral prostatectomy (TURP)
- Transurethral or interstitial thermotherapy
- Interstitial laser prostatectomy
- Urethral stents
- Open prostatectomy

TURP is the 'gold standard' treatment for bladder outflow obstruction due to benign prostatic hyperplasia. The bulk of the prostate is reduced endoscopically. The prostate is excised using a wire loop. The bladder is irrigated with glycine. The chips of prostatic tissue are washed from the bladder and an irrigation catheter is inserted. Obstruction is reduced and urinary symptoms considerably improved in over 90% of patients. Absorption of the irrigation fluid can result in acute hyponatraemia – the TUR syndrome. The possible complications of TURP are shown in **Table 23.6**. Postoperative retention occurs in about 5% of patients. Retrograde ejaculation occurs in about 80% of patients. Post-prostatectomy incontinence is a transient phenomenon in many men but becomes a

Complications of TURP		
Early	**Intermediate**	**Late**
Primary haemorrhage	Secondary haemorrhage	Bladder neck stenosis
Extravasation	Retrograde ejaculation	Urethral stricture
Fluid absorption (TUR syndrome)	Erectile dysfunction	
Infection		
Clot retention		
Epididymo-orchitis		
Incontinence		

Table 23.6 Complications of transurethral prostatectomy (TURP)

persistent problem in about 5% men. Risk factors for post-prostatectomy incontinence include:

- Preoperative incontinence
- Neurological disease
- Previous pelvic or prostatic surgery
- Large benign prostate

About 75% of cases are due to sphincter damage and 15% due to detrusor abnormality. Conservative management improves symptoms in 50% patients.

Prostate carcinoma

Prostate cancer is the most common cancer in men accounting for nearly a quarter of all new male cancers. There are about 35,000 new cases per year in the UK. Although there has been a rise in prostate cancer incidence over the last 20 years, this has not been reflected in mortality rates. It is more common in northern Europe and North America and rare in far east Asia. It is uncommon before the age of 50 years. It is found at post-mortem in 50% of men older than 80 years. About 5–10% of operations for benign disease reveal unsuspected prostate cancer. Much of the increased incidence can be attributed to the incidental discovery of prostate cancers following TURP and, more recently, the use of prostate specific antigen (PSA) testing.

Pathology

Prostate cancer is an adenocarcinoma usually arising in the posterior part of the gland. About 70%, 20% and 10% arise in peripheral, transition and central zone, respectively. Spread occurs through the capsule into perineural spaces, bladder neck, pelvic wall and rectum. Invasion into the seminal vesicles is associated with distant spread. Lymphatic spread is common. Haematogenous spread occurs to axial skeleton.

Tumours are graded by the Gleason classification. It is based on the glandular and cellular pattern of the tumour. It combines the two most common architectural patterns of cancer within the sampled specimen. Each of the two most common patterns is assigned a grade from one to five. A Gleason sum score is reported as the two scores added together.

Clinical features

Early low-grade disease is often asymptomatic. About 60% of patients present with symptoms of bladder outflow obstruction. Approximately 10% of cancers are identified as an incidental findings at TURP. The remainder present with bone pain, cord compression or leuco-erythroblastic anaemia as a result of metastatic disease. Renal failure can occur due to bilateral ureteric obstruction. With locally advanced tumours, the diagnosis can be confirmed by rectal examination. Features include a hard nodule or loss of the central sulcus.

Investigation

Transrectal ultrasound is the most important diagnostic investigation. It can confirm the diagnosis and an ultrasound-guided transrectal biopsy can be performed. Pelvic CT or MRI is useful in the staging of the disease. PSA is a kallikrein-like protein produced by prostatic epithelial cells. A serum level of 4 ng/mL is the upper limit of normal. A level greater than 10 ng/mL is highly suggestive of prostatic carcinoma. However, it can be also be raised in BPH. Serum PSA is a useful marker for monitoring response to treatment. Bone scanning will detect the presence of metastases. A bone scan is unlikely to be abnormal if the patient is asymptomatic and the PSA level is less than 10 ng/mL.

Management

More men die with than from prostate cancer. Treatment depends on the stage of the disease, the patient's age and his general fitness. For local disease the options are observation, radical radiotherapy or radical prostatectomy. For locally advanced disease the options are radical radiotherapy or hormonal therapy. Hormonal therapy is the mainstay of treatment for metastatic disease.

Radical prostatectomy

Radical prostatectomy involves removal of the entire prostate gland. The seminal vesicles are removed with the prostate gland. Care is taken to preserve the peri-prostatic plexus of nerves. The urethra is anastomosed to the base of the bladder. Radical prostatectomy is associated with improvement in mean survival compared to simple observation and a 50% reduction in risk of metastatic disease. However, erectile dysfunction occurs in 50% patients and about 3% develop stress incontinence.

Hormonal therapy

About 80% of prostate cancers are androgen dependent for their growth. Hormonal therapy involves androgen depletion and it produces good palliation until tumours 'escape' from hormonal control. Androgen depletion can be achieved by:

- Bilateral subcapsular orchidectomy
- LHRH agonists – goseraline
- Anti-androgens – cyproterone acetate, flutamide
- Oestrogens – stilbeostrol
- Complete androgen blockade

Urinary retention

Retention of urine can be acute or chronic. Chronic retention can be associated with either low or high intravesical pressure.

Acute retention

Acute retention usually presents with an inability to pass urine for several hours. It is usually associated with lower abdominal pain. The bladder is visible and palpable and tender on palpation. Causes of acute retention include:

- Bladder outflow obstruction
- Faecal impaction
- Urethral stricture
- Acute or chronic prostatitis
- Blood clot in the bladder
- Retroverted gravid uterus
- Post operation
- Spinal anaesthesia
- Spinal cord injury
- Urethral rupture
- Anal pain
- Drug induced – anticholinergics, antidepressants

Management

The immediate management of acute retention is urethral catheterisation. A catheter is passed using a full aseptic technique. Urethral analgesia can be achieved with lignocaine gel.

The gel should be massaged into the posterior urethra and a catheter not passed for at least 5 minutes. A 12 to 16 Fr gauge Foley catheter (usually with 10 mL balloon) is then inserted. The catheter should pass easily into bladder. The balloon should not be inflated until urine is seen coming from the catheter. A drainage bag should be attached and the volume of urine drained recorded. Female catheters should only be used in women. If the catheter fails to drain a significant volume of urine, reconsider the diagnosis. An attempt at a 'trial without catheter' can be made at 48 hours. If difficulty is encountered in passing the catheter:

- Do not use force
- Do not inflate the catheter balloon until urine has been seen in the catheter
- Do not use a catheter introducer unless adequately trained in its use

If unable to pass a urethral catheter the use of a suprapubic puncture is desirable. If an appropriate technique of catheterisation is used then complications are rare. False passages and urethral strictures can occur if there is significant trauma to the prostate or urethra. Minor degrees of haematuria can occur but usually clears spontaneously. Post obstruction diuresis has been described but is usually self-limiting. It occasionally requires intravenous crystalloid volume replacement. There is no evidence to support gradual decompression of the bladder.

Chronic retention

Chronic retention is usually relatively painless. High intravesical pressure can cause hydronephrosis and renal impairment. It can present as late-onset enuresis and may also present with hypertension. Low pressure chronic retention presents with symptoms of bladder outflow obstruction. Patients with chronic retention and renal impairment need urgent urological assessment.

Pain and swelling in the scrotum

Testicular tumours

Testicular tumours are one of the commonest malignancies seen in young men. There are about 1500 new cases per year in the UK. The incidence has doubled in the past 25 years. The two main type of tumour are teratomas and seminomas. They have a roughly equal incidence and have a peak age of presentation of 25 and 35 years, respectively. The highest incidence is seen in caucasians and is five times higher than other ethnic groups. Risk factors for the development of testicular tumours include:

- Cryptorchidism
- Testicular maldescent
- Klinefelter's syndrome
- Family history

The classification of testicular tumours is as follows:

- Seminomas
- Teratoma differentiated
- Malignant teratoma intermediate
- Malignant teratoma undifferentiated
- Malignant teratoma trophoblastic
- Yolk sac tumours

Treatment for testicular cancer is very effective. Nearly all men are cured by surgery, chemotherapy and radiotherapy. In those with disease localised to testis, the 5-year survival is more than 95%. Even in those with metastatic disease at presentation, cure rates of 80% have been reported.

Clinical features

Testicular tumours usually present with a testicular swelling or lump. The amount of pain is variable, but it is often minimal. Patients occasionally present with gynaecomastia. Seminomas metastasise to para-aortic nodes. Teratomas metastasise to the liver, lung, bone and brain. Patients may present with symptoms of metastatic disease, usually abdominal or back pain or respiratory symptoms.

Investigation

The diagnosis can often be confirmed by testicular ultrasound. A pathological diagnosis is made by performing an inguinal orchidectomy. There is no place for scrotal exploration and a testicular biopsy. The disease can be staged by thoraco-abdominal CT scanning (**Table 23.7**). Tumour markers are useful in staging and assessing response to treatment, α-fetoprotein (αFP) is produced by yolk sac elements and is not produced by seminomas. Beta-human chorionic

Royal Marsden staging of testicular tumours		
Stage	**Definition**	
I	Disease confined to testis	
IM	Rising post-orchidectomy tumour marker	
II	Abdominal lymphadenopathy	A – Less than 2 cm
		B – 2–5 cm
		C – More than 5 cm
III	Supra-diaphragmatic disease	O – No abdominal disease
		A, B, C – Abdominal nodal disease
IV	Extra-lymphatic metastases	
L1	Less than three lung metastases	
L2	More than three lung metastases	
L3	More than three lung metastases one or more greater than 2 cm	
H+	Liver involvement	

Table 23.7 Royal Marsden staging of testicular tumours

gonadotrophin (βHCG) is produced by trophoblastic elements and elevated levels are seen in both teratomas and seminomas.

Management

In most cases, initial surgical treatment is by radical inguinal orchidectomy. The spermatic cord is divided at the deep inguinal ring before the testis is mobilised. Testis-preserving surgery may be possible or may be necessary in those with synchronous bilateral tumours or a tumour in a solitary testes.

Seminomas are radiosensitive. Stage I and II disease is managed by inguinal orchidectomy plus radiotherapy to the ipsilateral abdominal and pelvic nodes. Stage II disease and above should be treated with chemotherapy. Teratomas are not radiosensitive. Stage I disease treated by orchidectomy and surveillance. Chemotherapy should be given to those with Stage II disease, those who relapse or have metastatic disease at presentation.

Contralateral intra-tubular germ-cell neoplasia occurs in 5% of men presenting with testicular cancers. As a result, it has been recommended that patients with testicular cancer should undergo contralateral testicular biopsies. Contralateral intra-tubular germ-cell neoplasia has a high-risk of progression to invasive cancer and irradiation of the testis should be considered. Patients should be offered storage of semen. High-risk patients include those with:

- Testicular maldescent
- Testicular atrophy
- Age less than 30 years

Scrotal swellings

Scrotal swellings can arise from above or from within the scrotum. The exact nature of a scrotal swelling can usually be determined by obtaining an accurate history and performing a thorough clinical examination. Extensive investigation is usually not required. The differential diagnosis of a scrotal swelling is shown in **Table 23.8**. To determine the nature of a scrotal swelling four things need to be assessed:

- Can you get above the swelling?

Differential diagnosis of a scrotal swelling	
Swelling not confined to scrotum	Swelling confined to scrotum
Hernia	Epididymo-orchitis
Infantile hydrocele	Testicular tumour
	Epididymal cysts
	Vaginal hydrocele
	Torsion testis

Table 23.8 Differential diagnosis of a scrotal swelling

- Can the testis and epididymis be identified separately?
- Does the swelling transilluminate?
- Is the swelling tender?

Testicular torsion

Testicular torsion is a common surgical emergency in adolescent boys. The peak incidence is in the second decade of life. A high insertion of the tunica vaginalis ('Bell clapper testis') predisposes to the condition. The abnormality is usually bilateral and the contralateral testis usually has a horizontal lie.

Clinical features

Testicular torsion usually presents with acute scrotal pain. However, it may present with acute abdominal pain and no testicular symptoms. Therefore, it is essential to examine the scrotum in all boys who present with acute abdominal pain. Urinary symptoms are uncommon. About 50% of boys have had previous episode of pain. Examination shows a tender high-riding testis often with a small hydrocele.

Management

Investigation is usually not required. Testicular torsion is a clinical diagnosis requiring urgent surgical exploration. The diagnosis is usually obvious. If the testis is infarcted then an orchidectomy should be performed. If the viability of the testis is in doubt, then the testis should be wrapped in a warm swab and observed. If the testis is viable, then both the ipsilateral and contralateral side should be fixed within the scrotum.

Approximately 60% of testes are salvageable. However, if patients are re-examined at 6 months after surgery, 10% of testes are found to be atrophic. The outcome is best in those operated on less than 6 hours since the onset of symptoms. Beyond 12 hours, salvage of the testis is less assured. Occasionally, long-term sub-fertility is a problem possibly due to an auto-immune response affecting both testes.

Epididymitis

Epididymitis is uncommon in adolescents and one should be wary about making the diagnosis at this age. Patients usually have a more prolonged history, the pain may not be severe and urinary symptoms may be present. Examination shows tenderness which is greatest over the epididymis. Treatment is with antibiotics.

Idiopathic scrotal oedema

Idiopathic scrotal oedema usually occurs in boys less than 10 years old. It presents with scrotal redness and oedema. Pain is slight and the testis feels normal. Management is conservative.

Torsion of a testicular appendix

Torsion of a testicular appendix presents with sudden testicular pain but often not severe. A hydrocele with a tender appendage (hydatid of Morgagni) is often apparent. If discovered during scrotal exploration, the appendage should be excised.

Varicocele

In the scrotum, the veins from the testis form the pampiniform plexus. This reduces to one or two well-defined veins in the inguinal canal. One testicular vein is formed at the deep inguinal ring. The left testicular vein drains into the left renal vein. The tight testicular vein drains into the inferior vena cava. Some venous drainage also occurs via the cremasteric vein into the inferior epigastric veins. A varicocele consists of dilatation of the veins of the pampiniform plexus.

Clinical features

Most varicoceles are detected in adolescence or early adult life. About 95% occur on the left side and are idiopathic. They are occasionally associated with left renal tumours. Most are asymptomatic. If they do cause symptoms, it is usually a vague or annoying discomfort. Examination shows the typical 'bag of worms' which reduces in size in the supine position. Varicoceles are occasionally associated with infertility but there is no evidence that surgery increased semen quality or conception rates.

Management

Varicoceles only need treatment if symptomatic. The veins can be ligated via either a scrotal or inguinal approach. Recently laparoscopic ligation has been reported. Recurrence can occur due to the collateral supply via the cremasteric vein.

Priapism

Priapism is a persistent erection of the penis. It is uncommon but early diagnosis and treatment is essential. Delayed presentation or treatment results in corporal anoxia and loss of erectile function.

Pathophysiology

Priapism can be either high or low flow. Low-flow priapism is more common and is due to venous stasis and ischaemia. Aetiological factors include:

- Intracavernosal injection
- Pelvic malignancy
- Blood disorders – sickle-cell disease, leukaemia
- Trauma – spinal cord injury
- Prolonged sexual activity
- Urogenital tract inflammation
- Drugs

High-flow priapism is uncommon and is due to the development of an arteriocavernosal fistula. This can follow blunt or penetrating penile or perineal trauma. Anatomically, it involves the corpora cavernosa only.

Clinical features

An adequate history and clinical features will allow differentiation of low-flow and high-flow priapism. Low-flow priapism presents with painful persistent erection. The penile shaft is firm and glans penis is usually soft. High-flow priapism is often painless. There is invariably a clear history of trauma.

Management

Aspiration of the corpora will distinguish the two types. In high-flow priapism, the blood is arterial. In low-flow priapism, the blood is dark and viscous and is similar to venous blood. Intracorporeal blood gas analysis can be useful to distinguish the two types. Early treatment is essential, preferably within 12 hours of the onset of symptoms. Low-flow priapism requires urgent aspiration and instillation of a vasoconstrictor. Aspiration alone is successful in only 30% cases. Phenylephrine can be used as the vasoconstrictor. This should be followed by a drainage procedure into:

- The glans penis (Modified Winter/Ebbehoj shunt)
- The corpora spongiosum (Quackel procedure)
- The long saphenous vein (Grayhack procedure)

Detumescence can be achieved in 70% of patients and maintenance of erectile function is present in about 40%. High-flow priapism requires closure of the arteriocavernosal fistula and can often be performed by an interventional radiologist.

Vasectomy

Vasectomy is one of the safest and most effective means of contraception. Approximately 100,000 vasectomies are performed in the UK each year. Approximately 1 in 6 men over the age of 35 years have had a vasectomy. Most are performed under local anaesthetics. The vas deferens is identified ligated and divided. Most surgeons excise a segment of the vas. Fascial interposition is more effective than ligation alone. Recovery is rapid and complications are rare.

Postoperative semen samples are required at 8 and 12 weeks after surgery. Two negative specimens are necessary before other forms of contraception can be abandoned. Failure can occur and pregnancy has been reported following 1 in 2000 vasectomies. Complications of vasectomy include:

- Bruising or haematoma
- Wound infection
- Epididymo-orchitis
- Sperm granuloma
- Chronic testicular pain

Reversal of vasectomy

About 5% of men subsequently seek vasectomy reversal. A vasectomy can be reversed by either a vasovasostomy or vasoepididymostomy. In experienced hands, vasovasostomy can result in a tube patency rates of greater than 90% but pregnancy occurs in no more than 50%. Outcome depends on several factors. The time since the vasectomy is important. Vasovasostomy is more likely to be successful if it is performed within 3 years of vasectomy. Greater success has been reported with microsurgical techniques.

Aspects of pelvic surgery
Gynaecological causes of acute abdominal pain

Ectopic pregnancy

An ectopic pregnancy is defined as a gestation that occurs outside the uterine cavity. It is seen in 1% of all pregnancies with 11,000 cases per year in UK. The incidence is increasing. The mortality is less than 1%. Risk factors include:

- Previous pelvic inflammation
- Infertility
- Tubal surgery
- Intrauterine contraceptive devise
- Previous ectopic pregnancy

The commonest site for an ectopic pregnancy is in the tubal ampulla. It usually presents with 6 to 8 weeks of amenorrhoea. The patient has lower abdominal pain and slight vaginal bleeding. Cardiovascular collapse and shoulder tip pain suggest a large intraperitoneal bleed. Examination will often shown abdominal and adnexal tenderness. The patient invariably has a positive urinary pregnancy test. Ultrasound will show an empty uterus and may identify the ectopic pregnancy. A intrauterine pregnancy on ultrasound almost invariably excludes an ectopic pregnancy. If the patient is shocked immediate laparotomy is essential. If there is no evidence of cardiovascular compromise, laparoscopy is the investigation of choice. The fetus can then be removed by laparoscopic salpingotomy or salpingectomy.

Pelvic inflammatory disease

Pelvic inflammatory disease (PID) is usually synonymous with acute salpingitis. It is an ascending sexually transmitted disease due to chlamydia (60%), *Neisseria gonorrhoea* (30%) and anaerobes. Untreated it can progress to a pyosalpinx or a tubo-ovarian abscess. It presents with lower abdominal pain and a vaginal discharge. Pelvic examination is uncomfortable. High vaginal and endocervical swabs are essential. If doubt over the diagnosis exists, consideration should be given to a diagnostic laparoscopy. PID often improves with antibiotics (tetracycline and metronidazole) and surgery is rarely required. PID increases the risk of infertility and there is a 40% chance of tubal occlusion after three episodes. It also increases the risk of ectopic pregnancy by a factor of six-fold. About 20% of patients develop chronic pelvic pain.

Endometriosis

Endometriosis is the presence of functional endometrial tissue outside the uterine cavity. It results from either retrograde menstruation or celomic metaplasia. It usually affects the ovaries, fallopian tubes and the serosal surface of the bowel. It is most commonly seen in women between 30 and 50 years. It presents with premenstrual lower abdominal pain. It may also cause back pain, intestinal obstruction and urological symptoms. Large 'chocolate' cysts may rupture causing acute abdominal pain. It is a cause of infertility. The diagnosis can be confirmed at laparoscopy. Hormonal therapy may improve symptoms and danazol is the first line treatment of choice.

Ovarian cysts

Ruptured ovarian cyst

Ovarian cysts are either functional or proliferative. They cause abdominal pain if they rupture, tort or infarct. Patients present with sudden onset of severe lower abdominal pain. The differential diagnosis includes PID or a ruptured ectopic pregnancy. Cysts may be palpable on bimanual examination. The diagnosis can be confirmed by transabdominal or transvaginal ultrasound or laparoscopy. Treatment usually involves ovarian cystectomy.

Functional cysts

Functional cysts are the commonest type of ovarian cyst (**Figure 23.7**). They present as follicular, corpus luteal or theca luteal cysts. They are benign and usually resolve spontaneously. They may be an incidental finding on a clinical or radiological investigation. Symptoms result from pressure or rupture. The differential diagnosis includes a tubo-ovarian abscess or ectopic pregnancy. Most regress in 6–10 weeks and surgery can often be avoided.

Mature cystic teratoma

Mature cystic teratoma accounts for 10% of ovarian neoplasms. They develop from totipotential cells and have well differentiated mesodermal and ectodermal elements. About

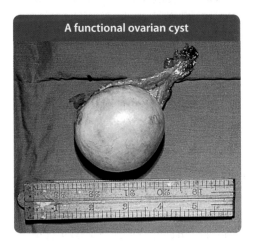

A functional ovarian cyst

Figure 23.7 A functional ovarian cyst

10% are bilateral. Cystic teratomas have a smooth capsule and may grow to 30 cm in diameter. They may contain mature elements including bone, hair and teeth (**Figure 23.8**). Functioning thyroid tissue may cause thyrotoxicosis (struma ovarii). Malignant transformation is rare. Treatment is by ovarian cystectomy.

Ovarian germ cell tumours

In adolescents and young women, the majority of ovarian neoplasms are germ cell tumours. Approximately 25% of these tumours are malignant. If they are functioning they can present with precocious puberty or early menarche. Tumour markers such as CEA, α-fetoprotein or β-hCG may be increased. CA125 is usually not raised in germ cell tumours. Types of malignant tumour include dysgerminoma and embryonal carcinomas. Treatment is usually by surgical debulking and chemotherapy.

Ovarian carcinoma

Approximately 6500 women are diagnosed with ovarian cancer in the UK each year making it the second most common gynaecological cancer and the fifth most common cancer in women. Ovarian carcinoma arises from either the ovarian or celomic epithelium. About 75% are serous and 20% are mucinous. Risk factors include:

- Advancing age
- Nulliparity
- Family history (BRCA1 and BRCA2)
- Possibly fertility drugs

Clinical features

The clinical features of ovarian carcinoma are often non-specific. Early features include urinary frequency and abdominal discomfort. Later features include distension, early satiety and anorexia. An abdominal mass and ascites may be present.

Investigation

The diagnosis of ovarian carcinoma can often be confirmed by abdominal and pelvic CT. The serum CA125 may be raised. In patients presenting with ascites with no obvious cause, cytology may show characteristic malignant cells. Ovarian carcinoma spreads by three routes – trans-celomic, lymphatic and haematogenous. The staging of the disease is surgical and 20–40% of patients are upstaged after surgical intervention. The International Federation of Gynaecology and Obstetrics staging of ovarian carcinoma is as follows:

- Stage 1 – Tumour limited to ovaries

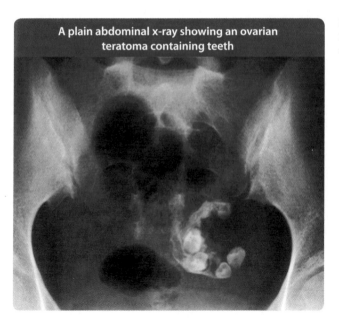

A plain abdominal x-ray showing an ovarian teratoma containing teeth

Figure 23.8 A plain abdominal x-ray showing an ovarian teratoma containing teeth

- Stage 2 – Involvement of one or both ovaries with pelvic extension
- Stage 3 – Involvement of one or both ovaries with extension beyond the pelvis
- Stage 4 – Involvement of one or both ovaries with distant metastases

Management

Thorough surgical staging should be undertaken of all patients. For Stage 1 disease a unilateral salpingo-oophorectomy should be performed if future fertility required. Otherwise Stage 1 disease should be managed with a total abdominal hysterectomy and bilateral salpingo-oophorectomy +/– omentectomy and peritoneal biopsies. For Stage 2 and 3 disease surgical debulking should be performed. This should be followed by chemotherapy. Platinum-based chemotherapy regimens are the most effective. The role of a second-look laparotomy and further debulking is controversial.

The role of screening for ovarian carcinoma is currently under investigation. There is currently no evidence for CA-125 or ultrasound screening of the general population.

Urinary incontinence

Incontinence can be defined as the involuntary loss of urine, causing social or hygiene problems that can be objectively demonstrated. It is a common and under reported problem that affects at least 4 million people in UK. It affects women more than men, particularly the elderly. It can be classified as:

- Stress incontinence
- Urge incontinence
- Overflow incontinence

Stress incontinence

Stress incontinence affects about 30% of women over 30 years. It usually develops after childbirth and symptoms worsen with age. Incontinence occurs with effort or exertion and is worse when upright. Urine loss is seen immediately after a rise in intra-abdominal pressure.

Urge incontinence

Urge incontinence is part of the overactive bladder symptom syndrome. Patients experience frequency, urgency and incontinence due to detrusor muscle overactivity.

Overflow incontinence

Overflow incontinence occurs in both sexes. Symptoms are often relatively few. Patients tend to dribble urine. Men often have a full and palpable bladder. Women often have abnormal anatomy or a vesicovaginal fistula.

Investigation

In the investigation of incontinence, the following investigations should be considered:

- Mid stream urine specimen
- Renal function
- PSA in men
- Renal ultrasound
- Flexible cystoscopy

Urodynamic assessment evaluates the function of the bladder and results should be interpreted with the clinical presentation. Assessment can involve:

- Frequency–volume chart
- Pad test
- Flow rates
- Residual volume by ultrasound
- Conventional cystometry
- Videocysturethrography – filling and voiding

Management

The manaagement of incontinence should start with general support. This involves specialist nurses using appliances, pads and catheters. Specific treatment will depend on the underlying cause.

Urge incontinence

The overactive bladder syndrome can be managed by behaviour change, drugs – anti-muscarinic agents, desmopressin and surgery. The surgical options include:

- Injection of botulinum toxin
- Neuromodulation
- Clam cystoplasty
- Detrusor myectomy
- Urinary diversion

Stress incontinence

Stress incontinence can be managed by physiotherapy, biofeedback, electrical stimulation and drugs – duloxetine. The surgical options include:

- Burch colposuspension
- Anterior colporrhaphy
- Marshall–Marchett–Kranz procedure
- Needle suspension of bladder neck
- Pubovaginal slings
- Periurethral bulking agents
- Implantation of artificial sphincters

Index

Note: Page numbers in **bold** or *italic* refer to tables or figures respectively.